Praise for LIFE OVER CANCER

"*Life Over Cancer* is the compilation of Dr. Keith Block's three decades of research and development of his optimal model of integrative cancer treatment. As chief of surgical oncology of a major medical institution, I have sent many patients to the Block Center. They experienced less treatment toxicity, improved treatment response, better quality of life, and improved outcomes. In my opinion, Dr. Block's clinic is unique and is the top integrative oncology center in the U.S. It is where I would go if I was ever diagnosed with cancer."
—*N. Joseph Espat, M.D., Professor and Chief, Surgical Oncology, Roger Williams Medical Center, Providence, Rhode Island*

"*Life Over Cancer* is a must-read for anyone combating this disease. It provides genuine hope, as well as the evidence, rationale, and instructions in how to live a healthier, fuller life with cancer, while providing a broader array of treatment options that improve quality of life."
—*Nick Vogelzang, M.D., Director, Nevada Cancer Institute, Las Vegas; Professor of Medicine, University of Nevada School of Medicine, Las Vegas*

"Here is cancer care as it should be: person-centered, integrated, individualized, and science-based. If you or your loved ones have been touched by cancer, or if you care for those with cancer, read this book."
—*Wayne B. Jonas, M.D., President and CEO, Samueli Institute; Director (1995–1999), Office of Alternative Medicine, National Institutes of Health*

"Keith Block is one of the great pioneers of integrative oncology. This important book is essential reading for patients and health professionals alike. Block's approach is indicative of much of the future of this critically important field of medicine."
—*Michael Lerner, Ph.D., President, Commonweal; Cofounder, Commonweal Cancer Help Program*

"*Life Over Cancer* provides the reader with an accessible and comprehensive program that combines the best of conventional cancer therapy with effective complementary interventions. It is this 'whole person' approach to patient care that Dr. Block brought to the University of Illinois Integrative Medical Education program, which he established in the mid-nineties. His dedication and efforts have transformed the school's medical education curriculum and inspired future physicians to view integrative medicine as a truly significant component of health care."
—*L. J. Sandlow, M.D., Senior Associate Dean for Academic & Educational Affairs, Professor and Head, Department of Medical Education, University of Illinois College of Medicine*

LIFE OVER CANCER

The Block Center Program
for Integrative Cancer Treatment

Keith I. Block, M.D.

Foreword by
Andrew Weil, M.D.

Preface by
Robert Newman, Ph.D.

BANTAM BOOKS

LIFE OVER CANCER
A Bantam Book / April 2009

Published by Bantam Dell
A Division of Random House, Inc.
New York, New York

Book design by Diane Hobbing

Bantam Books is a registered trademark of Random House, Inc., and the colophon is a trademark of Random House, Inc.

Library of Congress Cataloging-in-Publication Data

Block, Keith (Keith I.)
  Life over cancer : the Block Center program for integrative cancer treatment / Keith Block ; foreword by Andrew Weil, preface by Robert Newman
      p. cm.
  Includes bibliographical references and index.
  ISBN 978-0-553-80114-9 (hardcover) — ISBN 978-0-553-90638-7 (ebook)   1. Cancer—Popular works.   2. Integrative medicine—Popular works.   I. Title.

RC263.B563 2009
616.99'406—dc22

                                        2008047806

Printed in the United States of America
Published simultaneously in Canada

www.bantamdell.com

10 9 8 7 6 5
BVG

DEDICATION

To my parents, Judge Jack and Shirley Block, who imbued me with vision, solid values, and the inner strength to hold to my convictions in order to overcome the myriad challenges I would face along the way.

To Penny, the love of my life and my partner in every way imaginable: Because of you this book and our work have been possible, meaningful, and worth every steep climb we have encountered.

To Carla, Shana, Ben, and Julie: You have often lived with the battle of cancer as a kitchen-table centerpiece and even from a young age recognized the value of our work. Your understanding has been a source of inspiration. May you each, your spouses, and our grandchildren live in a healthier world with better answers.

And to my patients through the many years, those of you who have won your battles and, sadly, those who have not: Your courage in the face of uncertainty has been an inspiring example of how to manage adversity. Because of you—your will, resolve, force of spirit, and, yes, your heart—I am forever changed.

A NOTE TO READERS

Before following any of the self-help suggestions and treatments described in this book, we strongly recommend that you give careful consideration to your particular condition and consult with your doctor or health care practitioner. Because everyone is different, it is important that the suggested techniques, treatments, or lifestyle changes referred to in this book be undertaken only with the guidance of your doctor or health care practitioner to make sure they are appropriate for your particular condition and circumstance and won't lead to any adverse interactions with other treatments you may be undergoing.

In the event you use any of the information in this book for yourself as part of a self-care program, the author and publisher specifically disclaim any and all types of liability, loss, or risk, personal or otherwise, that is incurred as a consequence, directly or indirectly, of the use and application of any of the contents of this book.

The anecdotes presented in this book are true and accurate. However, except when requested, the names and some identifying details have been changed to maintain anonymity. Further, each individual's experience might be attributable to factors other than the ingredient itself. As such, results may not be typical and your results may vary.

This book recommends botanicals, nutrients, and other ingredients that have been shown in scientific studies and literature to potentially help fight diseases and promote health. Many of these scientific findings, however, are relatively recent, and more research is needed to fully investigate and understand their ultimate usefulness for cancer patients.

CONTENTS

FOREWORD

*L*ife *Over Cancer* sets the course for what I believe is the future of successful cancer treatment. This indispensable guide helps patients and their families understand and navigate their treatment options in order to develop a multifaceted, individualized plan for renewed health and recovery.

The message of *Life Over Cancer* is simple yet profound: the person diagnosed with cancer can take specific measures to reverse the course of the disease and keep it from returning. By judiciously combining conventional treatments with natural agents, fitness regimens, stress care strategies, and other noninvasive modalities, Dr. Block believes—and his clinical work demonstrates—that people with cancer can realize optimal health, a better quality of life, and lifelong remissions. This model for care is based on his thirty years of pioneering work in integrative oncology, of living on the front lines of cancer treatment. Dr. Block has developed an essential profiling system to individualize treatments in order to counter the tumor's unique molecular fingerprint, while making the microenvironment inhospitable to future cancer growth. His program includes research on drug-nutrient and drug-herb interactions, and a relentless search for strategies and interventions to reduce drug toxicity and improve treatment outcomes.

Life Over Cancer creates an organized model from Dr. Block's deep experience in integrative oncology. As the "father" of this field, and as a clinician, researcher, and educator, Keith is a leading figure in its present growth and evolution. In all of my years in integrative medicine, I have not seen a model with this level of sophistication that so thoroughly addresses the needs of cancer patients.

I have devoted the past thirty years to developing, practicing, and teaching others about the principles of integrative medicine. In 1994, I established the Program in Integrative Medicine, now the Arizona Center for Integrative Medicine, a Center of Excellence of the University of Arizona College of Medicine. Its main work is the education of physicians, medical students, and other health care providers, and one of its initiatives is to develop a fellowship in integrative oncology. Keith is an essential part of our faculty precisely because we want tomorrow's doctors to be able to offer the kinds of care described in *Life Over Cancer*.

I believe in Keith's program and would go to the Block Center if I were facing a diagnosis of cancer. It is where I have sent and will continue to send my friends and family members. For many years, the Block Center was the only facility practicing true integrative cancer treatment. Today, a few others exist, but the Block Center continues to set the standard by which all other integrative cancer care facilities should be measured.

Life Over Cancer is the program every cancer patient deserves in order to have the best chance for recovery and restoration of health.

Andrew Weil, M.D.
Tucson, Arizona
October 2008

PREFACE

For the past twenty-five years, I have been a molecular pharmacologist, professor, and cancer researcher at the University of Texas M. D. Anderson Cancer Center. As co-director of the Pharmaceutical Development Center in the Department of Experimental Therapeutics, I oversaw a $40 million facility with dozens of researchers, focusing on the development and application of new drugs for the prevention and treatment of cancer. In all my years in this field, however, I have never seen a model as comprehensive, as well-developed, and as strategically sound, as the Life Over Cancer (LOC) program.

Modern medical research seeks to find and exploit differences between healthy and diseased tissues so that we might be better able to discover the "Achilles' heel" of cancer and thus the possible pathway to a cure. We have typically sought to find the *one* intervention that will eradicate the *one* underlying defect responsible for the proliferation of this disease. Our "magic bullets," however, often fail us. Not because they haven't hit and perhaps even crippled their intended targets, but because the tumor cell now begins to use multiple survival strategies, the existence of which we may not even have been aware.

I regard this as an important reminder to those of us distant from the patient's bedside. We need to step back from the research bench and realize that the battle against cancer is not so much against a single defect in a protein or cancerous mutation, as it is a war on many fronts that must be engaged with every weapon we have at hand.

And therein lies the wisdom of *Life Over Cancer.* Dr. Keith Block details a strategic, multidimensional, personalized approach to treating cancer that reprograms the biochemical and molecular environments of his patients by selectively targeting *multiple* defects as well as *multiple* pathways. Preliminary evidence suggests that by adhering to the full Block model, treatment toxicity can be decreased, life quality improved, and even therapeutic benefit enhanced.

Life Over Cancer embraces all that modern oncology has to offer and seeks to improve it by making us—for we are all susceptible to cancer—better able to withstand the hardest battle many of us will ever face. The integration of surgery, radiation, chemotherapy, molecular therapies, and well-researched plant and herbal science, together with the benefit of exercise, reduced stress, and other important health-promoting strategies, has already resulted in better cure rates as well as improvements in the quality of life of cancer patients. Dr. Block's individualized approach to patient care and the Block Center's patient survival studies reinforce the benefits of integration and provide an important basis for future research.

This long-awaited book puts forth a full systematic plan designed to eliminate disease and also optimize total health and well-being. It is a critical road map for people who are lost, a virtual Mapquest for the mind, body, and soul of cancer patients. In addition, it is a living testimony to Keith's three decades of research, education, and clinical work in the world of integrative oncology. I am in awe . . . really.

Robert A. Newman, Ph.D.
Professor of Cancer Medicine (Pharmacology)
Codirector, Pharmaceutical Development Center
Department of Experimental Therapeutics
University of Texas M. D. Anderson Cancer Center
Houston, Texas

RETAKING CONTROL OF YOUR LIFE

You have cancer."
  A doctor has uttered three of the most dreaded words you can hear. A moment before, you were a husband, a wife, a teacher, an accountant. Now, suddenly, you are a *patient*. In the ensuing panic, disbelief, fear, and grief, you run a real risk of losing your identity to the disease and seeing it take over your life, as has happened to countless cancer patients before you. But it is possible to choose a different path, a path of discovery, action, and self-advocacy. You can choose life over cancer.

It is not easy. It requires strength, courage, and an independent spirit. But time and again I have seen patients marshal these survival qualities to face the greatest challenge of their life. You can, too.

In choosing life over cancer, you must consciously and purposefully embrace life and reject the disease every single day. To do so, and to greet each day with authentic hope and conviction, you need the right tools, including sound information about the full range of cancer therapies, both conventional and complementary, and strong, sophisticated forms of support.

In this book, I will explain these tools and how to use them as you set out to reclaim your health. You *can* take charge of your treatment and your life. You *can* beat the odds. But more than that, you can recover from it with not only your life but also your health.

Why Is Cancer So Hard to Cure?

In 1971, President Nixon declared war on cancer. Almost forty years and billions of dollars later, that war is far from won. Cancer remains the second-leading cause of death in the United States and is poised to become the nation's leading killer. Races and walks for "cures" are being scheduled for many years into the future. For although we can treat, and even drive into submission, a few distinct cancers—pediatric cancers, for instance, have a much higher survival rate than they did two generations ago—the most common and lethal cancers remain difficult to cure unless they are caught very early, and sometimes even then the prognosis is grim. It is sobering that some of the most vaunted new targeted molecular therapies, billion-dollar medications such as Avastin and Erbitux, extend life span by mere months, on average, if at all. Obviously a "successful" cancer treatment is measured quite differently than are treatments for other diseases. In contrast, cardiovascular disease is not the killer it once was: in the same fifty years during which the age-adjusted mortality rate for cancer has remained about the same, that for cardiovascular disease has fallen by about two-thirds.

What is it about cancer that enables it to survive despite surgery to excise it, radiation to burn it, and chemotherapy to poison it?

We have only recently begun to grasp the nature of this disease. Cancer is not an isolated group of errant cells waiting passively to be annihilated by a wonder drug. Instead, it is caused by a cascade of genetic and molecular glitches. That's why cancer does not present a single target for a magic bullet; a tumor is merely the most obvious symptom of an altered, unbalanced system. And that's why both the new targeted therapies and the older weapons of surgery, radiation, and old-line chemotherapy so often fail to prevent the spread or recurrence of the disease:

they neither pick up renegade cancer cells, strengthen the body's biological balance, nor reach all of the underlying molecular accidents that initiated cancer in the first place. As a result, even if the original tumor is gone, this biological imbalance creates an environment for cancer to recur: tumor cells use the body's own healthy resources to grow and multiply. This means that cancer is a systemic disruption and perversion of the body's resources and mechanisms. Because cancer will try to use every bit of your body's biochemistry to proliferate, you must strengthen every biochemical defense possible to defeat it.

The Block Center for Integrative Cancer Treatment

I am a medical doctor who has treated over fifteen thousand people with cancer at our medical center in Evanston, Illinois. I have spent thirty years developing a comprehensive program to treat cancer patients. Based on an individually tailored approach to integrative medicine, it blends treatments from different disciplines ranging from diet and exercise to mind-spirit techniques, natural medicines, and standard chemo and radiation.

This program is based not only on my own clinical experience and research but also on the research and experience of other experts in oncology, nutrition, botanicals, mind-body medicine, and therapeutic exercise, many of whom are staff members at our center. *Life Over Cancer* reflects our understanding of cancer's multiple causes and means of surviving. It is based on new understanding of how treatments interact with each other, with your body, and with the cancer itself. It is designed to create a foundation of general wellness from which cancer can be treated more effectively and with fewer side effects. We combine the best of conventional medicine—including chemotherapy, radiation, surgery, and biologic and targeted therapies—with the best of complementary medicine, encompassing state-of-the-art anti-cancer nutrition, herbs, supplements, physical exercise, and mind-body techniques. Because no two people are alike, the integrative program is individually tailored through detailed profiling to each patient's specific disease, biochemistry, molecular fingerprint, personal needs, and healing philosophy. The result is a program that transforms lifestyles while reprogramming patients' biochemical environments.

This approach to wellness lets cancer patients live longer and more rewarding lives. As an example, two recent studies found that our patients with either metastatic breast cancer or metastatic prostate cancer, diseases with a grim prognosis, lived roughly twice as long and were far more likely to reach the five-year survival milestone than similar patients receiving only conventional treatments, as I will discuss in Chapter 1.

Many of our patients carry on their daily lives as if they were managing a chronic illness such as diabetes. In fact, I encourage you to begin thinking of your cancer as an illness you can live with or, even better, one you can overcome. I have treated many patients with widespread metastases who were pronounced "incurable" by their doctors but who, with this program, recovered. These survivors testify to what can happen with an integrative approach to treating and managing cancer: no matter what the diagnosis, there are patients who prevail over whatever odds they have been given.

You Have More Options Than You Think

I will never forget how alone and afraid I felt during my own trials with serious illnesses. Soon after I began medical school, I was stricken with bleeding ulcers. I kept losing weight, and became terrified of what would happen if the condition grew worse. Desperate, I turned to antacids, stuffing bottles of them under the car seat and sucking on them throughout the day.

Finally, finding no relief, I saw a doctor. After a brief examination, he told me that if my condition worsened, my only option would be surgery followed by a long and painful recovery. Even then, he warned, I might not be cured. I was stunned that the doctor had so little to offer. Surely there must be other options. But where to find them?

As I began my search, I identified a variety of natural therapies that seemed to improve my condition. But when I combined some of them, it was disastrous. For example, I found that fasting and exercise both made me feel better, so I did both at the same time. Then, while jogging, I felt light-headed and faint. I collapsed and was nearly mowed over by a stream of bikers and other joggers. Eventually, I was able to successfully blend natural medicines and dietary and lifestyle changes in a way that enabled me to get my ulcers under control.

The experience of sitting helplessly at the other end of a stethoscope made a lasting impression on me. Shocked at the scarcity of therapies and how little the standard tools of medicine had to offer, I resolved to become a doctor who offered his patients more—much more—than what I had received. I have devoted my career to that goal.

By the time cancer patients arrive at my center, many feel listless, overwhelmed, weary, or depressed and anxious. After only a few weeks, however, they find their fatigue subsiding and their spirits rising. Many are able to tolerate treatment with few side effects. Some benefit from therapies that had previously failed. When you and I work together through this book, your overall health and quality of life have the potential to be better than you ever thought, giving you a foundation of general wellness from which you can combat your cancer.

You Can Beat the Statistics

Bombarded with doom-and-gloom statistics, you may feel overwhelmed trying to muster enthusiasm for life. So forget all the talk of "survival rates." *They do not apply to you.* All statistics, by definition, apply only to groups, not individuals. Researchers use them to determine whether a therapy works or not, and physicians use them to help make choices among different therapies. But as an empowered individual, you should not use statistics to dictate *your* chances of survival.

Two of my earliest patients (whose real names I do not use) avoided "becoming a statistic." I was just finishing my training when Sam, an executive, came to see me. He had heard that I was researching the clinical use of nutrition as a therapy to fight malignant disease. Sam had prostate cancer that had metastasized to his bones. He lived in constant pain, unable to find any real relief. Sam had made good use of the macrobiotic diet and other alternative treatments, but even those brought him no respite from his pain. Desperate, he pleaded with me to help him fight his disease, as I had done for myself with my ulcers. There was nowhere else for him to turn, he said. His doctors had hit him with the dreaded "nothing more can be done" edict.

At about the same time, Ira came to see me. He was also suffering from advanced prostate cancer that had spread to his bones. Chemotherapy had made him so sick he quit in the middle of his first cycle. After we talked in my office about possible treatments, he fished a bottle of sleeping pills from his pocket and set it on my desk. "Be honest with me, Dr. Block," he said. "I need to know if you can help me. Because if you can't, I'm going to check into a hotel and put myself and my family out of misery."

In medical school, we were taught that in some circumstances extraordinary measures can be used to save a patient's life. This is known as clinical urgency: when there are no more treatment options and the patient is suffering or terminal, a physician is duty-bound to roll up his sleeves and take almost any rational action he can think of. Ira and Sam were textbook cases of clinical urgency. I talked it over with my wife, Penny, who is also my partner and cofounder of the Block Center for Integrative Cancer Treatment. We decided to put our long-held convictions into action and do everything possible—to go beyond what other doctors had done—to help these two men reclaim their lives and health.

Our work with Ira and Sam became cornerstones of our Life Over Cancer program. Like so many of the patients who followed them to Evanston, Ira and Sam had both been told by their doctors that there was no hope; other cancer centers had turned them away as beyond help. Yet, after following our early program, which further refined the diet and therapeutic changes he had made, Sam ended up living eleven productive and pain-free years. Ira lived eight years. Scans showed that each had experienced complete remission of his cancer.

They proved to represent many of the thousands of patients we've seen since 1980. Most arrive with disease that has already spread, or metastasized, to areas in the body distant from the original tumor. Most have been through chemotherapy two times or more and are dealing with recurrent and relapsed disease, a stage when most fatalities occur. A tragic number have heard the same dreaded words from their doctor: "There is nothing more that can be done." Yet, after following the Life Over Cancer program, many exceed the expectations of their original doctors—and not by months but by years. That is why I urge you to ignore survival rates, remission rates, and other statistics. *They need not apply to you.*

That is especially so if you are one of the lucky ones. It may seem odd to pair the words *lucky* and *cancer,* but all the advice that follows applies just as much to patients who are at the beginning of their journey—that is, to those who have been diagnosed for the first time with a primary tumor and in whom the cancer has not spread. As I am sure your doctor has told you, you have every reason to remain optimistic. For one thing, surgery alone is often effective against a contained solid tumor. For another, today's chemotherapy agents and high-tech radiation treatments are allowing more and more people to survive cancer. By combining these mainstream therapies with those in this book, your chances of joining their ranks are even greater.

It's time to begin our journey together.

CHAPTER I

WHY INTEGRATIVE CARE WORKS

Cancer is one of the ultimate challenges any of us can face. I tell my patients that it is like being forced to climb Mount Everest: your trek to recovery requires the same committed focus and fitness of body and mind. Many of my patients tell me this analogy not only captures how overwhelmed their illness makes them feel but also reinforces two key ideas. First, to surmount your illness, just as to climb Everest, you need know-how, planning, and preparedness. Second, all mountains are ascended one step at a time, and all illnesses are conquered one step at a time. Every new health-promoting behavior you adopt is a victory. Every improvement in your symptoms, no matter how small, is an important step toward the summit of health.

The first point: preparedness is a key to successful cancer therapy. If I dropped you onto the summit of Everest, you would be lucky to survive a few hours in the intense cold and low-oxygen atmosphere. In the same way, unprepared cancer patients often lack the reserves to carry them through treatment. Of course, no rational person would ever let himself be plopped beneath the summit of Everest unprepared. You need training, proper equipment, and time to study the routes and learn the terrain *before* starting your trek. En route, you pace yourself and set up camps along the way to acclimatize yourself to the altitude. If you're smart, you also enlist an experienced guide, one who helps you navigate the trickiest terrain.

So it is with cancer. Ascending Everest is analogous to the *attack phase* of cancer therapy—the conventional treatment for debulking, or shrinking, the primary tumor. The better and smarter the preparation, the more likely you are to complete this treatment. Don't worry if there is only a little time between when you receive your diagnosis and when you begin treatment such as surgery: even a little preparedness can go a long way. With an experienced guide offering strategies complementary to your chemotherapy, radiation, and surgery, treatment will be less debilitating and more effective.

If the attack phase is successful in shrinking or eliminating the primary tumor, you've achieved either a partial remission or a complete remission. This is like reaching the summit of Everest. What next? More often than not, nothing. Former medical thinking viewed successful completion of the attack phase ("we got it all") as almost synonymous with a cure. But even with remission after surgery and chemo, some residual undetectable cancer cells likely remain. It has been estimated that approximately half of all cancer patients in remission actually have metastases, malignant cells that have broken off the original tumor, traveled through the bloodstream to far-flung sites in the body, and begun the insidious process of growing into another dangerous tumor. Just because you have achieved remission through elimination of the primary tumor does not mean you are home free. Cancer is not like an infection, where you wipe it out and move on. It is a *chronic condition* that needs constant vigilance. While conventional cancer treatments often remove much of the disease burden—and it is critical to remove tumor bulk from your body—that is only half the battle. Even when the primary tumor is eliminated, micrometastases may already have migrated to and seeded other parts of the body. These dormant cells can rear up and reestablish themselves.

That's why for my patients, complete remission does not

mean the end of treatment. Instead, it means the start of the *containment* or *growth control phase*, when we focus on stopping or slowing further growth of any residual disease (visible tumors) or invisible metastatic cancer cells. Post-treatment is a time to be particularly aggressive.

To continue the Everest metaphor, a successful climb is not only about summiting but also about getting back down. This is where climbers often err because the potential for catastrophe—treacherous ice patches and wrong turns that send you plunging into an abyss—is so great. Similarly, for a cancer patient it is critical to look past the summit of clear scans and remission so that your preparedness carries over into the post-treatment, or *remission maintenance,* phase.

Unfortunately, this is the most neglected phase of cancer treatment. Conventional cancer treatment does little to prevent cells from regrouping, proliferating, and forming new tumors. It also does little to help patients recover from persistent side effects and potentially life-threatening complications of attack-phase treatments. But with the right strategy these effects can be avoided or overcome: we have tools—especially diet, nutritional therapy, and experimental and off-label drug use—that can delay or block the return of cancer.

Now cancer patients part ways with mountain climbers. When mountain climbers return to base camp, their ordeal is over. They have triumphed. Not so with cancer patients who have reached the summit (achieved remission) and descended safely (kept metastatic cells in check). With cancer, you must remain attentive to self-care, taking an active role in your continued health. Rather than waiting passively for the results of your next scan or checkup, you can actively seize control of your future. This will likely entail making changes in what you eat, how you stay fit, and how you balance life's stressors, but I can just about guarantee that the small investment will yield a huge return: not only will this new way of life decrease your risk of relapse, but it will decrease your risk of diseases other than cancer, too, and make you feel better, stronger, and more empowered every day.

The Beginnings of Life Over Cancer

Cancer entered my life long before I went to medical school. As a teenager, I watched my grandmother, my grandfather, and an uncle all die of cancer. They all suffered great pain toward the end, not just from the disease but from the treatments they endured. It was as if the quality of their lives were irrelevant, as if it no longer mattered how they felt once their doctors had proclaimed that there was nothing more that could be done. Though I had no medical training, I couldn't believe there was nothing more that could be done—at least to improve their quality of life as they underwent treatment.

I remember sitting at my grandmother's sickbed, watching helplessly as her cancer progressed and she became increasingly frail and thin. Her body was betraying her, but so were her physicians. Only sixteen, I was undergoing intensive physical training for high school football. I wondered: why weren't her caregivers encouraging her to exercise? Logic told me that keeping her muscles active might help her resist some of the wasting syndrome she suffered.

After my grandmother passed away, I kept thinking about all the things I might have done had I been her doctor. (This was one of the experiences that motivated me to become a doctor.) I was certain she could have lived the remainder of her life, even with her cancer, with far more awareness, dignity, and well-being had she been given a whole other level of care. This experience also made me resolve to be a different kind of doctor, one who did more than run tests and administer standard treatments. I wanted to tend to my patients' emotional and physical well-being, too.

That resolve only grew stronger. As a resident, I sometimes followed an attending physician as he made his rounds at the hospital. One day I was following a doctor who was notoriously a morning person, beginning his rounds at 6:30 A.M. sharp, regardless of the patients' sleep schedule. His first stop that chilly dawn was the bedside of a Chicago bus driver in her mid-forties. Admitted the previous night, she had an advanced case of cancer. This physician, whom she had never laid eyes on, was the first doctor to speak to her. He sailed into the room and woke her up. With no preamble, he declared, "I am sorry to tell you that you have colon cancer, and it will probably take your life shortly." He turned with a squeak of shoe leather and left the room, followed by his entourage.

I stayed behind, unable to move a muscle, rooted to the spot where I'd stood as the attending pronounced judgment. The color had drained from the face of this poor woman, and her jaw was slack from the shock. Her entire body appeared frozen in terror. And no wonder. She had just been awakened in a strange bed in a strange hospital by a man who coldly informed her that she was doomed. I found myself in shock as well—not by what he'd said, but how. I stayed with her for over an hour, returning for long periods in the days and weeks that followed, doing what I could to restore her shattered will to live.

When I founded the Block Center for Integrative Cancer Treatment in 1980, I knew it would be essential to provide an environment of hope and authentic caring. We would of course offer the best treatments from mainstream oncology to shrink or eliminate tumors. Although I was intrigued by anecdotal reports of success with purely alternative therapies, there was not enough solid evidence of their effectiveness to employ them alone. In the Life Over Cancer plan, it is crucial to eliminate the bulk of the tumor, freeing the body's natural defenses for the job of ridding the body of residual or microscopic disease. We recognized that it was asking too much of our body's immune system and other anti-cancer defenses to destroy or even shrink large, established tumors. It was clear to me that with rare exceptions, patients need and can benefit from established conventional therapies.

But conventional cancer treatment, while necessary, is not sufficient. Also crucial are nutrition (the quickest and surest way to affect one's biochemistry), natural medicines (since, with a few rare exceptions, the pharmaceutical industry has not produced a true cure for any cancer), exercise, and mind-spirit care (including support and therapy to alleviate the terror associated with cancer treatment). These would be among the most important components of the care we offered. Just to be clear, we use nutrition, exercise, and mind-body treatments to enhance standard cancer treatments, not replace them.

The term did not exist then, but our approach was the first truly *integrative* cancer treatment in North America. Through innovative interventions and therapies, custom-tailored to the clinical, psychological, biochemical, and molecular characteristics of each patient, we treat the whole person, not just the cancer. Throughout, patients are active participants in their care, as we explain what we are prescribing and why, and what they need to do to have the greatest chance of success.

The Life Over Cancer program was not set in stone in 1980. We have continuously made changes as we learned from patients' experiences, and adopted novel treatments supported by the burgeoning medical literature in cancer therapy, both mainstream and complementary. Full-time staff members stay on top of the latest research, as well as plan and conduct studies of new therapies. As a result, the Life Over Cancer program has improved with time as we've learned in the clinic what works and what doesn't, and as research breakthroughs have emerged. Put simply, if a new treatment holds promise and is safe and effective, we consider including it.

Way back in 1984, I discussed some of our cases of advanced metastatic cancers at a cancer seminar at the University of Chicago. I showed X-rays indicating that the disease had spread to many distant sites in the body—yet these patients had all experienced regressions of their disease and were still alive, many years later. That astonished these specialists. Indeed, a number of patients who have been referred to our center and were considered "hopeless" or "terminal" have stunned even me as they lived and thrived years longer than expected. It was a few years after this talk that I first pointed out that false hopelessness—which some practitioners may implant in the minds of patients—is fully as dangerous as the "false hope" that some alternative therapeutic claims may stimulate.

No matter how impressive, however, anecdotes are not proof of the effectiveness of the Life Over Cancer program. Starting in the mid-1980s, therefore, we devoted ourselves to collecting voluminous data on two groups of our sickest patients—those with metastatic breast cancer or prostate cancer—in order to determine whether the Life Over Cancer program of intensive integrative oncology helps cancer patients live better and longer lives compared with patients relying solely on the best mainstream treatments.

Evidence of Longer Survival

In ninety women with metastatic breast cancer, the disease had spread to the liver, lungs, brain, bones, or other organs. (Why one kind of primary tumor metastasizes to one set of organs while another kind spreads to a different set remains one of the enduring mysteries of cancer biology.) This is called stage IV metastatic breast cancer. All the women participated in the full Life Over Cancer (LOC) program, including our tailored diet, supplements, exercise, and mind-spirit programs. Eighty percent of them received multiple chemotherapy regimens after they came to us; this was sometimes their third, fourth, or even fifth round of chemo. We compared the survival of our patients with those from other studies conducted by leading researchers in the United States in which the patients received hormonal and/or chemotherapy treatments. Our breast cancer patients lived roughly twice as long as patients getting standard treatments alone as we reported in a study published in 2009 in *The Breast Journal.* Our median survival was thirty-eight months, compared to fifteen to twenty-three months in the comparison studies of other stage IV patients. Moreover, *our patients were 33 percent more likely to be alive at five years than patients getting standard treatment alone.*

This edge held even in women with the worst metastases. Our patients with bone metastases lived almost twice as long (forty months versus twenty-three months) as non-LOC patients with bone metastases receiving standard therapy. Our patients with liver metastases lived ten months longer (twenty-three months versus thirteen months) than non-LOC patients with liver metastases receiving standard therapy. Our patients with lung metastases lived more than twice as long (forty-three months versus eighteen months) as non-LOC patients with lung metastases receiving standard therapy. In sum, our metastatic breast cancer patients on the Life Over Cancer program had doubled survival times, increased five-year survival rates, and dramatically better long-term outcomes than patients on standard therapy alone.

We also studied twenty-seven men with metastatic prostate cancer. The disease had spread to their bones or visceral organs, meaning they had stage D_2 cancer. All received the standard treatments, called combined androgen blockage, from either our center or their original oncologist to halt production of the male hormones that stimulate the growth of prostate cancer. The patients also all received a drug designed to block the further spread of the cancer. In addition, they received our whole package of integrative treatments, including our dietary plan, select nutritional supplements, a therapeutic exercise program, and a mind-spirit regimen for psychological and spiritual well-being. We compared our patients' results with results for stage D_2 patients from four different studies who underwent treatment at leading cancer centers such as the Johns Hopkins University Medical Center and to patients whose cancer was less advanced (stage C, having spread from the prostate to the local surrounding tissue, but not to the bones or other organs).

The results? Our Life Over Cancer patients lived, on average, twice as long as stage D_2 patients getting standard treatments alone. For the latter, median survival at the four cancer centers averaged thirty months. The median survival time of patients in the Life Over Cancer program was sixty months. In other words, *Life Over Cancer patients had a median survival twice as long as patients getting standard care alone.* Since "median" means that half the patients lived longer than that amount of time and half lived shorter, fully 50 percent of the Life Over Cancer patients were alive five years after diagnosis. Only 26 percent of prostate cancer patients receiving just standard hormone treatments survived five years. Moreover, 20 percent of our metastatic prostate cancer patients lived more than ten years.

How did the Life Over Cancer patients—all stage D_2—fare

compared with patients whose disease had not spread as far? They lived twenty months longer than a group that included equal numbers of stage C and stage D patients. Median survival in the mixed group ranged from thirty to just under forty months, so our median survival was over twenty months longer. *Thus, our patients lived considerably longer than patients who, as a group, were far less sick.*

We recently have begun collecting data on other cancers. Nearly 70 percent of lung cancer patients who come to the Block Center are stage IV, compared with 38 percent of lung cancer patients nationally. In other words, they are sicker than most. Nevertheless, the median survival time that we observed is about twice what is usually expected. As you can imagine, our clinical and research staff are encouraged by these treatment outcomes. These are among the most compelling studies to date supporting the potential role integrative oncology can play in the lives of cancer patients. Our next research steps are underway to extend and expand these findings using randomized trial designs.

Your Blueprint for Recovery

The Life Over Cancer program can be effective, and can reach into so many aspects of your life, because cancer is not merely a tumor. It is an underlying condition. It is based on abnormal patterns driven by genetics and lifestyle. It reflects changes in your body all the way down to the microscopic and molecular levels, changes that began long before you had any symptoms of cancer—indeed, long before cancer was diagnosed or even detectable. It therefore makes no sense to think of cancer as a tumor. That is merely its most obvious manifestation. A whole slew of physiological processes are also out of whack—sufficient to allow malignant cells to arise, grow, and proliferate uncontrollably.

Although only limited progress has been made in treating cancer, biologists have made tremendous strides in understanding its origins and development. Cancer can begin in any of several ways. Toxic chemicals from the air we breathe, the water we drink, the smoke we inhale, or the food we eat can alter the DNA in a single one of our cells and cause a genetic mutation. Or the unstable and highly reactive molecules called free radicals, generated by normal metabolism, can damage DNA, also giving rise to mutations. Alternatively, cancer can arise by chance: DNA in our cells is forever making copies of itself, and if the copy is flawed, the resulting cell can start down the path to malignancy.

Normally, the body's defense systems eliminate mutated cells by causing them to commit suicide and through other mechanisms. If mutations overwhelm the body's defenses, however, the mutated cells will proliferate uncontrolled until they are numerous enough to form a solid tumor or a blood cancer. Even more perniciously, cancer can hijack many of the body's own mechanisms to create an environment that actually nurtures a tumor's growth and spread. The Life Over Cancer program emphasizes strengthening your anti-cancer biology: unless the body's physiological defenses prevent the growth and spread of malignancies, they are likely to return sooner or later.

Tumors affect the body in many devious ways. Chemicals they release can cause abnormal blood clots. They can take over and pervert the body's metabolism of carbohydrates, fat, and protein, a theft of nutrients that can lead to loss of appetite, weight loss, nutritional wasting, and fatigue. Tumors can alter the body's hormone levels, causing depression, weight gain, and the loss of lean body mass and skeletal muscle. Many of the complementary therapies included in the Life Over Cancer program combat these insidious effects of cancer—for obvious reasons. If you suffer from fatigue, for instance, you may not be able to endure the arduous process of cancer treatment. If appetite loss and the erosion of lean muscle tissue lead to the wasting syndrome called cachexia, you may survive your cancer but succumb to its side effects. And if you develop depression, you are more likely to have a poor response to chemotherapy; indeed, studies estimate that one-third of cancer patients abandon chemotherapy, most of them suffering from psychological distress or physical debilitation. Little wonder, then, that depression and hopelessness seem linked to high rates of recurrence and premature death in patients with some types of cancer.

I hope this makes clear the futility of trying to cure cancer solely by destroying tumors. Tumors are merely a manifestation of a broader condition, and painful experience has shown that far too often they reappear, with even greater resilience, if the systemic condition that nurtured them is not treated. That is why the fixation on eliminating tumors, which has dominated cancer care for well over half a century, has brought dismal results for so many patients. Yes, surgery or radiation can remove the tumor, but unless you change the environment that nurtured it in the first place, malignant cells that remain behind can simply pick up where they left off. Sometimes that happens alarmingly quickly: studies of postoperative cancer patients show that when a surgeon cuts close to a tumor to remove it, growth signals associated with wound healing can sometimes be unleashed, triggering any residual malignant cells to grow and develop into a new tumor. To reduce this risk, when the location of the incision permits, the surgeon will use a wider incision to remove the tumor.

The good news is that the Life Over Cancer program can reduce the physiological imbalance and deprive the malignant cells of the resources they need in order to thrive. That will allow your biochemical and physiological systems to return to health, and you to recover.

The Three Targets of the Life Over Cancer Program

The Life Over Cancer program consists of changes you will need to make in three areas. Let me explain them briefly; each is covered more thoroughly in the three parts of this book.

▶ Improving Your Lifestyle

First, you will need to adopt changes in how you live, including changes in what you eat, how you stay fit, how you handle stress, and how you sleep. Each of these can enhance or undermine your health. Each time you choose a certain food or physical activity or experience unrelieved distress, you are influencing your health. By making more healthful lifestyle choices at any point along your journey—including after you have been diagnosed with cancer, and even after you have completed conventional therapy—you improve the odds that your body will be able to combat cancer. A low-fat, plant-based diet; aerobic, flexibility, and strength exercises; and stress-reducing activities are the basic ingredients of sound health. Whatever your condition and whatever your stage of cancer, implementing these measures can be crucial toward improving your health.

▶ **Boosting Your Biology**

Second, you will need to strengthen your anti-cancer biology, the physiological environment that either encourages the growth and spread of malignancies or thwarts them. While targeting the tumor directly is obviously essential, if you do so in a way that leaves untouched the biochemical environment that supports it, then recovery is likely to be short-lived. This internal biochemistry includes levels of oxidation and inflammation, the state of your immune system, and levels of growth signals. While the standard tools of modern oncology are certainly good at removing tumors, they often fail to prevent the spread or recurrence of cancer. In part, that's because they ignore the environment that supports the cancer.

▶ **Enhancing Your Treatment**

In addition to helping you make changes in how you live and in the environment that supports your cancer, the Life Over Cancer program targets the tumor directly, through surgery, chemotherapy, radiation, and molecular-targeted therapies. This, of course, is the focus—really, the sole focus—of conventional treatment. But the Life Over Cancer program goes further. In some cases, I advise experimental options, off-label use of approved drugs, and natural medicines, all of which can sometimes shrink or eliminate tumors. In addition, I will explain which aspects of diet, supplements, fitness regimens, and mind-spirit interventions will complement these therapies, minimizing their toxic or debilitating side effects and increasing their effectiveness.

The Life Over Cancer program works for two main reasons. First, therapies and interventions are chosen to complement

INTEGRATIVE CANCER CARE

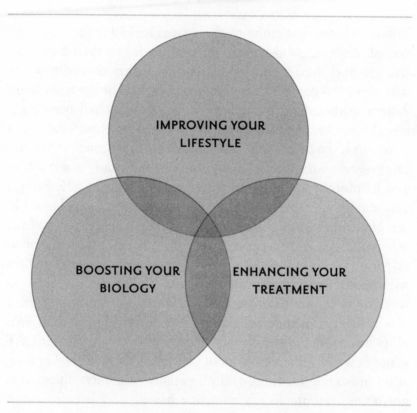

each other, with diet increasing the chance that a tumor eliminated by radiation will not return, for instance, and nutritional supplements as well as specific mind-spirit techniques making it less likely that you will become too nauseous and debilitated from chemotherapy to continue. Second, the plan can be individualized to fit each person's disease and situation.

This may all seem a little abstract, so let me describe how individualized Life Over Cancer plans worked for two of my patients. Delores and Marlene (not their real names) each had breast cancer when they came to the Block Center for Integrative Cancer Treatment. By explaining how these two very different women battled their cancers using individualized versions of the Life Over Cancer program, I hope to give you the insight and inspiration you need to face and overcome your own illness.

Delores: Counteracting the Typical American Lifestyle

When Delores first came to the center in 1999, she was a reserved, mellow, good-humored woman who worked a nine-to-five job and lived a sedentary lifestyle. In her mid-forties, she was about 50 percent over her ideal weight. She ate a standard American diet, high in sugar and fat. Delores had been diagnosed with localized breast cancer. When we first saw her, a year after diagnosis, she had already undergone a mastectomy—after which her surgeon told her they had "got it all"—and six months of a chemotherapy regimen called CMF. Being a "good patient," she had followed her doctor's game plan without question. But as she began reading about nutrition and the role it could play in keeping cancer from recurring, she came to us for advice on how she might fortify her biological defenses without committing to a full program. When we later ran blood work to assess her risk of recurrence, the results indicated there was already evidence of high tumor activity. Less than two years after surgery, her cancer was back. Even worse, her CAT scan showed four small spots of cancer on her liver, a dire situation indicating far-flung and potentially fatal metastasis. (It is not quite accurate to say someone has died of breast cancer. Death is caused by metastases of the original tumor that have spread to a vital organ.) Delores decided to begin the full Life Over Cancer program immediately.

After studying a patient's medical records, my first step is always a full assessment of his or her lifestyle, diet, fitness level, and mind-spirit strengths. In Delores' case, this showed that beneath her cheerful and controlled manner, she was beset by extreme anxiety. Interviews revealed that she believed this anxiety, like the physical effects of her disease, was beyond her control. Throughout her life, she had downplayed the importance of her own needs compared with the needs of others; indeed, she panicked at the mere thought of doing anything that might disrupt the routine and emotional equilibrium of her family, even something that might save her life.

Next, I tested Delores' "biochemical terrain," as I call it. Blood tests showed high levels of oxidative stress, probably a result of both her cancer and her chemotherapy. Her immune function was low, also due to the chemo. Levels of the stress hormone cortisol were abnormally low, too, which meant that Delores would have a hard time sustaining her energy and other crucial bodily resources. Other tests detected high levels of insulin and growth hormones, essential to the spread of cancer, and common in people who are overweight.

Now that we knew her situation, our first step was to attack the tumors in her liver. I chose a three-drug chemotherapy combination frequently used to treat breast cancer, referred to as CAF, which was at that time the standard treatment. The delivery method, however, was decidedly non-standard. Instead of the usual large and highly toxic dose, we used a slower, graduated process called fractionated infusion. By administering her chemo in a slow, steady dose, we helped avoid known side effects of the CAF drugs, including damage to the heart. To further avoid side effects, Delores took detoxifying supplements to help her body flush out toxic chemo metabolites. Finally, to enhance Delores' sensitivity to the drugs and reduce the likelihood that the tumor cells would develop resistance to treatment, I advised melatonin and fish oil.

As Delores began her chemotherapy, our staff helped her to make changes to her lifestyle. She adopted a semi-vegetarian diet low in animal fats and high in vegetables, whole grains, legumes, and fruit. I believe there is no better diet for general wellness (my wife, Penny, and I both follow this diet for prevention and optimal health, and have raised our four children on it), and such nutrition is especially crucial to anyone living with cancer and its treatments. Delores supplemented this diet with a protein-rich drink that helps maintain nutrients and repair tissue. Because obesity is associated with a poorer prognosis for cancer patients, we started Delores on gentle strengthening exercises while enhancing her aerobic capacity, with the goal of a healthier weight and increased muscle mass. Being fitter lowered her insulin levels (which greatly improves the prognosis for breast cancer patients), allowed her to better withstand the rigors of chemotherapy, and, not incidentally, helped her feel better, lifting her out of depression.

To counter her anxiety, Delores learned "relaxed breathing" exercises, which helped her break the chain of panic felt whenever she dwelled on her condition. She also learned biofeedback so she could observe and become confident about her newfound ability to control what she had thought were inevitable responses to stress. A religious person, Delores also practiced prayerful meditation. This enabled her to tap into a source of calm and strength. Cognitive training helped her adjust her priorities and embrace the things she had to do to preserve her health.

Next we focused on strengthening Delores' anti-cancer biology. As mentioned above, tests showed high levels of oxidative stress, low immune function, low cortisol levels, and high levels of growth hormones. Tumors thrive in these conditions, so it was obviously necessary to get them back to healthful levels. To combat the oxidative damage, possibly a result of her prior chemotherapy, I recommended a twice-daily 8-ounce glass of a vegetable-fruit drink rich in phytochemicals (phytochemicals are the powerful healing compounds found in plant pigments), equivalent to a dozen servings of vegetables. She also began taking Siberian ginseng to normalize cortisol production and immune function. To support normal insulin production, I placed her on the supplement taurine.

We were now ready to introduce complementary therapies and natural medicines aimed at enhancing the efficacy of standard cancer treatments. I started Delores on a Chinese herbal formula composed of ginseng, astragalus, cinnamon, and other ingredients that we have found helps patients maintain energy levels. I also recommended micronutrients (cancer patients need to avoid standard multivitamins, as too much iron, copper, manganese, and high levels of vitamins B_1 and B_{12} can promote cancer). These included antioxidants, fish oil capsules that support a healthy inflammation response, and a formulation containing extracts from six types of medicinal mushrooms thought to support immune function. Since Delores' breast cancer was estrogen-receptor-positive, I also gave her calcium d-glucarate, a compound that research suggests may support normal metabolism of estrogen, the hormone that can latch on to estrogen receptors and trigger tumor-cell proliferation. After her chemotherapy and full integrative program knocked out her liver tumors, Delores regained and, in fact, greatly improved her overall health. However, as is commonly the case with metastatic disease, her cancer eventually began to show signs of returning. The integrative lifestyle program seems to have kept it at bay, since it was a full three years before it came roaring back (usual survival after diagnosis of liver metastases was a little over a year at that time). This time, metastases covered 80 percent of her liver.

But because we had stretched her survival, we were now able to turn to a new conventional therapy. Molecular analysis showed that the molecule HER2/neu studded the surface of Delores' tumor cells, similar to the way that estrogen receptors stud the surface of many breast cancer cells. Herceptin, a new molecular target therapy, had just received FDA approval for treating HER2/neu-bearing tumors. Thus, in 1999, Delores became one of the first U.S. patients to receive Herceptin outside a clinical trial. Had we not been able to keep her cancer at bay with her integrative program, she might have missed this chance. Once again, conventional therapy knocked out her liver tumors, and her full program continued to support her health.

Just as important as enhancing the potency of treatment is preventing what can be its serious side effects. I therefore gave Delores a micronutrient, coenzyme Q_{10} (coQ_{10}), an amino acid supplement, L-carnitine, as well as a plant extract of hawthorn, all to support her heart muscle. (Adriamycin in the CAF therapy as well as Herceptin can damage heart muscle tissue.) Despite receiving Herceptin for four years and undergoing several more rounds of chemotherapy, Delores' last heart scans before she discontinued Herceptin were completely normal.

As Delores progressed through treatment I adjusted the dosages of coQ_{10}, L-carnitine, and hawthorn extract. When the common side effect neuropathy (which Delores experienced as numbness in the fingers) occurred, Delores began taking the botanical supplement ginkgo biloba and lipoic acid as nervous system supports. Delores went on to survive seven years beyond the few months she had been given when her liver mets were found, living well and getting to see her children graduate from college.

Marlene: Overcoming Mistrust

Marlene faced a very different set of challenges. She was an exercise addict, a competitive bodybuilder, and, in her own words, "a mountain climbing fanatic" who began her day at 5:45 A.M. by lifting weights for nearly two hours. She worked two jobs. Too busy to cook, she had made fast food and sugar the centerpieces of her diet, ingesting a steady stream of cookies and sugary sodas as she powered through her grueling schedule. In order to fuel this frenetic lifestyle, she drank an average of eight cups of coffee a day and smoked heavily.

Marlene was in her mid-forties and in peak physical condition when she found a large lump in her breast. An extraordinary capacity for denial, as well as severe apprehension about doctors, kept her from having the lump examined for nearly six months. Eventually she saw her physician and learned she had cancer. Five days later she underwent a modified radical mastectomy that removed her breast and lymph nodes. Because of her deep mistrust of the medical world, at five in the morning the day after the surgery she struggled out of her hospital bed, pulled out her IV, got dressed, and demanded to be released.

Her pathology report was not encouraging. The tumor was 4.5 centimeters in diameter, and ten of thirteen lymph nodes examined showed evidence of cancer. At a follow-up visit her doctor told her, "I'm sorry, but you will die from this disease." This fatal pronouncement stirred Marlene's rebellious spirit. She read everything she could find about cancer treatment. She began a strict macrobiotic diet. Happening on a description of our center, she made an appointment to see us. As she put it, she felt she "had to trust somebody."

Marlene received a full, individualized assessment upon her arrival in 1996. Although she appeared to be in good physical condition and of normal weight, her detoxification capacity was greatly reduced, likely due in part to her history of smoking. We did not need to conduct a formal psychological assessment to see that Marlene had a strong aversion to medical settings: she experienced extreme anxiety whenever she underwent any type of exam (we therefore used relaxed focused imagery before each exam to calm her). Our assessment revealed a woman truly panic-stricken at a perceived loss of control over her body and her life. Furthermore, she suffered from an underlying depression that deprived her of a sense of pleasure in being alive.

Tests of Marlene's biochemical terrain found high levels of stress hormones. While having too low a level of cortisol, as Delores had, is associated with a decline in vitality and generalized enervation, chronically high levels of the stress hormone cortisol are associated with poor outcomes. Marlene also had high oxidation levels (a reflection of smoking and stress) and inflammation (probably in part from excessive exercise). Unlike Delores' tumor, Marlene's was estrogen-receptor-negative, an indication that something other than this hormone was fueling cellular proliferation.

We first targeted Marlene's lifestyle. I focused on a balanced fitness regimen, advising her to add stretching and flexibility. I encouraged her to continue hiking but to reduce high-impact exercises such as excessive weight lifting, which can promote inflammation. I advised her to relax her overly rigid version of the macrobiotic diet in order to get important nutrients such as omega-3 fatty acids (found in fish oils) and lycopene (found in tomatoes, which were not part of her strict macrobiotic diet). By widening her food choices, I hoped, she would reap an added benefit: obsessive dietary attitudes can keep you from really enjoying food, with the result that you absorb fewer nutrients.

In the mind-spirit area, we worked with Marlene to help her master her anxiety, recapture pleasure in her life, and alleviate depression. Training with our staff in cognitive therapy allowed her to identify what triggered her anxiety around any medical encounter and calmly prevent these events from tipping her into an anxiety attack. She learned to focus on the pleasurable aspects of her life and to enter the highly focused state of self-hypnosis, where she was able to conquer much of her fear just prior to each medical encounter by inducing her body's relaxation response at will. Most important, Marlene learned that there are many acceptable ways of living between the opposing poles of utter failure and perfection, something that let her enhance relationships with family members, who in turn provided invaluable support as she dealt with cancer.

Now it was time to attack her cancer directly. At first, Marlene refused to even consider chemotherapy. I worked hard to gain her trust, speaking to her at length about my patients' experiences, and explained that the severity of her disease made chemotherapy imperative to prevent progression and advanced disease. I reassured her that, bolstered by our supplement program, I believed that she would be able to tolerate chemo with little discomfort and few side effects. She finally agreed to begin chemotherapy.

As with Delores, we opted for a CAF regimen. To minimize her anxiety, I obtained a portable chemo pump that she could wear in a fanny pack. It allowed Marlene to receive the CAF through the fractionated infusion method, as Delores did, and it also made her less anxious than she would have been stuck in a chair getting chemo. She actually received CAF while taking walks. This helped her regain a sense of control. Marlene experienced no side effects and, over the six months of chemo, never missed a meal.

To complement this treatment, I recommended a Chinese herbal concoction that promotes energy levels. Marlene also took macronutrients that support appetite and immune function and protect the gut wall, which can be damaged by chemo. She took an antioxidant, a formula of fish oil and curcumin (a turmeric extract) for a normal inflammatory response, and silymarin (a milk thistle extract) to promote healthy liver function. Because tests showed Marlene had low levels of essential phytochemicals (such as the anti-cancer compound lycopene), I also started her on a phytochemical drink.

Let me pause for a moment to underline how individualized Marlene's and Delores' treatments were. Marlene took silymarin; Delores did not. Delores took immune-enhancing mushrooms;

Marlene did not. Delores took Siberian ginseng for her stress response; Marlene did not. The differences were not confined to supplements. Persuading Marlene to relax her strict macrobiotic diet and exercise regimen proved extremely helpful, but such an approach would have been inappropriate, even dangerous, for Delores with her high-fat, high-sugar diet. In fact, it is probably a misnomer to refer to *the* Life Over Cancer program. There are as many Life Over Cancer programs as there are patients, with each program customized to a patient's unique biochemical, social, psychological, and biological characteristics.

Today Marlene has completely restructured her life. She is successfully balancing work, relaxation, and relationships and is following an improved diet and sensible exercise regimen. She says that although she wouldn't have wished for cancer, her "life after cancer is richer than it was before." In 2008, over twelve years after her surgeon told her she would die from the disease, Marlene is healthy and completely free of malignancy. Her complete remission is impressive, a true testament to the Life Over Cancer program and Marlene's terrific spirit.

Your Turn

I hope these two stories have given you a sense of how the Life Over Cancer program is customized—tailored to fit your needs and your situation. Some elements, such as a diet rich in vegetables and fruits, apply to everyone. Others, such as the precise supplements you should take to make your internal biochemical environment as hostile as possible to cancer, vary from one person to another. This book will allow you to create an individualized program, one that is much more effective than the standard one-size-fits-all therapies offered by much of conventional and complementary medicine. It's time to dive in.

CHAPTER 2

FORMING YOUR
WINNING TEAM

Cancer is not something you want to face alone. Processing information, making decisions, and taking appropriate action are just too overwhelming without support. As anyone with the disease knows, cancer can be such a stressful experience that patients struggle to maintain clarity, equanimity, and inner peace. Decision making is far more difficult when you're overwhelmed with tension and anxiety. That is why assembling your personal "A-Team" should be among your top priorities. Whom you choose to see you through will affect your quality of life and your chances of attaining and sustaining a full remission.

The purpose of the A-Team is to help you meet the major challenges of cancer. The right friends and loved ones can promote your health and well-being just by their presence, screening intrusions that would otherwise distract you from the information you have to process, listening sympathetically to your fears and hopes, and enhancing your sense of equanimity amid the storm of emotions incited by a diagnosis of cancer. They can relieve stress by providing meals, helping out with transportation or child care, scheduling relaxation or recreational time, helping you explore treatment options, following up on diagnostic reports. Your A-Team can bring you clarity, coherence, and peace of mind as you move toward recovery.

The members of your A-Team must be capable of providing you with five basic forms of support—emotional, practical, informational, coaching, and decision-making. You therefore need to pick people whose personalities and coping styles make them well equipped for a particular role. Someone able to listen empathetically and constructively, without denying the validity of your feelings or imposing their own, is the kind of person you want providing emotional support. Someone whose strength is more intellectual, rational, and logical is better suited to providing informational support. Let me explain what each form of support entails, and suggest the kind of person best suited to provide it.

1. Emotional support. Think of the people in your life who are best equipped to help you feel less overwhelmed and more empowered. In all likelihood, your emotional supporter will be someone who has been a loving friend or relative for many years—a spouse, lover, sibling, or close friend. It might be someone who has provided support during another crisis in your life. It should be someone you think of as a "comforter," someone you can count on for emotional solace, someone who can provide a safe and nonjudgmental space for you to express your feelings. It should be someone you feel you can confide in, someone with whom you can share your darkest thoughts. Whom did you turn to when your heart broke or when a setback at work made you feel worthless? Who served as a confidant when you felt alone or confused? Although this may well be an old friend or relative, you may find that a nurse or doctor can provide emotional support, too. Don't underestimate the value of this. There is an abundance of evidence that "psycho-oncology" can profoundly impact your quality of life, immune competence, response to treatment, and even survival. One 1995 study, for instance, found that breast cancer patients who had a confidant had a 10 percent better seven-year survival rate than those with no confidants. The seven-year survival rate for women with two or more confidants was 20 percent higher.

2. Practical support. Cancer can be such an all-consuming disease that it becomes difficult to take care of the nuts and bolts of daily existence. The person you want in this role is one I call the go-getter. He or she (or they—some patients have more than one person fill each role on their A-Team) will keep you supplied with food, supplements, and medications and might shop for groceries and prepare or buy your meals. This person gets you to your appointments, car-pools your children, and organizes regular R&R such as evening walks. Think of people who are whizzes at organizing—and generous enough to give of themselves—and so can give you a hand arranging for and keeping track of transportation, child care, and therapy sessions, as well as keeping designated family members and others updated on your condition. Since one of the possible functions of the go-getter is to accompany you to the doctor, he or she should be good at listening and taking notes, since medical consults can involve complex scientific rationales that are tough to understand and assimilate even for people who are not emotionally drained by a diagnosis of cancer. Of course, this does not mean you should abdicate this role. If you feel more empowered by taking notes and asking questions of the doctor, then you should certainly do so. This role—taking notes and accompanying you to medical appointments—is so crucial that it is also part of the third form of support.

3. Informational support. In this age of the computer, it is all too easy to drown in the flood of information about cancer available to anyone with an Internet connection. Indeed, the first thing many patients do when they are diagnosed with cancer is rush home and Google "non-Hodgkins lymphoma," "estrogen-receptor-negative breast cancer," or whatever their diagnosis happens to be. Thanks to reliable sites such as that of the National Cancer Institute (NCI), much of what you find will be enormously valuable, even reassuring, boosting your confidence and helping you regain a sense of control over your disease and treatment. It can also make you feel empowered to actively participate in making treatment decisions; more and more patients, when they visit their oncologist, go armed with a printout of a scientific paper. Information can help dispel feelings of hopelessness and helplessness.

But it can also bring on information overload. Faced with the quantity of information, its complexity, and, perhaps worst of all, possible contradictions—with a study from one cancer center concluding that treatment A is better than treatment B, and a study from another group concluding that B is more effective than A—some cancer patients simply shut down. (And that's even without being barraged by your second cousin Millie telling you that when her hairdresser had your form of cancer she underwent a completely different therapy and is doing fine twenty years later.) Especially right after your diagnosis, when you are likely to be emotionally fragile and confused, you need someone calm, organized, and smart enough to wade through and filter this information.

The person on your A-Team who provides informational support need not have a scientific degree, let alone be a medical professional, but must be able to grasp and assimilate new and complex information. Ideally you would pick someone with a high degree of scientific literacy, someone who can not only comprehend and translate medical terminology but also untangle, synthesize, and present complex scientific data. Your "researcher" should be able to differentiate between strong and weak evidence and to interpret the relevance of a study to your situation. Indeed, this role is demanding enough that many patients turn to someone other than close friends or relatives to fill it. But do not assume that you have to go this route. I have seen many patients whose researcher has no scientific training, but who performs the role with enormous effectiveness.

In order for the researcher to give you the help you need, you need to determine how much information you are comfortable with. Not everyone wants to hear all about the molecular markers that indicate the probability that Erbitux will be effective against colon cancer. I have seen patients wither when supplied with sheets of scientific studies. Others revel in details.

Don't assume your physicians know your preferences. They may give you more or less information than you want, or they may try to get you more involved in treatment decisions than

WHAT LEVEL OF INFORMATION SUITS YOU BEST?

To figure out what level of information you are most comfortable with, ask yourself these questions:

• Would you rather choose among different treatment options your doctor presents, or leave the decision to him or her? If the former, do you want your researcher to take the lead role, or just be there to support you when you make the decision?

• Do you work better with group discussion and input, or do you prefer to go off on your own, read all you can, and make a decision alone? If the former, you need a researcher who will actively gather information and discuss it with you at whatever length you desire.

• Are you accustomed to asking your health care providers many questions about your tests and treatment? If you want to ask questions but feel too shy, this is obviously something your researcher—or your go-getter—can do.

• Are you comfortable asking your doctors questions, or do you prefer to keep quiet and trust that they know what they're doing? If the latter, you probably do not want a researcher who, even unintentionally, undermines that trust by challenging the doctors' decisions.

• Do you want your doctors to decide on the treatment plan without presenting the scientific basis for that choice, or do you want a detailed rundown of why they are recommending X rather than Y? If you want the rundown, you will benefit from a researcher who can not only listen carefully and take notes on what the doctor says but also dig for the supporting information—as well as any contrary information that may exist.

you want to be or dictate to you their decision when you want to have input. You need someone to guide the discussions with your doctors, someone who can ask them to "please avoid statistical data" or "please present the data without distorting it but emphasizing the most positive potential." (For instance, saying that 60 percent of patients with your cancer won't respond to a chemo regimen is mathematically equivalent to saying 40 percent will. Many people very much prefer to hear the latter.) With your researcher, prepare questions such as these:

Why do you advise this treatment at this time?

What are the possible side effects?

What will you do to counteract side effects?

Will you support my use of complementary strategies such as hypnosis before surgery to reduce my anxiety, playing tapes during surgery or in the recovery room, and using supplements during chemotherapy?

After each visit, determine whether you feel satisfied with the type and amount of information you got. If you think things could have gone better, work with your information person to refine your questions and approach. Don't be afraid to follow up an office visit or hospital procedure with a phone call if you left with questions unanswered.

You don't need to have a different person for every function. Some A-Team members may be able to perform two or even three. And as you saw, either the go-getter or the researcher can accompany you to the doctor and ask questions. But you and your team will need to determine what is a reasonable set of responsibilities, given their schedules, energy, and availability.

4. **Integrative coach.** It is also helpful to have someone acting as your "integrative coach," to help you implement the Life Over Cancer program. This person pushes you to attend support group sessions and keep up your exercise regimen, and generally keeps you on track toward recovery. The integrative coach

can be someone who reminds, reinforces, coaxes, and even inspires you to go a little further in your commitment to healing. While the strategic planner, your fifth A-Team member, is concerned with the overall program and in particular the medical treatments you receive, the integrative coach is devoted to making sure you carry out your program at home.

You will notice that none of the people I am recommending for your A-Team are physicians, let alone oncologists. If you are reading this book, chances are you already have an oncologist. There is great value in continuity of care, so changing doctors is never something I recommend lightly. But there is no question that you need someone you are comfortable with, who takes your concerns and questions seriously. Do rely on the researcher on your A-Team to make sure your treatment is in line with the best science; if your oncologist says that you "are not a good candidate" for a treatment that has been shown in rigorous studies to be effective, ask why. As you will see in the chapters that follow, I always tell patients that they must inform their physician of what supplements they are taking and what other integrative practices they are following. For many of my patients, the protocol I recommend is actually carried out by an oncologist near their home. It is not exactly news that some physicians are somewhere between wary and antagonistic about integrative care; if yours is, you will need to decide if that is something you can live with or whether you need to find another oncologist. Do not feel that you will be insulting the doctor you leave; all that matters here is giving yourself the best chance at getting well and staying well. But rest assured that much of the Life Over Cancer program can be carried out by you and you alone, no matter who your doctor is.

5. **Strategic planner.** That brings me to the final member of your A-Team: someone with in-depth knowledge of cancer medicine, someone who can help guide you in your decision making. Ideally, this person will be a physician who specializes in integrative cancer treatment. I call this person the "strategic planner." He or she will act as a conduit or liaison between the A-Team and your medical team. When you're with your strategic planner, you

want to have your research and questions organized beforehand (ideally by the researcher); you do not want to drop a mountain of information in the strategic planner's lap. At the Block Center, we handle much of the strategic planning with our patients and their A-Teams, even helping patients receive treatment elsewhere.

You may well find you have needs I have not thought of. Make sure to articulate any concerns as they arise—your needs will fluctuate as you move through treatment and recovery. And do stop occasionally to express your genuine gratitude for the special care your A-Team generously provides.

Dynamics of the Recruiting Process

I hope the descriptions above of the role each member of the A-Team will play give you some ideas about the people in your life who might best fill them. It is only natural to think first of the people closest to you, but it is not always the case that your family or best friends are the best candidates for the A-Team. I frequently advise patients that it is important to recognize that their family and friends have been hit by shrapnel from the explosion that the patient herself has suffered. Very often, your closest family members and friends will be experiencing emotional distress themselves, as they struggle to empathize with you in your predicament and confront their own fears of mortality.

You're entitled to be very selective about your A-Team. As much as possible, these individuals should be compatible with your priorities, beliefs, and values. You want people who will listen without judging you, who will voice their opinions when asked, but respect yours, who are committed to helping you, who will be there for you if times get tough, who will encourage and support your choices. The most effective teams have regular discussions to get everyone's input, even if over the phone or by e-mail. By listening attentively to your A-Team members, you are not unlike a president with a cabinet. Once you have made a decision, as long as it is made with a sound mind, your team's role shifts to supporting that choice. For in the end, decisions about your health and well-being are yours and yours alone to make. You are the leader. With that in mind, the following questions should help you avoid picking the wrong people:

For the comforter: Do you think you'll be able to handle my emotional ups and downs, or perhaps explosions, and help me emerge from my deep funks? Can you listen without feeling compelled to resolve or purge me of all my distress?

For the go-getter: Are you comfortable with my asking you to perform various tasks, even if they seem repetitive or mundane (e.g., cooking, transportation)? Will you admit it if you feel overloaded?

For the researcher: Are you willing to spend at least a couple of hours per week digging through the Internet and Medline? Are you confident about your ability to explain the scientific results?

For the integrative coach: Are you willing to push me while being sensitive to my vulnerabilities? Will you be okay if I object and reject or even yell back?

For the strategic planner: Are you comfortable with me disagreeing with or questioning the proposed plan? Will you abide by my thinking on what's best? (Ultimately, the patient has veto power over any proposed plan.) Do you think you can support me without judgment? Without being obtrusive or disrespecting my need to do things my way? Do you think you can support my adhering to the Life Over Cancer dietary, exercise, supplement, mind-spirit, and other guidelines without skepticism or argument?

There are no rules about whom to choose, no rules about the length of their term in "office." Which brings me to my next point: "un-recruiting" can, not surprisingly, be trickier. If you sense that any member of the team is undermining your position or your priorities, or is simply unable to fulfill his or her role, you should find a replacement. If someone is not working out, you must feel free to make changes without worrying that you are hurting the person's feelings. This should be understood by all team members from the start. In fact, it may be a good idea to have someone, possibly the integrative coach, help you periodically evaluate whether the team is meeting your needs. He or she can also smooth out any needed transitions.

Other Sources of Support

If your circumstances make it difficult to recruit the A-Team that I describe, I urge you to seek out a professionally facilitated, structured support network. Support resources, including support groups, are available through reputable online forums as well as in face-to-face programs. Community organizations, including religious congregations, may be able to provide assistance. The medical social work department at your local hospital may also be able to guide you to support resources.

Another possibility is to start your own cancer blog or website to describe your cancer journey. Not only is this a good way to keep family and friends informed, but it enables you to receive meaningful emotional support from afar. An easy-to-use Web service for doing this can be found at CaringBridge.com.

For more suggestions, particularly on finding support that matches your individual needs and personal style, please refer to the section called "Reconnecting" in Chapter 11.

CHAPTER 3

WHERE ARE YOU NOW? QUICK-START MAPS FOR USING THIS BOOK

Some of you may need immediate answers and want to begin implementing the Life Over Cancer program right away before reading the whole book. The quick-start maps below will allow you to get started now. Once your immediate situation, such as impending surgery or a chemo decision, has passed, however, I urge you to read the entire book. In your battle against cancer, you'll be grateful for every tool in your tool kit.

As I've noted, the Life Over Cancer plan targets cancer in three main areas, or spheres:

1. Lifestyle (your general health, physical activity, emotional state, diet/nutrition)
2. Biology (your internal makeup, blood chemistry)
3. Disease treatment (type of treatment based on molecular tumor-tissue analysis, scans, labs)

Each of the quick-start maps will lead you to the most pertinent information within each of these targets for your situation.

I've grouped many of the recommended treatments into two levels. "Your Self-Care Program" contains medical, dietary, supplement, herbal, or other treatments that you can choose and implement on your own, even if you are unable to come to the Block Center. Much of the Life Over Cancer program is like this. Nonetheless, you should inform your doctor— general physician, oncologist, or integrative physician—of any treatments you adopt. While all have been designed with safety in mind, there may be rare circumstances in which an interaction or interference with other treatments you are undergoing is possible. I advise that you find a supportive and knowledgeable physician to assist you with your integrative program and make sure it is completely safe for you. Please also read on page 45, "How to Choose Supplements for Your Life Over Cancer Program." Even if you are unable to come to our center in Evanston or locate another integrative cancer specialist, this book will provide the information and practical advice you need to implement many integrative treatments on your own.

"Medical Partnership" strategies are diagnostic procedures or treatments that require a doctor. For instance, there are tests that you can't order or interpret on your own, treatment decisions that depend on the results of the tests, and therapies such as chemotherapy regimens and infusions of vitamins or other nutrients that you cannot do on your own. Throughout this book I'll make clear which are Self-Care Program strategies and which are the Medical Partnership strategies.

Quick start for patients about to undergo surgery

Treatment support diet: Chapter 6, page 132, to build up your strength before the operation

Exercise training: Chapter 8, page 199, to increase muscle mass and strength

Relaxation techniques: Chapter 11, page 230, to reduce anxiety and prepare mentally for surgery

Inflammation: Chapter 15, to make your internal biochemistry as hostile as possible to the spread of cancer cells from the original tumor and reduce postoperative pain and swelling

Immune building: Chapter 16, to strengthen your natural defenses against infection and the spread of malignant cells

Banking tissue: Chapter 22, page 452, so you have a sample of cells that can be tested for vulnerability to new chemotherapies or molecular targeted therapies

Tumor profiling: Chapter 22, page 452, to determine which molecular agents your tumor is particularly susceptible to

Quick start for patients undergoing, or about to undergo, chemotherapy or radiation

Diet: Chapter 6, for overall health and strength to weather the treatments and for ways to avoid or manage common side effects such as nausea and loss of appetite. Review Treatment Support diet, page 132.

Physical care: Chapter 9, to gain strength and stamina you'll need during treatment, and for fitness regimens that work when treatment leaves you weak or debilitated

Mind-spirit: Chapter 12, to prepare psychologically for treatment and learn techniques to reduce side effects

Chemotherapy support: Chapter 23, to find strategies to control chemotherapy side effects

Chemosensitizing: Chapter 24, to make malignant cells more vulnerable to chemo or radiation

Radiation support: Chapter 25, to reduce debilitating side effects and increase effectiveness

Quick start for patients who have recently completed treatment (surgery, chemotherapy, radiation) and want to avoid a recurrence (first year after treatment)

Diet: Chapter 5, for the foods and natural supplements that reduce the risk that any remaining cancer cells will proliferate

Physical care: Chapter 8, for a basic fitness program you can follow throughout your whole life

Mind-spirit: Chapter 11, to find a new normalcy, maintain healthy sleep patterns, and manage anxiety

Growth control and containment: Chapter 26, to keep malignant cells from growing

Immune-building: Chapter 16, to improve immune activity, mopping up residual cancer cells

Oxidation: Chapter 14, to reduce development of aggressive cancer cells that could become a problem in the future

Quick start for patients who have had to stop treatment due to complications and need to rebuild strength in order to resume treatment

Diet: Chapter 6, to counter wasting and loss of strength and stamina

Fitness: Chapter 9, to build up strength

Mind-spirit: Chapter 12, to revitalize emotional stamina and attain healthy sleep patterns

Rehabilitation: Chapter 27, for an intensive all-around rebuilding program

Inflammation: Chapter 15, to overcome inflammatory changes that promote muscle wasting

---

Quick start for patients who have been told there is no conventional treatment option

Diet: Chapters 5 and 6, to maintain ideal weight and gain strength

Fitness: Chapters 8 and 9, to regain as much strength as possible, which you will need for any unconventional treatments you choose

Mind-spirit: Chapters 11 and 12, to keep anxiety and depression at bay

Growth control: Chapter 26, to reduce factors that promote tumor growth

No stone unturned: Chapter 28, for experimental therapies that open new doors to hope

---

Quick start for patients who have achieved a complete remission (one year or more after finishing treatment) and want to avoid a recurrence

Diet: Chapter 5, to keep your internal environment hostile to a recurrence

Fitness: Chapter 8, to retain strength and endurance

Mind-spirit: Chapter 11, to manage stress

Oxidation: Chapter 14, to reduce a major disruptive factor that can promote development of aggressive cancer cells

Remission maintenance: Chapter 29, for an all-around program

Quick start for family and friends, those who are at high risk for cancer or other chronic diseases, and for those interested in prevention and optimal health

Diet: Chapter 5, for a diet high in health-promoting vegetables, fruits, whole grains, proteins, and fats, and low in refined sugar and inflammatory fats

Fitness: Chapter 8, for help in designing an exercise program that addresses core fitness needs

Mind-spirit: Chapter 11, for stress management strategies that you can use on a daily basis

Supplementation: Chapters 14, 15, 18, and 19; read sections up to Medical Partnership

Chemoprevention: Chapter 29, to learn about foods and phytochemicals that may lower cancer risks, and about ways to reduce toxic exposures in your environment

---

How to Choose Supplements for Your Life Over Cancer Program

Many patients have come to my office with a shopping bag full of supplements that they are taking without any rhyme or reason. The Life Over Cancer program is different: there is a specific reason for taking each type of supplement, and a specific situation in which you should take it. Do not go through this book and make a list of all the supplements you see mentioned, and then attempt to purchase and take them all. Taking too many supplements or taking excessive dosages can definitely be harmful to your health. Some supplements may also interfere with conventional drugs essential to your treatment.

You should be working with an integrative medical or nutritional practitioner to individualize your supplement regimen, help determine the optimal dosages, and avoid unwanted drug interactions.

Here is a guide based on the three spheres of the LOC program:

Sphere 1 (Lifestyle):
Supplementation is based on the Healthy Dozen Power foods (see Chapters 4 and 5). To get proper amounts of these twelve important types of food into your diet you have two options:

Option 1. Take a shake or complete formula that includes members of all twelve food groups

Option 2. Take the following three types of supplements:
A multivitamin/mineral formula designed for cancer patients (see Chapter 5, page 116)
Fish oil
A "green drink" or vegetable/fruit drink

Sphere 2 (Biology):
The purpose of supplementation in this sphere is to transform your biochemistry to make it more difficult for cancers to grow. You will first assess different aspects of your internal terrain through laboratory tests or a questionnaire, including oxidation, inflammation, and glycemia, among other factors. Then take the following types of supplements:

1. A broad-spectrum formula that gently normalizes all or most of the terrain factors (see Chapter 13)
2. Two or three of the focused supplement formulas for the terrain factors that are most problematic for you

Sphere 3 (Disease Treatment):
Sphere 3 chapters are organized around the phases of care: you
will typically be taking one to three formulas at any one time. It
is especially important that you work with an integrative practitioner in the crisis, attack, and containment phases. Since you
will usually be taking multiple medications in these phases, help
is essential to avoid supplement-drug interactions.

The Life Over Cancer Website:
www.lifeovercancer.com

The Life Over Cancer website is an integral part of this book. I
and my colleagues have chosen this method to provide docu-
mentation and resources because of the speed with which new
information on cancer treatment is emerging. Rather than wait
for a new edition of the printed book, we can provide updated
studies and resources as soon as we begin to make use of them
at the Block Center. The website includes:

- Complete reference notes for each chapter, keyed to the superscript numbers in the text, with a description of how to
  use the PubMed online database to retrieve articles and abstracts

- Updates on new and ongoing studies being conducted at the
  Block Center, and new and cutting-edge treatments available globally

- Resources to support your Life Over Cancer program, such
  as books that teach meditation techniques and guided imagery tapes to help you get through treatment

- Sample meal plans and recipes for the Life Over Cancer diets

- A directory of labs that conduct procedures such as tissue
  banking and chemosensitivity testing

- Sources for herbal and other supplements discussed in the book, and a discussion of how to choose high-quality supplements

- A directory of other integrative cancer centers and individual practitioners

Look for the icon (i) in the text.

SPHERE I

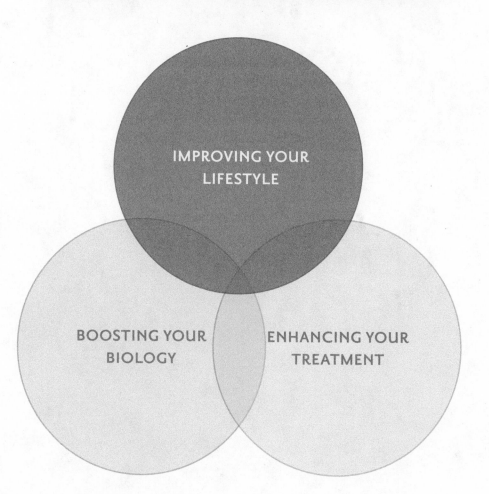

IMPROVING YOUR LIFESTYLE

BOOSTING YOUR BIOLOGY

ENHANCING YOUR TREATMENT

CHAPTER 4

THE ANTI-CANCER DIET

Since much of what you do to overcome cancer—surgery, radiation, and chemotherapy—requires highly technical expertise, you may be surprised that a thoroughly mundane activity like eating can also be a powerful anti-cancer treatment. But that is exactly what I tell my patients at our first meeting: the Life Over Cancer nutrition program fights cancer. It boosts your energy so you have the stamina for radiation and chemo; it deprives the tumor of compounds it feeds on; it fills you with nutrients that keep malignant cells in check.

And it epitomizes the integrative approach to cancer. Remember my point in Chapter 1 that the Life Over Cancer program embraces the best conventional therapies? The nutrition program, our clinical experience suggests, can both increase the efficacy and diminish the toxicity of conventional treatments, allowing you to derive even greater benefit from them. And unlike surgery, radiation, and chemo, which you don't have much control over, the nutrition program lets you take an active role in your treatment and recovery. Research has shown the importance of committed personal involvement in the successful outcome of integrative programs, as I'll discuss in Chapter 10.

Whether you read five-thousand-year-old texts of Chinese medicine or the latest scientific studies, it is clear that nutrition can exert a profound influence on the course of disease—and on recovery from that disease. The Japanese, for instance, have long had a diet rich in vegetables and fish and low in meat, refined sugars, and high-fat foods. They also have long had lower cancer rates than in the United States and better survival.[1] Men in Japan and the United States are equally likely to have very early prostate cancer, for example—the kind that never causes clinical problems. But men in the United States have much higher rates of advanced prostate cancer. This suggests that while whatever causes prostate cancer is equally prevalent in both populations, something in American men fuels its growth. Similarly, early studies found that Japanese women diagnosed with early-stage breast cancer lived much longer than women in the United States. In both cases, scientists suspect that diet explains much of the differences—especially since when Japanese people move to the United States and adopt a Western diet (less seaweed, more burgers), their cancer rates approach those of Americans.[2] Sadly, the Japanese no longer have to emigrate to the United States for a Western diet. Now that their consumption of meat, eggs, and dairy products has climbed, so have their death rates from breast and prostate cancer.[3]

What's wrong with the standard American diet?

Like most of you, I was raised on it. When I was in a hurry, I'd wolf down a greasy burger and wash it down with colored sparkling sugar water. Snack time called for a rich milk shake, cake, candy, cookies, chips, or donuts. Lunch and dinner meant saturated fats in the form of fried chicken, beef, pizza, and french fries. Little did my parents or I know that this fare is packed with the wrong fats, the wrong proteins, and the wrong carbohydrates. It's no wonder nutritionists commonly abbreviate the Standard American Diet as SAD.

At least, they're wrong if you don't want to feed your cancer. I lay out the danger of the standard American diet later in this chapter, but here's a preview. If you eat too much dietary fat and refined carbohydrates, you run the risk of increasing body fat and weight while weakening your immune system and increasing oxidative stress, inflammation, and blood levels of substances that promote tumor growth and angiogenesis (new blood supply to tumors). Diets high in fat tend to cause more

DNA damage, which allows mutations to accumulate in the cells that make up tumors. The more mutations, the more aggressive the cancer and the more likely it is that malignant cells will survive chemo and radiation and travel through the bloodstream to seed distant sites of your body with cancer. It is no surprise, then, that cancer death rates are generally lower in populations that follow low-fat, vegetable-rich diets.

Is the LOC Diet Macrobiotic?

Beginning in the late 1970s, the correlation between low cancer rates and a traditional Japanese diet led the alternative medicine community to investigate the macrobiotic diet as a cancer treatment. What we in the United States call a macrobiotic diet is actually a Westernized version of the traditional Japanese diet. It emphasizes whole grains, vegetables (especially cruciferous ones such as cabbage and broccoli), and fish, with limited fruits. I discovered its healing properties as a medical student when it helped me overcome ulcers and migraines. After that experience, I began combing the scientific literature for information on whether the macrobiotic diet might reduce the risk of cancer or improve its prognosis. There is a lot of evidence that it does, as you'll learn in this chapter, and research on the potential of the macrobiotic diet to improve outcomes in cancer continues to this day. My clinical practice with cancer patients began on a foundation of macrobiotic counseling, and I continue to embrace many of its core tenets.

However, I also found that the macrobiotic diet as it was being followed by people in the United States was often missing quite a bit in the way of nutrition that can fight cancer. As I saw more patients with advanced cancers in our clinic, I became more concerned with its potential for misapplication. In fact, forms of the macrobiotic diet advised by some, but not all, practitioners can lead to outright malnutrition in patients with advanced cancers, with disastrous results. I thus became convinced of the need to make adjustments in the diet so that it could be more easily adapted to the cultural background of the person following it, and could allow for more relaxed food choices in particular circumstances. When it comes to designing diets for patients with serious illnesses such as cancer, quantifying a regimen and fine-tuning it to the needs of each patient is important. Eventually Penny and I supervised a team of university dietitians to make a systematic, clinically relevant adaptation of the macrobiotic diet in order to take advantage of recent advances in nutritional science.

As a result, although the Life Over Cancer nutrition program has its roots in the macrobiotic diet, it is strategically different. In addition to incorporating what nutrition researchers have learned about phytochemicals (compounds naturally found in plants), fats and oils, and the disease-fighting properties of plant pigments, it is specially adapted for the wide range of nutritional stresses that cancer patients encounter. From the early days of my practice, I regularly combed science journals for new research on nutrition and cancer. (Now, though, the literature is so voluminous that keeping up is a full-time job—a telling commentary on the importance of nutritional science in cancer. So I've added researchers with expertise in nutrition to our clinic staff.) It wasn't only what I was reading that convinced me that certain foods can inhibit cancer while others can encourage its survival and spread. I also began seeing hints of that in my patients. Before they came to me, many had cancers that had gone into remission but then recurred; other patients had experienced only partial remission despite the best conventional treatments; still others had not responded and had extremely poor prognoses. Yet after making dramatic changes in their diet, along with a full integrative program that included conventional treatment, a surprising number beat the odds, even going into sustained remission. While I in no way suggest that these recoveries are the result of diet alone, I certainly believe it is a major factor.

Ed: The Power of Diet

Ed Hanley was the patient who first opened my eyes to the power of diet. In 1979, Ed, then sixty-two, was diagnosed with what appeared to be a slow-growing prostate cancer. Doctors believed it could be controlled with diethylstilbestrol (DES), but by 1982 Ed's cancer had become aggressive, with metastases spreading to his pelvis, forehead, and ribs. Ed was given no meaningful chance of surviving. In desperation, he visited the Block Center for Integrative Cancer Treatment in July 1983. Disillusioned with DES and concerned about the side effects of other conventional treatments, he told me he wished to use only natural methods to treat his disease. "If we try the diet but the disease gets worse, I may be willing to reconsider your advice to start other conventional therapy," he said. "But let me try the diet first."

I asked Ed to eliminate cancer-promoting foods and adopt a diet based on plant proteins, deep-ocean cold-water fish, fruits, vegetables, and whole grains. By September 1984, a bone scan and biopsy of his prostate revealed that he was in complete remission. Not only was his body rid of visible disease, but his energy level, mood, sleep, alertness, and concentration had all improved. "It's just amazing how good I feel," Ed told a reporter in 1985, four years after receiving a virtual death sentence. Ed lived for two decades free of cancer. In his eighties, however, cognitive decline and other problems caused him to stop following the Life Over Cancer program, and within a couple of years both his prostate cancer and bone metastases had recurred. Ed died in October 2004.

I mentioned in Chapter 1 giving a seminar at the University of Chicago in which I presented the cases of six stage D_2 prostate cancer patients, all of whom had bone metastases and all of whom survived much longer than anyone (especially the specialists they first saw) expected. Ed was one of them. Since these six survivors had all followed the Life Over Cancer nutrition program, the cases raised the serious possibility that metastatic prostate cancer should not be treated by conventional means alone but that diet should play an integral role. More than two decades after I presented these cases, research is showing the benefits of an anti-cancer diet. A 2006 study published in *Integrative Cancer Therapies,* for instance, followed prostate cancer patients whose disease had recurred after standard treatment. Adopting a plant-based diet, along with stress reduction, significantly slowed the men's steep rise in prostate-specific antigen (PSA), a marker of tumor growth, showing that this intervention slows that growth.[4] A 2008 study in the prominent journal *Urology* also showed that the increase in PSA was slowed after just three months of a diet low in saturated fat and protein from meat and dairy products and high in vegetables.[5] This is consistent with what we have seen with patients in the clinic for many years.

In fact, there is an especially strong case for using diet to thwart prostate cancer. Many men with the earliest stages of this disease decline treatment and opt for "watchful waiting," in which a physician periodically monitors their PSA levels and clinical signs to see if the tumor is growing or spreading. To give these men another noninvasive option could make a big difference in their outcome. After all, if you are not receiving radiation or chemo, at the very least you want to have "natural medicines," anti-cancer biochemicals derived from food, turning watchful waiting into active participation.[6,7]

How Diet Affects Cancer

Diet affects cancer both directly and indirectly. Nutrients directly impact the mechanisms by which cancer cells grow and spread. They indirectly help control the cancer by changing the surrounding biochemical conditions that either encourage or discourage the progression of malignant disease. The bottom line is that what you eat can spell the difference between conquering your disease and having it rage out of control.

Here are some examples of findings from recent studies that support the importance of diet in fighting cancer:

• Diets high in fat and refined carbohydrates make you more likely to become overweight, which in turn increases your risk of tumor recurrences.[8] Obese men are at significantly greater risk of developing more aggressive prostate cancer.[9]

• Dietary fats can impair the body's anti-cancer defenses by depressing the activity of natural killer (NK) cells, while a low-fat diet markedly increases NK activity.[10,11,12] Natural killer cells play a key role in preventing metastasis.

• Obese breast cancer patients are two to four times more likely to experience a recurrence than women of normal weight.[13]

• For every additional 10 percentage points of calories derived from fat in the diet of newly diagnosed breast cancer patients—by going from 25 percent to 35 percent of calories from fat—the risk of recurrence approximately doubles.[14] An increase of 10 percentage points is alarmingly easy: just add 4 ounces of beef, 4 ounces of mozzarella cheese (about the size of three 9-volt batteries), a cup of ice cream, or four pats of butter to your daily intake and you're there.

• High intake of many dietary fats is linked with higher rates of cancer recurrence, lower rates of survival, or both.[15] At the American Society of Clinical Oncology meeting in 2005, I listened to a stunning presentation of a randomized controlled study of 2,400 breast cancer patients. It found that those who adopted a diet in which 20 percent of the calories came from fat (the U.S. norm is more like 35 percent) had a 24 percent lower rate of relapse. The lowered risk of relapse was particularly great for the 42 percent of women with the more dangerous estrogen-receptor-negative breast cancers. Because these women have fewer good conventional options, this is an especially important finding.[16]

Despite this overwhelming evidence for the benefits of a healthy diet when you are fighting cancer, that is not what mainstream medicine recommends. Yes, when it comes to cancer *prevention*, the American Cancer Society recommends a diet that is heavy on fruits, vegetables, whole grains, and low-fat proteins while restricting unhealthy fats, refined carbs, and fatty red meats. So far, so good. Yet the standard advice for patients with cancer—that is, those for whom prevention didn't

work—is "all you can eat."[17] Cancer patients are told to get all
the calories they can, from butter, margarine, high-fat dairy
products, mayonnaise, eggs, meat, hard and soft cheese, ice
cream, and peanut butter. The rationale is that a fat- and calorie-
packed diet prevents or combats cachexia, the "starvation response" seen in cancer patients. It does not. But this response
is hardly universal; only some patients become cachectic, and
only at certain points in their treatment. The reality is that
there are far more patients for whom "all you can eat" is exactly the wrong prescription: it makes them fill their plates
with animal protein, saturated fats, unhealthful omega-6 fats,
and refined carbohydrates, all of which have tumor-promoting
properties.[18] In fact, a 2007 study reported in the *Journal of the
American Medical Association* found that stage III colon cancer patients who ate the least meat, fat, refined grains, and
desserts had half the mortality risk of those who ate the most
of these foods.[19]

I don't want to pick on mainstream cancer groups—in my
five years as vice president of the uptown Chicago chapter of
the American Cancer Society (ACS), I saw firsthand the good
intentions of everyone involved. Nonetheless, the disconnect
between the ACS's cancer-*prevention* dietary advice and its
cancer-*fighting* dietary advice is hard to justify. Even laypeople
can see that. A number of my patients have said to me, "My
doctor used to advise that I should eat fruits and vegetables and
avoid too much meat and fat so I wouldn't get cancer. Now that
I got a diagnosis of cancer, I'm supposed to eat cheesecake, milk
shakes, and cream sauce. That doesn't make sense." They're
right: it strains credulity to think that the very foods you are
told to minimize in order to reduce your risk of developing
cancer should be dietary staples once you have cancer. The
cheesecake-and-cream-sauce advice also ignores the growing
scientific evidence of the tumor-promoting potential of the standard American diet. To a great extent, the foods recommended
for cancer prevention are also the foods that seem to suppress
cancer after it's diagnosed. In most cases it is reasonable to use
prevention studies as a guide for how patients should eat, especially in cancers where healthy diets reduce risk.

Maryann: Two Decades of Health

One of my earliest breast cancer patients was Maryann, a forty-four-year-old chemist and single mother bringing up three teen-agers when she was diagnosed with breast cancer in 1983. "I was numb," she says. "You never think it's going to happen to you. I didn't know what to do, so I basically went with the rec-ommendation of the doctor" for a modified radical mastectomy. Since the cancer had spread to several lymph nodes, her oncolo-gist prescribed radiation followed by chemotherapy. Maryann refused the radiation, fearing its side effects, but agreed to the six cycles of standard chemo. No one on her medical team gave her any nutritional guidelines. Still, she did fine for three years. Then a bone scan revealed numerous metastases throughout her rib cage and spine; she was told she had one year to live.

The shock sent Maryann to our clinic. She refused chemo, telling me that the earlier rounds had caused vomiting, fatigue, and hair loss. Although I told her that the experience for most of my patients on our program is a reduction in side effects, she would not be swayed. Based on her scans and medical history, I felt she had time to explore other options, and so I encouraged but did not immediately insist on chemotherapy, although I did explain her risks with and without it. "For the time being," I told her, "let's see how you respond to a natural, complemen-tary approach."

I laid out a low-fat, high-fiber diet consisting mainly of whole grains, fruits, vegetables, and legumes, plus foods rich in anti-cancer nutrients such as shiitake mushrooms, sea vegetables, ginger, and green tea. Maryann eliminated all dairy, meat, and refined sugars and never looked back. Within weeks, she expe-rienced a major boost in energy and overall well-being. Four months after her first visit, a bone scan showed a reduction of the cancer in her spine, and scans every few months kept show-ing reductions or the outright disappearance of metastatic spots on her ribs and spine. Sixteen months in, Maryann appeared to be in complete remission. As I write, twenty-two years after Maryann walked into our clinic with bone metastases, she re-mains cancer-free—and still adheres to the cancer-fighting diet.

An important caveat: diet alone should never be regarded as the answer to cancer. We have had a number of patients who ended up at our door after attempting a diet as their only cancer treatment. Although some show improvement, especially in the short term, an experience like Maryann's is more the exception than the rule. At the risk of sounding like a broken record, let me say again that combining conventional treatments with complementary therapies in an integrative system buys the best odds for a successful outcome. It is said that all truth goes through three stages. First, it is ridiculed. Second, it is violently opposed. Third, it is accepted as self-evident. I predict that the relevance of a truly healthy diet for cancer, now opposed by many, will one day be accepted as self-evident.

Nutrition 101

To stay alive, humans need a diet that contains three things: protein, carbohydrates, and fats. But not all proteins are equal, nor are all carbohydrates or all fats. Your sources of protein, carbohydrates, and fat matter whatever your state of health, but especially when you are battling cancer. In addition to these big three, your body needs micronutrients—vitamins, minerals, and phytochemicals—to maintain normal biochemistry and metabolic stability, including the biochemistry that affects immunity, inflammation, detoxification, oxidation, and normal cell growth, all of which affect the development of cancer. Let's examine each of these four—fats, carbohydrates, proteins, and micronutrients.

▶ **SAD Facts About Eating Bad Fats When You Have Cancer**
Diets high in fat tend to cause more DNA damage. That allows malignant cells to accumulate ever more mutations, which in turn make it more likely that they will escape the effects of chemotherapy and radiation.[20,21] Result: more aggressive cancer. In addition, a diet high in fat can weaken your immune system[22] while increasing inflammation,[23] angiogenesis,[24] and blood levels of tumor-promoting growth factors.[25] This is likely

why people eating the standard American diet have a higher rate of cancer and a worse prognosis than populations that adhere to low-fat, vegetable-rich diets such as the traditional Japanese diet or the Mediterranean diet.

In addition to limiting your overall intake of fat, you need to watch the kind of fat you eat. As I said, not all fats are equal. Steer clear of cancer-feeding trans fats, found in partially hydrogenated oils, which occur rarely in nature: primarily, they are manufactured for processed foods. Partially hydrogenated fats have been shown to promote the progression of colon cancer: colon cancer patients who habitually consumed foods high in hydrogenated fats had twice the risk of having a mutation in a gene called p53, which has been linked with more aggressive, radiation-resistant cancer.[26] In 2006, the federal government required food manufacturers to indicate on labels, and fast-food restaurants to make available on flyers or menus, how much trans fat a product contains. As a result, many manufacturers are phasing out this unhealthy fat. But until and unless they do, stay away from anything containing partially hydrogenated fats: margarine, most commercial baked goods, much fast food, processed food such as packaged crackers and imitation cheese products, potato chips, french fries, vegetable shortening, commercial peanut butter, and instant foods such as some microwave popcorn and cake or biscuit mixes. Again, check the labels.

Fully hydrogenated fats, a newer product, lack harmful trans fats but are commonly combined with less healthy oils to make them more spreadable, so they are not a good choice.

Saturated fats, though natural, are no better. Found in animal products such as meat and dairy, they are notorious for increasing the risk of cardiovascular disease such as strokes and heart attacks. But they also suppress immune function,[27] slow down the body's ability to detoxify,[28] and increase levels of oxidation.[29] Small wonder, then, that the higher your consumption of butter and lard—the richest sources of saturated fat—the higher your risk of dying from breast, prostate, rectal, colon, and lung cancer, as a 1991 study found.[30] Other research has found that men with prostate cancer who had the highest intakes of saturated fat were three times more likely to die from their disease than those whose diets were lowest in saturated fat.[31] A 2008 study in the *International Journal of Cancer* found that men who ate the least saturated fat were half as likely to have their prostate cancer recur after their initial treatment.[32] And breast cancer patients with the highest consumption of saturated fat were twice as likely to die from their disease as women with the lowest intakes.[33] To put some numbers on that, for every increase of 5 percentage points in the calories obtained from saturated fat (going from 10 percent to 15 percent, for instance, which is as easy as adding two slices of bacon, 2 tablespoons of cream, or 1 ounce of cream cheese to your daily diet), the risk of dying from breast cancer increased by 50 percent.[34] As someone who has been diagnosed with cancer, you therefore need to keep your saturated fat intake to a minimum. What's a minimum? Some researchers say men should get no more than 10 percent of their calories from saturated fat. For anyone with aggressive or advanced cancer, I recommend 5 percent. That means little to no coconut oil, palm oil, lard, butter, cream, regular ice cream, cheese, other whole milk products, steak, hamburgers, and other land-animal products. If you are eating 2,000 calories a day, 5 percent is 100 saturated-fat calories, which is the amount in two pats of butter or 4 tablespoons of sour cream.

Unsaturated fats pose the lowest health risk, but some are better for you than others. Omega-3 and omega-9 fatty acids are the most beneficial,[35,36] omega-6s the least.[37] Why? Omega-3s can reverse tumor metastasis[38] as well as a tumor's resistance to radiation or chemotherapy,[39] and may also enhance the effectiveness and minimize the toxic side effects of some chemotherapy drugs.[40] Omega-6 fatty acids, on the other hand, are essential (healthy people need about four times as much omega-6s as omega-3s) but can be less beneficial for cancer patients.[41] Although the body transforms omega-3s into prostaglandins that quell inflammation, omega-6s are turned into pro-inflammatory fatty acids.[42] Inflammation can make your internal environment more hospitable to cancer cells; for one thing, it stimulates the formation of new blood vessels—the process called angiogenesis—that allows tumors to grow and spread.[43] Omega-6s can also stimulate the production of tumor-promoting growth factors, and activate a cancer-promoting gene called *ras*-p21, which leads to uncontrolled cell replication and tumor growth.[44] A diet rich in omega-6s therefore creates an ideal biochemical environment for the growth of cancer. Moreover, if the body is processing lots of omega-6s, it cannot process enough omega-3s; it's as if these metabolic pathways, or "fat tracks" as I call them, must both pass through the same narrow tunnel. If more omega-6s are getting through, fewer omega-3s can, which means you will not get the benefits of omega-3s I described above.[45] Finally, omega-9s appear to have profound anti-cancer effects, including suppressing the breast cancer gene HER2/neu, the molecular target of the blockbuster drug Herceptin.[46]

Omega-3s are found in fish and in walnut and flaxseed oils. Omega-9s include monounsaturated fatty acids such as those in olive oil. Omega-6s, including linoleic acid and arachidonic acid, are found in corn oil and animal fats, respectively. I feel that a ratio of 1:1 or 1:2 omega-3s to omega-6s is appropriate for most people with cancer.[47] Unfortunately, a standard American diet has twenty times as much omega-6s as omega-3s. To bring that ratio into a healthier balance, eliminate unhealthy fats by avoiding deep-fried foods, processed meats, bacon, pepperoni, sausage, batter-coated foods, breaded shrimp, fish sticks, chicken nuggets, onion rings, tacos, french fries, sauces, gravies, margarine, mayonnaise, salad dressings, commercial peanut butter, milk shakes, regular ice cream, corn oil, safflower oil, and sunflower oil. Minimize or eliminate altogether beef, milk, cheese, pork, whole eggs, and poultry, which are rich sources of the omega-6 arachidonic acid. Even skinless chicken has significant amounts of arachidonic acid and could induce the production of inflammatory molecules that can drive the growth and progression of cancer.[48] For a source of animal protein, you are better off with fish, which is high in omega-3s. You can also get omega-3s from canola, flaxseed, and walnut oils; healthy seeds such as pumpkin or sesame; and nuts, especially walnuts. Egg whites are fine, but if you are going to eat an occasional yolk, be sure it is from omega-3-fed chickens. Some leafy green vegetables and many algae and sea vegetables contain omega-3s. Omega-9 fats are found in olive and canola oils, almonds and Brazil nuts, and avocados. But don't overdo even healthful fats, since fat quantity can override fat quality regardless of the source; fats are all high in calories and may contribute to weight gain if eaten in excess.[49] And weight gain is definitely problematic: a study presented at the annual Frontiers in Cancer Prevention Research meeting in 2007 found that breast cancer patients who were obese were twice as likely to die from their cancer as normal-weight patients, and that an 11-pound weight gain after cancer diagnosis translated into a 14 percent increase in mortality risk.[50] Obesity also increases mortality from endometrial cancer and from prostate cancer, as reported in a 2007 article in *Cancer*, and very obese colon cancer chemotherapy patients have an increased mortality risk.[51]

▶ **SAD Facts About Eating Refined Carbohydrates When You Have Cancer**

Compared with normal cells, cancer cells have a sweet tooth: they consume between ten and fifty times more glucose than surrounding healthy cells.[52] In addition, the faster a tumor's proliferation, the more glucose it consumes. Experiments have shown that when lab animals are injected with an aggressive cancer, they have much higher survival rates if they have low or normal blood sugar than if they have high blood sugar; glucose enables the cancers to grow with reckless abandon.[53] These and many similar findings suggest that controlling your blood sugar can make a substantial difference in controlling the course of your cancer.[54] (I explore these connections in greater detail in Chapter 18, on glycemia.)

What raises blood sugar? The chief dietary culprits are refined carbohydrates.[55] But refined carbs don't stop there. They also cause the insulin resistance that characterizes type 2 diabetes, in which both insulin levels in the blood and blood glucose levels are abnormally high. Unfortunately, insulin fuels a number of cancers, including those of the breast and colon.[56] And now we come full circle: insulin not only is a potent stimulator of tumor growth but also increases cancer cells' appetite for glucose—creating a vicious cycle of sugar "bingeing" and growth stimulation.[57] It comes as little surprise, then, that in a 2002 study published in the *Journal of Clinical Oncology*, women in remission with the highest insulin levels were twice as likely to develop a recurrence of breast cancer, as well as three times as likely to develop metastases, as women with lower glucose levels.[58]

Notice that the culprits here are *refined* carbohydrates. Just as with fats, there are good carbs and bad carbs, an important distinction that the recent fad for low-carb diets ignores. Carbohydrates represent your most important source of energy and calories; they add bulk and satisfaction to meals. Most important for our purposes, they are a major part of traditional diets associated with low cancer rates and high cancer survival.[59] Eating whole grains is not the same as eating refined sugar, white bread, cookies, crackers, potato chips, and pastries. The latter contain empty calories that raise insulin and blood sugar. Whole grains such as brown rice, buckwheat, whole-grain bread, wild rice, rye, quinoa, whole-wheat pasta, and barley, on the other hand, are rich sources of complex carbohydrates, phytochemicals, amino acids, essential fats, and fiber.

That is why complex carbohydrates play a starring role in the Life Over Cancer nutrition program. Their fiber dilutes, binds, inactivates, and removes carcinogens, cholesterol, bile acids, and various toxic substances.[60] Fiber also smoothes out levels of glucose and insulin, keeping these tumor feeders in check.[61] These effects help explain why breast cancer patients who eat more whole grains have higher rates of survival than patients whose diets are full of refined carbs and low in fiber.[62]

So avoid refined carbohydrates: white sugar, honey, high-fructose corn syrup, cookies, cakes, pastries, white bread, crackers, potato chips, french fries, commercial waffles, candy, donuts, and many dry breakfast cereals (juice-sweetened cereals listing whole grains as a primary ingredient are okay, but those with added sugar, evaporated cane juice, or honey are likely to raise your levels of tumor-fueling blood sugar and insulin). Instead, emphasize whole grains such as those above, as well as complex carbs such as vegetables, legumes, beans, and fresh fruit. If you crave something sweet, try dried fruit, rice syrup, barley malt, agave, kiwi sweetener, stevia, FruitSource, or maple syrup.

► **SAD Facts About Eating Animal Protein After a
Cancer Diagnosis**

Habitual consumption of red meat has been linked with cancers
of the colon, lung, breast, esophagus, larynx, stomach, kidney, endometrium, ovaries, and prostate.[63] For our purposes, however,
an even greater concern—since almost all of you reading this far
already have cancer—is that meat affects your chances of surviving with cancer. Every daily serving of red meat, liver, and bacon
doubled the risk of breast cancer recurrence, according to a 1998
study;[64] that is, eating two servings a day was associated with four
times the risk of recurrence.

What's wrong with meat?

- For starters, it is typically high in iron, which causes your
body to generate highly reactive molecules called free radicals.
These are the culprits causing DNA damage (which leads to
treatment-resistant mutations) and promoting an environment
conducive to tumor growth.[65]
- Red meat and poultry are packed with arachidonic acid, an
omega-6 fat we met above. Arachidonic acid is converted to inflammatory molecules that fuel tumor growth and metastasis.[66]
- Meat (as well as dairy, which we'll get to below) contains
cholesterol, which is bad news for people with cancer.[67] High
levels of serum cholesterol are associated with more deadly
metastases, whereas lower levels of LDL ("bad") cholesterol
have been linked to better patient outcomes.[68] Furthermore, the
more cholesterol cancer cells absorb, the more resistant they become to chemotherapy drugs such as Adriamycin (doxorubicin), found a 1996 study.[69]
- Diets rich in meats and dairy boost the level of estradiol.
This hormone can stimulate the growth of tumors, especially
those of the breast, ovaries, uterus, and cervix. In contrast,
high-fiber, vegetable-rich diets lower estradiol levels.[70]

For all these reasons, dietitians at the Block Center recommend that patients with advanced cancer lean toward a more
vegetarian diet,[71] with the exception of small amounts of fish,
egg white, and supplemental whey. In place of animal protein,

add vegetable protein: legumes, soy foods, seitan ("wheat meat"), nuts, and seeds. When you eat fish, limit your serving to a 4-ounce portion (about the size of the palm of your hand). Emphasize deepwater, northern ocean fish such as salmon, cod, haddock, mackerel, and sardines. By removing meats and most other animal products from your diet, you will keep your levels of tumor-sustaining iron, cholesterol, and estradiol in check.[72]

Unfortunately, everything I just said about meat also pertains to dairy products, which can also increase levels of cholesterol and tumor-stimulating growth factors and cause digestive problems in some chemotherapy patients. And dairy products are bad news for people with cancer for additional reasons.

• Dairy products contain high amounts of calcium, which can tie up the body's store of vitamin D. Although more research is needed, free vitamin D appears to be crucial in controlling cancer cell division. Astonishingly, epidemiological studies are showing that in northerly latitudes with long winters, survival of breast and lung cancer is much lower in patients diagnosed in the short days of winter than in the summer; recent evidence implicates low levels of vitamin D from sunlight. Although most milk is fortified with vitamin D, other dairy products are not, and supplementation may be necessary to overcome high calcium levels in those whose diets are high in dairy.[73]

• Whole milk and full-fat dairy products contain high quantities of saturated fat; almost half the calories of whole milk come from fat, mostly saturated, as do about one-third the calories in low-fat milk. Saturated fat can raise cholesterol levels. And just because low-fat milk is lower in fat than whole milk doesn't mean it's really low. Only skim-milk products have zero saturated fat. Saturated fat can also increase the likelihood of abnormal blood coagulation, which can cause major problems for people with certain cancers.[74]

• Milk contains significant levels of lactose and other sugars, which can raise your blood sugar[75] and, if you develop insulin resistance, insulin as well.[76] In addition, many chemotherapy drugs produce temporary lactose intolerance, so consuming lactose can cause you abdominal pain and digestive disturbances.[77]

• Even the protein content of milk raises concerns. Milk protein is 80 percent casein, which accelerates the growth of tumors and metastasis in lab animals.[78] The other 20 percent is whey, which helps inhibit cancer.[79] Whey is a good source of protein, but it should be taken as a supplement rather than in milk.[80] I encourage shakes made of whey and berries mixed with rice or soy milk for patients who need protein or calorie supplements.

• Keep in mind that the natural purpose of cow's milk is to make a newborn calf grow. As such, nature packed milk with compounds that raise blood levels of growth-stimulating factors such as estrogens, insulin,[81] insulin-like growth factor 1 (IGF-1),[82] and polyamines[83]—not only in the calf but also in you. The hormones and growth factors are supposed to stimulate growth of normal cells,[84] but they act the same way on malignant ones, making them proliferate even faster. IGF-1 is a potent tumor-growth stimulant that can be particularly dangerous for patients with hormone-sensitive cancers such as prostate and breast cancers.[85] For instance, high dairy intake has been linked to poorer survival in patients with cancers of the upper digestive tract and with laryngeal cancer, as well as prostate cancer (whereas fish was linked with better outcomes).[86] Milk may cause problems for prostate cancer in particular because excessive calcium consumption ties up the body's vitamin D, which is needed to keep prostate cancer growth in check.[87] As a cancer patient, you do not want your diet to work at cross-purposes with your treatments by fueling cancer growth.

You may be wondering, *If I don't drink milk, where will I get my calcium, which is needed to build and maintain strong bones?* Adults ages nineteen to fifty need 1,000 mg per day, and those over fifty need 1,200 mg. People at risk of osteoporosis should get 1,500 mg.[88] But you can reach these goals through supplements as well as calcium-fortified soy milk, oat milk, or orange juice; canned sardines with bones or canned salmon; and vegetables and legumes such as collard greens, spinach, turnips, cooked beans (white, soy, navy, and great northern), kale, okra, beet greens, firm tofu prepared with nigari, and bok choy. A cup of collards has a bit more calcium, and a cup of spinach a bit less, than a cup of skim milk, while a cup of cooked beans has about half as much as skim milk.[89] If fortified milk has been your major vitamin D source, remember that you need vitamin D as well, either from healthful sun exposure (avoid being outdoors without sunscreen for longer than about fifteen to twenty minutes at midday) or from supplements (a total of 800 to 2,000 IU daily is probably wise for most cancer patients).[90]

In sum, I advise all of my patients that they are better off reducing or even avoiding dairy: whole, low-fat, and skim milk, yogurt, cheese, ice cream, and ice milk. Nonfat organic yogurt with live active cultures and occasionally skim milk are okay when you are transitioning to the Life Over Cancer program, but I am not convinced that you need them for long. Instead, have soy milk, rice milk, oat milk, or almond milk. You can even find rice-, almond-, and soy-based cheeses, soy yogurt, and dairy-free ice creams. Pick those that are sweetened or contain brown rice syrup, agave, or a fruit sweetener rather than sugar, honey, molasses, or evaporated cane juice.

▶ **SAD Facts About Poor Intake of Micronutrients After a Cancer Diagnosis**

Most Americans are overfed but undernourished. We consume too many calories, primarily in the form of fat, sugar, and animal protein, and too few vitamins, minerals, and phytochemicals. For the first time in human history, you can be overweight but undernourished. A recent survey by the U.S. Department of Agriculture, for instance, found that 70 percent of men and more than 80 percent of women consumed less than two-thirds of the RDA for one or more nutrients.[91] In particular, most of us are not getting enough vitamin E, vitamin B_6, calcium, magnesium, and zinc. Maybe that shouldn't be surprising in a country where a president argued that ketchup should be considered a vegetable and about one in four "vegetable" servings are french fries.[92]

Actually, when it comes to a diet that can help you in your battle against cancer, the problem is even worse than the USDA found. RDAs, after all, were never intended to apply to people with disease, but only to prevent outright malnutrition. When you have cancer, you need even larger quantities of many nutrients. Worse, there are no RDAs for phytochemicals. These natural compounds are not to be underestimated. They can modulate tumor growth by affecting the workings of the genes that regulate cell division,[93] the production of inflammatory biochemicals[94] and tumor blood vessels,[95] and cells' suicide mechanism (or, as it is more properly called, programmed cell death, or apoptosis).[96] No wonder phytochemicals have been called "gene therapy with food."[97] At the same time that scientists are fathoming how phytochemicals work on the molecular level, they are also finding effects where it counts—in matters of life or death. Studies find that eating large quantities of vegetables improves the survival rates of patients with lung cancer and breast cancer.[98]

You do not need to learn chemistry to identify foods containing the most powerful phytochemicals: many are plant pigments. The red pigment lycopene, found in tomatoes and some other red fruit, is a member of the group of antioxidants called carotenoids. It appears to inhibit prostate cancer.[99] In a 2002 randomized study, patients awaiting surgery to remove the prostate ate a daily tomato concentrate containing 30 mg of lycopene (the amount in 1⅓ cups of tomato juice) for a few weeks after their initial diagnosis. When their prostates were compared with those of prostate cancer patients who had not upped their consumption of tomato products or lycopene supplements, those in the first group had smaller tumors and lower PSA levels.[100] That raises the intriguing possibility that lycopene can play an important supporting role in "watchful waiting" after a diagnosis of prostate cancer, taming the malignancy so that you die of old age before it ever threatens your life. A 2005 randomized trial with prostate cancer patients showed that a supplement of lycopene along with phytochemicals from soy and milk thistle increased the time it took for levels of the tumor marker PSA to double, from 445 days in the placebo group to 1,150 days in the supplement group.[101]

Mom was right when she told you to eat your broccoli: it and other cruciferous vegetables (including cabbage, watercress, collards, brussels sprouts, kale, mustard greens, and turnips) contain a veritable pharmacopoeia of phytochemicals with important cancer-fighting properties. All cruciferous vegetables contain sulfides and thiols, which can help the body remove chemical toxins. Broccoli contains sulforaphane, which blocks the growth of late-stage breast cancer cells, a 2004 study found, through a mechanism very similar to that used by certain cancer drugs.[102] Sulforaphane also activates enzymes that help carry the toxic metabolites of drugs and other substances out of the body;[103] this makes broccoli very appealing as a means of recovering from the toxic side effects of chemo. Cruciferous vegetables also contain indole-3-carbinol, which may block metastasis and also alter the metabolism of estrogen in a way that decreases the ability of this hormone to promote breast cancer.[104] Phenethyl isothiocyanate (PEITC), also found in cruciferous vegetables, induces cancer cells to commit suicide.[105]

The earliest direct evidence about these compounds came from animal experiments. When mice were injected with mammary tumor cells, those fed diets rich in cabbage and collards had fewer than half the lung metastases of control animals.[106] When prostate cancer cells were injected into mice, sulforaphane—the broccoli compound—inhibited their growth by causing the cells to commit suicide.[107] Research on human applications is now under way.

The red-purple color in berries comes from the pigments called anthocyanins. Like lycopene, these reds are also antioxidants. Those in elderberries, for instance, are taken up by the cells lining blood vessels, where they protect those cells from the mutation-inducing effects of free radicals.[108] A raspberry phytochemical, ellagic acid, is also a potent antioxidant, and has been shown to inhibit growth of breast and cervical cancer cells in test tube experiments.[109] Berries also contain phytochemicals that inhibit the activity of a protein called VEGF (vascular endothelial growth factor).[110] VEGF helps tumors grow the tiny blood vessels they need to survive, so targeting it should inhibit the growth and spread of cancer cells.[111] That's what some very smart pharmaceutical scientists think, at least: the new colorectal cancer drug Avastin targets VEGF. A number of other anti-VEGF compounds are in drug companies' pipelines.[112] But nature got there first.

Other phytochemicals seem to play a role in overcoming chemoresistance, in which malignant cells are impervious to chemotherapy. Quercetin, found in brightly colored fruits and vegetables such as apples, kale, and red onions, appears to re-sensitize breast cancer cells that have developed resistance to multiple chemo drugs, making them vulnerable to doxorubicin, a 1994 study found.[113] What seems to happen is that quercetin and related compounds block the activity of a protein that pumps toxic chemo agents out of the cancer cell as quickly as they can get in. As a result, the chemo drug gets in and stays in, reaching levels lethal to the cell.[114]

At this point, you may be wondering why you can't just go out and buy bottles of lycopene, sulforaphane, and quercetin pills, rather than get these phytochemicals in actual foods. One reason is that these compounds only scratch the surface of the chemical richness of the plant kingdom. There are countless phytochemi-cals out there, of which only a small fraction have been identified, let alone had their physiological effects nailed down.[115] What sci-entists have most consistently correlated with less aggressive can-cers and higher survival rates is not individual micronutrients but

ANTIOXIDANT SCORES OF VARIOUS FOODS[119]	
Food	Total Oxygen Radical Absorbance Capacity
Kale, spinach, strawberries, blueberries, blackberries, cranberries, raspberries	>100
Prunes, plums, red peppers, beets, brussels sprouts	60–100
Garlic, onions, pink grapefruit, cherries, tomato, lettuce, corn	20–60
Potatoes, sweet potatoes, yellow squash, cucumbers, string beans, celery, apples, bananas, pears	<20

whole foods.[116] Yes, the Life Over Cancer nutrition program recommends dietary supplements. But its basis is real food.

There are so many fruits and vegetables to choose from that you might not know where to start. Just choose a diversity of colors and varieties—vegetables, legumes, whole grains, seeds, and fruits. Buy organic when you can. Some data suggest that organic produce contains considerably more antioxidant compounds called phenolics than produce grown with toxic pesticides and fertilizers.[117] In one study, organic strawberries inhibited growth of breast cancer cells more than conventionally grown ones.[118] In general, load up on foods high in antioxidant capacity, as shown in the table above.

Why Diet Alone Is Not Enough

You must have seen many of the above recommendations before. Eat your fruits, veggies, and whole grains, minimize fat, avoid sugar . . . this is how everyone is supposed to eat to stay healthy and reduce the risk of disease. But you already have cancer. You need to overcome appetite-destroying anxiety, withstand debilitating treatments, replenish key micronutrients (especially vitamins B_1, B_2, B_{12}, C, E, and K, niacin, and folic acid)[120] depleted by chemo, and, most of all, win your battle against the disease. In other words, you need to do more.

Having cancer and being treated for it increase your body's needs for micronutrients, far beyond what the RDAs call for.[121] As I mentioned above, the RDAs are set with healthy people in mind and are the minimum they need to maintain health. Your nutritional needs are greater. In one double-blind randomized trial reported in the *Journal of Urology* in 1994, for instance, patients with bladder cancer received either a supplement containing the RDAs for all vitamins and minerals or the RDA supplement *plus* extra zinc and vitamins A, B_6, C, and E. Result: 91 percent of the RDA-only group suffered a recurrence of their cancer within five years. But only 41 percent in the RDA-plus group did, even though everyone received the same immunotherapy.[122] Similarly, although the Japanese consume a great deal of fish, those taking fish oil supplements following a bone marrow transplant for leukemia had a better survival rate and fewer complications than patients eating the standard Japanese diet alone.[123]

Just as an intake of micronutrients greater than the RDAs can help in your recovery from cancer, so it can help you better withstand the side effects of treatment. Radiotherapy and many chemotherapy drugs use free radicals to kill tumors; this raises the body's need for antioxidants[124] such as vitamins C and E, selenium, or green tea catechins, all of which can play key roles in promoting good health and recovery from advanced cancers. In fact, a 2007 study in the journal *Nutrition and Cancer* found that head and neck cancer patients who had the highest intake of beta-carotene-containing foods had fewer side effects and fewer recurrences than those whose diets included less beta-carotene.[125] Other studies have also shown lower mortality or recurrence rates for patients who had high dietary antioxidants. And if you have undergone surgery of the stomach or small intestine, you can suffer temporary loss of digestive functioning, leading to deficiencies of certain micronutrients. Most people who have undergone extensive stomach surgery will eventually develop a vitamin B_{12} deficiency[126] and require monthly injections of this vitamin in order to avoid anemia and a degeneration of the central nervous system leading to neuropathy.

The bottom line is that diet alone cannot deliver the nutritional power needed by patients undergoing treatment for cancer. Dietary supplements, in tandem with the diet I have been outlining, are therefore the only practical solution. Supplements that are based on whole plants are likely to be safer, as well as more in line with current scientific results on diet and cancer, and thus more effective. So whenever possible, I encourage formulations that are prepared with whole plants.

One concern you may hear about supplements is that they may interfere with chemotherapy or radiation that works by generating free radicals that kill the cancer cell. Logic might suggest that if you are flooding your system with antioxidants, they may mop up the free radicals before the latter can kill the malignant cells. I will discuss this in Chapters 4 and 24, but for now let me simply say that in a 2007 review of randomized controlled trials that my research staff and I published in *Cancer Treatment Reviews* we found no evidence of any such inhibition. In 2008 we published a paper in *International Journal of Cancer* that showed antioxidants appear to help relieve several chemo side effects.[127]

The trick is to balance your intake of these nutrients in a way that will support your ability to combat disease. A number of vitamins and phytochemicals act synergistically with anti-cancer drugs, making the combination more effective than either alone.[128] The reason is that different micronutrients hit cancer through different mechanisms. When these elements are combined, they can more readily outfox the cancer. (Oncologists apply the same principle when combining chemotherapy drugs.) So, for example, we know that soy protein blocks certain tumor-fueling enzymes,[129] while omega-3 fats[130] and green tea compounds[131] block others. Take all three, and you're hitting cancer from multiple angles.

I can't emphasize enough how important it is to take an integrative approach, combining nutrients in a way that attacks your cancer from all sides.[132] Consider "bad" estrogens, which promote estrogen-dependent cancers, such as some breast cancers, endometrial cancer, and ovarian cancer. It makes sense to use whatever means possible to keep them to a minimum. Diet can do just that. Fact 1: High-fat diets can send blood levels of harmful estrogens soaring.[133] Fact 2: Too little fiber reduces the excretion of harmful estrogens from the colon, so more estrogens are reabsorbed back into the bloodstream.[134] Fact 3: If your diet is too low in cruciferous vegetables, your body won't be as efficient at breaking down those harmful estrogens—so once again they build up in the blood and help fuel the growth of such estrogen-dependent cancers.[135] Notice how fat, fiber, and cruciferous vegetables all have their own unique impact on blood estrogen levels. Attend to all three components, and your body becomes much more capable of ridding itself of harmful estrogens. By the same token, however, if you ignore one of these components, the beneficial effects of the other two diminish: if you eat a high-fat diet, for example, even getting lots of fiber and cruciferous vegetables to promote excretion and breaking down of estrogens may not keep up with the resulting high levels of estrogens.

This shows why it's important to think not in terms of a single magic bullet, but in terms of combinations of nutrients and foods, which are much more likely to have an impact on your disease.[136] This goes for diet and supplements, too. Supplements will not counteract the harm of a poor diet. Without a strong dietary foundation, even the best efforts to use supplements will fall flat. As our center's dietitians tell patients, making a few minor changes in your diet is not likely to help you beat your cancer. Neither will taking a bucketful of supplements while you continue to consume a cancer-fueling diet. If you take an omega-3 supplement but eat fast foods on a regular basis, you cancel out the benefits of the omega-3s: there are too many factors in junk foods that promote the very effects that omega-3 would otherwise stifle. The supplement just can't keep up.

I hope I've convinced you of three things: (1) a healthy diet like the one outlined above is crucial to winning the battle against cancer, (2) whole foods should supply the lion's share of micronutrients, and (3) food alone cannot give you, a cancer patient, enough of these micronutrients. That points to my final dietary recommendation: obtain the additional micronutrients you need not in the form of a different pill for each micronutrient but as what I call powerfoods, which take aim at cancer in multiple ways.[137] The spice turmeric, for instance, hits at least forty-five molecules that allow malignant cells to proliferate or metastasize.[138] The grape phytochemical resveratrol hits thirty-four. Green tea compounds hit thirteen, and milk thistle, ginger, and pomegranate all hit the same molecular targets that the aptly named targeted chemotherapy drugs, such as Avastin and Erbitux, do.[139] But to get enough turmeric, resveratrol, and the rest, you'd have to eat curry and guzzle grape juice until you exploded. In contrast, concentrates such as the "green drinks" often sold in health food stores containing the right ingredients give you therapeutically beneficial amounts of these natural compounds in just a few servings.

Now that you know the general aims and principles of the Life Over Cancer nutrition program, let's work out a diet for your particular needs.

CHAPTER 5

THE LIFE OVER CANCER CORE DIET PLAN

You can use the preceding chapter to get started on eating in a way that improves your odds in the battle against cancer. Now I want to get even more specific, offering you food guidelines and sample meal plans that make up the Life Over Cancer core diet plan. Chapter 6 will describe adjustments you may need to make when undergoing treatment, experiencing cancer-induced weight loss, or in remission.

The best way to get started is to dive right in and quickly make as many changes as possible. This way you don't lose momentum, and you will be encouraged to stick with it by how good you start feeling. Changing your diet gradually may work for some, but it runs a greater risk of slipping back to old eating patterns, since the rewards are slower and less obvious. We often find that patients who transition more gradually struggle to take the next step, whereas people who jump into a healthful eating plan find that they feel so much better, they have little trouble sticking with it for the long haul.

While you might not be able to follow in the footsteps of one of my early patients, Joe Horcher, it is instructive to see commitment at work. After Joe's first visit with me, he went home, where his wife was cooking an elaborate roast for dinner. Joe said, "Honey, throw out the roast—we're going vegetarian!" With this attitude Joe succeeded in making the dietary changes necessary to conquer his metastatic prostate cancer (you will read about Joe's success in Chapter 18).

Just so you know what you're getting into, you can follow the core diet plan with meals built around Lemon-Scented Asparagus Risotto, Brown Basmati Rice with Cashews and Currants, Risotto with Corn and Roasted Peppers, Cold Sesame Noodles with shiitake, green onions, and a hint of dark sesame oil and shoyu, or Herbed Mediterranean Rice with Chickpeas and a splash of raspberry vinaigrette (you can find all these recipes on the LOC website). You can complement the grain with a protein dish such as Grilled Striped Bass with Lemon-Mustard Marinade, a stir-fry of tofu or tempeh and vegetables over brown rice, Bean Burritos, Sweet and Sour Salmon with Wild Rice and Peapods, Rainbow Trout Dijon, Grilled Tuna Salad, Curried Yellow Split Pea Soup with Squash and Raisins, or Fresh Fish Baked with Ginger and Garlic. Accent the meal with vegetables, preferably two or more varieties, such as Asparagus with Chinese Black Bean Sauce, Cucumber Cilantro Salad, or Hot Thai-Style Broccoli. For dessert, try Pumpkin Tart with Glazed Pecans, Apple Crepes with Caramel Sauce, Anise Cookies with Pignoli, Steamed Cranberry Pudding, or Lemon Poppy Seed Cake. Recipes for all of these can be found in cookbooks noted on the LOC website.

Practical Advice for Getting Started

This chapter contains four practical guides that will help you implement a successful program:

1. A Food Selection Guide. General dietary advice for helping you choose specific foods and food groups that help alter your internal biochemistry from cancer-promoting to cancer-inhibiting.

2. A Quantity Guide. Consuming enough food is vital to those undergoing treatment, as surgery, chemotherapy, and radiation are all stressful for the body. Too, weight loss is common among many facing the challenge of cancer—it's more commonly found in people with advanced cancers of the colon, ovaries, pancreas, stomach, esophagus, and lung, though it can occur with any malignancy.[1] The physical wasting syndrome, known as *cachexia*, is as disabling to the spirit as it is to the body, and can lead to an irreversible decline: rapid weight loss alone can predict poor survival in people with cancer.[2] For any of you who have gone through life trying to lose body fat, cancer-related weight loss at first may seem like a positive rather than a negative. When left unchecked, however, the eventual effect of this process on one's overall functioning and quality of life can quickly turn into a nightmare.[3] That is why both the quality and the quantity of what you eat are paramount.

3. A Meal Planning Guide. A sample daily meal plan, a starting shopping list, and cookbook recommendations. The Life Over Cancer website provides more meal plans, as well as recipes. If you need help structuring meal plans, you can consult one of our professional dietitians, who are available for in-person or telephone consultations, as noted on the website.

4. A Powerfoods Supplement Guide. Since it is difficult to get protective levels of phytochemicals and other micronutrients from food alone, I recommend concentrates from the twelve powerfood families.

Here's a summary of your core nutritional needs and how to meet them.

Need: Cancer-Fighting Phytochemicals
• **Recommendation 1:** Eat a rainbow of vegetables, emphasizing brightly colored ones (pigments contain cancer-fighting phytochemicals), leafy greens, and cruciferous vegetables such as broccoli, onions, and garlic. Choose locally grown and organic whenever possible. Try to get a mix of root vegetables, leafy green vegetables, and sea vegetables. Fruits should be limited to no more than two or three servings per day.

Need: Energy-Sustaining Foods
• **Recommendation 2:** Consume plenty of whole grains, the richest source of complex carbohydrates and fiber, which provide a slow, sustained supply of fuel for your daily activities while reducing fuel for your cancer.[4] Select unrefined and minimally processed foods. Eat small amounts throughout the day (grazing) to reduce hunger and food cravings or if you are experiencing blood sugar swings;[5] three meals with two or three snacks are ideal, though one less or one more is fine.

TIP: To reduce cravings for sweets and junk foods, try consuming whole grains at every meal. Build your meal around whole grains such as brown rice, oats, barley, millet, quinoa, buckwheat, whole-wheat bread, and whole-wheat pasta.

Need: Cancer-Fighting Proteins
• **Recommendation 3:** Consume plenty of legumes (lentils, chickpeas, beans), soy foods, fish, and occasional omega-3 eggs. These choices have cancer-fighting properties, contain many of the nutrients found in meat, and are an excellent source of the

complex carbohydrates and soluble fiber that help regulate and control blood sugar.[6]

TIP: To satisfy meat cravings, try grilling, barbecuing, or baking salmon, halibut, tuna, or haddock steaks. Try seitan or tofu hot dogs, veggie burgers, vegetarian bacon, and vegetarian cold cuts.

Need: Reduce Dairy Products

• **Recommendation 4:** Replace milk with rice, soy, oat, or nut beverages. For cheese, substitute cheeses made with soy, rice, hazelnuts, or almonds. Try soy or rice ice creams flavored with fruit or rice syrup.[7]

Need: Healthy Sweets

• **Recommendation 5:** Use fruit and small amounts of unrefined, healthful sweeteners to satisfy cravings for sweets. Choose foods made with rice syrup, barley malt, agave, kiwi sweetener, stevia, FruitSource, or maple syrup.[8]

Need: Essential Fats

• **Recommendation 6:** Limit total fat intake and shift to foods high in omega-3s and omega-9s such as deep-sea fish, olives, avocados, nuts, and flax and other seeds. Eliminate trans fats.

Need: Adequate Intake of Healthy Fluids

• **Recommendation 7:** Drink water and three to five cups daily of green tea plus other fluids and herb teas. Green tea is even better for rehydrating than water.[9] It contains many antioxidants and anti-cancer phytochemicals, and the caffeine levels of tea are not high enough to hinder rehydration.

BEFORE YOU DIVE IN

If you have diabetes: Keep in mind that improving your diet, increasing exercise levels, or losing weight may decrease your need for insulin or other diabetes medications. Be sure to communicate with your doctor and nutritionist as you proceed with making changes to your diet.

If you have food allergies or sensitivities: Exercise caution in adding foods to your diet. The food charts in this book do not have space to accommodate cautions about all the types of food that some readers may be unable to tolerate.

If you are taking Coumadin (warfarin) or other medications that can be affected by food: Be sure to consult with your doctor or pharmacist about precautions you may need to take in altering your diet.

To meet the seven specific food recommendations above, I suggest specific foods that inhibit or at least do not promote tumor growth, and rate them as follows:

OK **for Every Meal** ★ ★ ★	Eat these as often as possible; they should make up the bulk of your diet. These are the highest-quality, minimally processed, most nutrient-packed and phytochemically rich foods and those that pack a special cancer-fighting wallop.
OK **for Daily Use** ★ ★	These are high-quality food choices that are also nutrient-dense but may have gone through some mechanical processing—grinding, cracking, pressing.
OK **for Occasional** **Use** ★	These are acceptable food choices; they can accent and add variety to your diet. However, I encourage you to choose two- and three-star foods whenever possible.

The most difficult part of the transition for many is passing up the traditional tastes and textures of animal foods, dairy products, and suboptimal sweets. So, in each of these categories I have also included half-star foods for rare or infrequent intake, such as poultry, skim milk, nonfat cheeses, and even some red meat. The omega-6 and saturated fat content of these foods can promote inflammation, oxidative stress, and spikes in blood sugar and insulin, which in turn can promote tumor growth. Remember, the half-star foods are only indicated in select circumstances. Overall, you are safer sticking to one-, two-, and three-star foods.

None or Rare ½ ★	These foods can be eaten when you are transitioning to the Life Over Cancer diet, during family events and celebrations, when you are traveling, or if no other choices are available.

How this works in your daily diet will become clearer as we consider each of the seven recommendations in the Food Selection Guide.

RECOMMENDATION I: EAT A RAINBOW OF VEGETABLES

★ ★ ★ OK for Every Meal

Beet greens	Carrots
Beets	Cauliflower
Bell peppers (use organic)	Collard greens
Bok choy (Chinese cabbage)	Daikon (Oriental radish)
Broccoli	Dandelion greens
Broccoli rabe (rapini)	Garlic
Broccoli sprouts	Fresh ginger
Brussels sprouts	Kale
Burdock	Leeks
Cabbage, green	Mushrooms
Cabbage, red	Mustard greens

Napa cabbage	Turnips
Onion	Watercress
Parsley	
Pumpkin (starchy)	**Sea Vegetables**
Rutabaga	Agar (kanten)
Salsify	Arame
Scallions	Dulse
Spinach (use organic)	Hijiki (hiziki)
Squash, winter (starchy)	Kelp
Sweet potatoes (starchy)	Kombu
Swiss chard	Laver
Tomatoes	Nori
Turnip greens	Wakame

★ ★ OK for Daily Use

Artichokes	Kohlrabi
Asparagus	Lettuce, leaf
Celery (use organic)	Lotus root
Corn (starchy)	Okra
Cucumbers	Parsnip
Eggplant	Peas (starchy)
Endive	Radish
Jerusalem artichoke (sunchoke)	Squash, yellow
Jicama	Zucchini

★ OK for Occasional Use

Diluted carrot or beet juice	Nonorganic vegetables
Lettuce, iceberg	
Low-sodium vegetable juice (canned or bottled)	

Fresh vegetables are excellent choices, but frozen and some canned can also be good sources of nutrients. Choose organic when available, especially for vegetables most contaminated with pesticides, such as bell peppers, potatoes, spinach, and celery.[10] I have designated these foods as "use organic" in the chart above. With canned vegetables (especially tomato products), try to find those without added salt.

Most vegetables should be only slightly cooked—steamed, baked, stir-fried, or lightly sautéed until tender but still crisp. Light cooking breaks down cell walls and makes many of their nutrients more available. For this reason, canned tomato products and tomato sauces are excellent sources of lycopene. (They can be prepared with a little olive oil, which helps lycopene absorption.)[11] Salads and raw vegetables as part of your vegetable intake are fine unless you suffer from digestive problems. If your white blood count drops very low while you are undergoing chemotherapy or radiation, restrict raw vegetables temporarily as an extra precaution against infection.[12]

Some vegetables, such as corn and squash, contain more carbohydrates and calories than others and thus can be substituted for whole grains. These are marked "starchy" in the table and are also included in the grain recommendations in the next section.

Be careful not to get into a vegetable rut. Variety is not only more pleasurable but better for your health, since it provides the widest possible range of anti-cancer, health-enhancing phytochemicals. I encourage you to get a mixture of the following five phytochemical vegetable groups throughout the day, or at least throughout the week:

Glucosinolate (cruciferous family: cabbage, broccoli, kale, brussels sprouts)[13]

Organosulfur (allium family: garlic, onions, scallions, chives)[14]

Lycopene (red vegetables: tomatoes, red bell peppers, pimento, paprika)[15]

Lutein (most dark leafy greens: spinach, kale, watercress)[16]

Carotene (orange vegetables: carrots, pumpkin, winter squash)[17]

RECOMMENDATION 2:
EAT LOTS OF WHOLE GRAINS

★ ★ ★ OK for Every Meal

Amaranth	Quinoa
Barley (Job's tears)	Rye berries
Brown rice	Spelt
Buckwheat (kasha)	Teff
Millet	Wheat berries
Oat groats (whole oats)	Wild rice

★ ★ OK for Daily Use

Breads, whole-grain	Noodles/pastas (whole-grain)
Brown rice cakes, plain	Oatmeal (old-fashioned rolled,
Bulgur	or steel-cut)
Cold cereal, whole-grain	Pita, whole-grain
Corn (kernels)	Popcorn (plain)
Corn grits	Pumpkin, cooked, mashed
Cornmeal (stone-ground	Squash, winter (acorn, buttercup,
ungerminated)	etc.), mashed
Corn on the cob	Sweet potato, cooked
Couscous (whole-wheat)	Tortillas, corn or whole-grain
Crackers, whole-grain	Yams, cooked
Flour, whole-grain	

★ OK for Occasional Use

White-flour products	White potatoes (waxy varieties
(unbleached, unbromated	preferred—red, Yukon gold,
preferred, since bromine may	boiling potatoes)
interfere with iodine absorption)	White rice

½ ★ None or Rare	
Grain products made with unhealthful sweeteners, butter, and/or partially hydrogenated fats	White baking potatoes (Idaho, russet)

Whole grains can be boiled, steamed, pressure-cooked, or sprouted. I recommend pressure cooking for certain ones, such as brown rice, rye berries, oat groats, and whole barley, to improve digestibility; purchase a stainless-steel pressure cooker with a safety valve and a good cookbook as a guide, such as Lorna Sass' *Cooking Under Pressure*. The high pressure softens the grains better than boiling, and grains do not lose nutrients to steam, as they do when boiled. Adopt brown rice as your staple instead of white rice. In fact, eat a variety of whole grains, including barley, oats, millet, and quinoa. Try some of the less common ones and you will be surprised (as I was) at how delicious these can be.

It is important to purchase breads and baked goods that are free from refined sweeteners (such as sugar, evaporated cane juice, or high-fructose corn syrup), contain no trans fats, are made with 100 percent whole wheat or other whole-grain flours (look for at least 4 grams of fiber per slice), and have a minimal amount of preservatives (chemicals with names you can't pronounce).

Gluten-containing grains should, of course, be avoided by people who are gluten-intolerant.

RECOMMENDATION 3:
CONSUME ADEQUATE, HEALTHFUL PROTEIN

★ ★ ★   OK for Every Meal

Legumes
Aduki beans (adzuki, azuki)
Anasazi beans
Black beans (turtle)
Brown beans (Swedish)
Chickpeas (garbanzo, ceci)
Fava beans (broad)
Kidney beans
Lentils (brown, green, red, coral)
Lima beans (butter)
Mung beans

Peas (green)
Pinto beans
Split peas (green, yellow)
White beans (canellini, great
northern, navy)
Tempeh
Tofu
Seitan
Soybeans
Edamame

★ ★   OK for Daily Use

Ocean and freshwater fish
(make sure freshwater fish come
from uncontaminated sources)
Anchovy
Bass
Bass, striped
Bluefish, Atlantic
Butterfish
Carp
Catfish
Char, arctic
Cod
Dorado
Dore
Flounder
Grouper
Haddock
Halibut, Greenland

Halibut, Pacific
Herring, freshwater
Herring, Pacific or Atlantic
Mackerel, Atlantic
Mahimahi
Monkfish
Orange roughy
Perch, ocean
Pike
Pollack
Redfish
Red snapper
Sablefish
Salmon
Sardines, canned in water or fresh
Scrod
Smelt
Snook

Sole

Sturgeon, Atlantic

Tilapia

Trout

Trout, lake

Trout, rainbow

Turbot

Walleye

Whitefish

Sushi (raw fish poses a small risk of bacterial contamination, so if you have a low white cell count, stick to cooked fish)

Veggie burgers

Egg whites, organic if possible

Whey protein (micro-filtered, lactose-free)

★ OK for Occasional Use

Shellfish

Clams

Crab

Crayfish

Lobster

Mussels, blue

Oysters, Pacific

Scallops

Shrimp

Squid (calamari)

Omega-3 whole eggs (limit to 2 yolks or less per week)

Vegetarian meat substitutes

Tuna (canned tuna is fairly low in mercury but fresh or frozen tuna has somewhat elevated mercury levels)

Swordfish (elevated mercury levels)

Mackerel, king (elevated mercury levels) or chub

½ ★ None or Rare

Non-omega-3 whole eggs (limit to 2 yolks or less per week)

Lean game (venison, ostrich, buffalo)

Textured vegetable protein (TVP)

Naturally smoked fish

Skinless, free-range white-meat poultry

Grass-fed beef

Protein comes from many sources. While I don't think it's necessary for you to follow a totally vegetarian diet, I do strongly recommend that you emphasize plant sources. While it's true that, unlike animal protein, no single plant protein contains all of the essential amino acids, you'll get adequate complete protein as long as you mix different types of plant proteins (such as legumes and whole grains), throughout the day and week—you don't have to eat them at the same meal.[18]

As you start on your adventure into this new way of eating, you may want to start by replacing meat with vegetarian products that look and taste similar. Try Tofu Pups, BOCA burgers, Gardenburgers, soy or rice cheeses, and so on.

Don't stop there: explore the healthful world of soy products that have been consumed in the East for thousands of years.[19] These are a healthful source of daily protein. Tofu and tempeh can be used in a wide variety of stir-fries and soups. They generally taste better with some seasoning and when combined with a crunchy texture from vegetables or rice. Occasional frying in a very small amount of high-quality oil such as grape seed or sesame can also make these foods quite enjoyable.

Another excellent plant protein source that has sustained vegetarian Buddhist monks for over a millennium is seitan, a meat substitute made from cooked wheat gluten. It resembles meat in taste and texture and can be used in stir-fries or fajitas.

Cookbooks, especially ethnic ones, are full of recipes for beans, from Italian soups and Middle Eastern hummus to Mexican-style burritos and Indian curries. Choosing precooked (canned) beans will save you preparation time, but dried beans are less expensive, are lower in salt, and lack the heavy metals that may leach into canned beans. If you are cooking dried beans yourself, put a 4-inch strip of kombu or alaria (a sea vegetable) in the pot with each cup of dried beans you simmer; that will add vitamins and minerals and may minimize the properties in beans responsible for flatulence. Herbs that counteract gas include parsley, cumin, ginger, fennel, and epazote (use leaves only). I like to pressure-cook my beans for easier digestibility. Don't salt the beans during cooking, because salt toughens the skins; you can add a pinch of sea salt in the last ten minutes.

Since beans can cause gas, introduce them gradually if you are not used to eating them, with ½-cup portions two or three times a week until they do not cause you any distress. (You can also try an enzyme product such as Bean-O, which minimizes gas-producing problems from beans, high-fiber foods, and cruciferous vegetables. Chewing thoroughly helps as well.)[20]

As far as animal sources of protein, I recommend fish as the mainstay to my patients. Prepare it healthfully by baking, steaming, grilling, barbecuing (see recipes on the LOC website), or sautéeing in a small amount of healthy oil. Like lower-fat fish, shellfish contain less omega-3 fats and are recommended for occasional use only. Because shellfish are scavengers, cleanliness is also a concern. As noted above, some fish in the "Occasional Use" category also have elevated mercury levels and should not be overemphasized in your diet.[21]

RECOMMENDATION 4: REPLACE DAIRY PRODUCTS WITH ALTERNATIVES

★ ★ ★ OK for Every Meal

Soy milk	Rice milk
Oat milk	Multigrain beverage
Almond milk	Vegan cheeses, casein-free

★ ★ OK for Daily Use

Soy or rice "Parmesan" cheese	Soy yogurt

★ **OK for Occasional Use**

Soy-based ice cream (fruit-sweetened only)
Rice-based ice cream (sweetened with fruit or brown rice syrup only)
Fruit sorbets and ices (no added sugar)

Casein-containing soy, rice, or almond cheese or yogurt (these products contain small amounts of the milk protein casein, but considerably less than dairy products)

½ ★ **None or Rare**

Low-fat cottage cheese, nonfat or very-low-fat cheeses

Low-fat yogurt or kefir
Pecorino Romano

I use dairy alternatives daily in my meal preparation: a soy beverage in my tea or coffee, multigrain "milk" in my morning muesli cereal, and veggie burgers with rice "cheese." When I'm fortunate enough to enjoy Penny's apple pie or blueberry crisp, I will treat myself to the cold, creamy texture of soy or rice "ice creams"—and yes, with a little time, they came to taste just like the real thing to me. Because these dairy substitutes vary in flavor and texture, I encourage you to try a number of different ones until you find those you are most satisfied with.

WHERE WILL I GET MY CALCIUM?

You need not be worried about getting enough calcium. There are a multitude of nondairy foods that either contain calcium naturally or have been fortified. Adults ages nineteen to fifty should get 1,000 mg of calcium per day; those over fifty need 1,200 mg, and people at high risk of osteoporosis should aim for 1,500 mg. Supplemental calcium can help you reach these levels; I recommend either calcium citrate or calcium carbonate. Here is the calcium content of common foods:[22]

Food Source	Calcium Content (mg)
Nondairy milks such as soy or oat, fortified, I cup	200–350 (check label)
Sardines, canned, drained, with bones, 3 oz	200–325
Collards, boiled, drained, I cup	265
Spinach, boiled, drained, I cup	245–290
Turnip greens, boiled, I cup	195–250
Salmon, canned, 3 oz	180
White beans, canned, I cup	190
Kale, cooked, I cup	95–180
Okra, cooked, I cup	125–175
Soybeans, cooked, I cup	175
Beet greens, cooked, I cup	165
Bok choy (Chinese cabbage), cooked, I cup	160
Tofu, firm and prepared with nigari, 3 oz	130
Navy beans, cooked, I cup	125
Great northern beans, cooked, I cup	120
Kelp (kombu), ⅓ cup (¼ oz)	65
Hijiki, ⅓ cup (¼ oz)	116
Arame, ⅓ cup (¼ oz)	98
Wakame, ⅓ cup (¼ oz)	108
Almonds, hulled, I oz (22 nuts)	75
Brazil nuts, I oz (6 nuts)	45
Sunflower seeds, hulled, I oz	33
Sesame seeds, ground, unhulled, I tbsp	100
Tahini (hulled sesame paste), I tbsp	85

RECOMMENDATION 5:
CHOOSE HEALTHY SWEETS—FRUIT

★ ★ ★ OK for Every Meal

Apples (organic)

Apricots (organic)

Blackberries

Black raspberries

Blueberries

Cantaloupe (organic)

Casaba melon

Cherries (organic)

Cranberries

Honeydew melon

Kiwi fruit

Kumquats

Mango

Papaya

Peaches (organic)

Pears

Plums

Pomegranates

Raisins (organic)

Raspberries

Rhubarb

Strawberries (organic)

Watermelon

★ ★ OK for Daily Use

Applesauce (organic)

Bananas

Dates

Figs

Grapes, red or green (organic)

Nectarines

Oranges

Pineapple

Prunes

Tangerine

Organic 100 percent unsweetened fruit juice (use in small amounts; may raise blood sugar)

Tart cherry

Pomegranate

Purple grape

Apple

Lemon

Light fruit-juice-sweetened spritzers

Organic 100 percent fruit spread (no sugar)

★   OK for Occasional Use

Nonorganic domestic fruit
Grapefruit (caution: grapefruit
and grapefruit juice can affect
drug absorption; also, extensive
use might raise estrogen levels, a
potential problem in estrogen-
sensitive cancers)[27]

Orange juice
Pineapple juice
Prune juice
Unsulfured dried fruits

When selecting fruit, always choose organic whenever you can. Some fruits are especially likely to have pesticide residues;[23] these are indicated in the chart above. If organic is not available, domestically grown fruit is often safer than imported fruit because there are fewer restrictions on chemical use in some other countries.[24] Washing produce well helps reduce some chemical residues.[25] Fresh fruits in season are preferable to more exotic, off-season imports. Remember, fruit does contain natural sugar, so try not to overdo your intake. Fruit-based cooked desserts that are low in fat are a healthful way to enjoy special occasions.

Below is also a list of preferred sweeteners. For example, I advise small amounts of agave syrup, which is high in inulin, to accent the flavor of tea.[26] This natural sweetener does not raise blood sugar as dramatically as white sugar (see the LOC website). Stevia is another natural, non-caloric sweetener.

RECOMMENDATION 5:
CHOOSE HEALTHY SWEETS—SWEETENERS

★ ★ ★   OK for Every Meal

Agave nectar
Stevia (non-caloric)

Lo han (non-caloric)

★ ★ OK for Daily Use

Barley malt	Rice syrup

★ OK for Occasional Use

Pure organic maple syrup	Sugar alcohols (sorbitol, malitol, erythritol)

½ ★ None or Rare

Honey	Molasses

RECOMMENDATION 6:
LIMIT FAT INTAKE AND CHOOSE HEALTHFUL FATS

★ ★ ★ OK for Every Meal

Extra-virgin olive oil (expeller- or
cold-pressed)
Avocado (whole)
Organic tree nuts and tree nut
butters (high in monounsaturated
fats):
    Almonds
    Chestnuts
    Pecans

Walnuts
Ground flaxseed
Organic raw or dry-roasted seeds:
    Pumpkin seeds
    Sesame seeds (unhulled are
    best)
    Squash seeds
    Sunflower seeds

★ ★ OK for Daily Use

Other organic oils (expeller- or cold-pressed):
- Avocado
- Canola
- Flax
- Grape seed
- High-oleic safflower
- High-oleic sunflower
- Peanut
- Rice bran
- Sesame
- Walnut

Other organic tree nuts and tree nut butters:
- Brazil nuts
- Cashews
- Filberts
- Hazelnuts
- Pistachios (not dyed)

Olives—green or black

Peanuts

Tofu mayonnaise (Nayonaise)

Canola mayonnaise (Vegenaise)

Earth Balance Spread or Spectrum Spread

★ OK for Occasional Use

Soy nuts

Organic macadamia nuts

½ ★ None or Rare

Coconut oil (high in saturated fat)

Soybean oil

Organic butter or ghee (preferably unsalted to ensure freshness)

Avoid

Partially hydrogenated fats and oils

Trans fats

Margarine

Lard

Corn oil

Cottonseed oil

Sunflower oil

Palm oil

As I've noted, emphasize omega-3s and omega-9s instead of less healthful fats. But even too much of a high-quality oil can throw off your biochemistry (see page 64). So savor fats and oils and use them sparingly. In this category, I even count high-fat foods such as avocados, nuts, and olives, since it is so important to control your fat intake.

Good-quality oils are very perishable; they go rancid easily. Keep oils, nuts, and seeds refrigerated. If possible, buy oils that are kept in a refrigerated case in the store and that have an expiration date stamped on them. Be sure to check them periodically to ensure they haven't gone out of date. And if an oil is past the use-by date or if it smells "off," discard it immediately.

It is important to note that not all oils can be used for cooking. Some oils have low smoking points; when they are heated to too high a temperature, a chemical change occurs and the oil breaks down and becomes unhealthful. The oils that dietitians at our center recommend for frying, baking, sautéing, and stir-frying are light sesame (not toasted), grape seed, canola, rice bran, and peanut. If available, use canola oil specially processed for cooking at high heat.

Small amounts of oil are used to accent the flavor and texture of food. You can use certain oils in very small amounts (even in drops) to greatly increase the flavor of dishes without impacting your fat grams. For example, toasted sesame oil adds a nutty flavor and complements spicy dishes. Almond and walnut oils add their nutty flavor and complement salads well.

RECOMMENDATION 7:
DRINK ADEQUATE, HEALTHFUL FLUIDS

★ ★ ★ **Important Several Times Daily**
(OK Near but Not During Every Meal)

White tea (contains small amount of caffeine)

Green tea (contains slightly more caffeine than white tea)

Filtered water

Peppermint (can aggravate heartburn in sensitive people)

Other herbal teas (try cooling your favorite variety in the fridge for hot summer days)

Red tea (rooibos)

Genmaicha (Japanese green tea with roasted brown rice; contains small amount of caffeine)

★ ★ **OK for Daily Use**

Black tea (limit to I cup per day; contains caffeine)

100 percent fruit juice, diluted (4 oz unsweetened juice and 4 oz water):

    Tart cherry

    Pomegranate

Purple grape

Apple

Lemon

Caffeine-free natural coffee-like beverages (Cafix, Pero, Teeccino)

Chamomile tea

Kukicha twig tea

★ **OK for Occasional Use**

Decaf coffee (Swiss water-processed)

Coffee

Postum

100% fruit juice, diluted (2 oz juice and 2oz water):

    Pineapple

    Prune

    Orange

½ ★ **None or Rare**

Decaffeinated coffee (processed with chemical solvents)

Tap water

Bottled water (from soft plastic containers)

Ice (from tap water)

Water, after oxygen, is the most essential nutrient; therefore, it is imperative to have safe, contaminant-free water. And since proper hydration of your body is a key to health, you should consume an additional 8 cups of fluids a day above what you cook with, and up to 10 cups if you have no problem with fluid retention, or edema, and are undergoing chemotherapy.

First, know your source. Many communities' water supplies and private wells are contaminated with heavy metals such as lead or arsenic, solvents, pesticides, nitrates and other chemicals, viruses or bacteria, and even traces of pharmaceutical drugs. Even common additives such as chlorine and fluoride have come into question as potential hazards in recent years.

Don't use water from the hot tap for cooking or drinking, since the hot water leaches more contaminants from the pipes. Let water from the tap run for thirty seconds to two minutes first thing in the morning to reduce contaminants and/or lead that leaches from lead-soldered pipes.

I am concerned about not only tap water but also bottled water. The conclusions of a four-year study that examined more than 1,000 bottles of 103 types of bottled water from many parts of the country raise the question of whether bottled water is any better than tap water, or even any different. The researchers found "one brand of 'spring water' whose label pictured a lake and mountains, but actually came from a well in an industrial facility's parking lot, near a hazardous waste dump, and periodically was contaminated with industrial chemicals at levels above FDA standards."[28] The government estimates that at least a quarter of bottled water is tap water and may contain significant contamination. There are also rising concerns with the actual safety of some of the plastic containers that water is stored in: small amounts of the chemical bisphenol-A (BPA), used to create the hard plastic polycarbonate, may leach into foods or beverages stored in polycarbonate containers, especially when the contents are acidic, high in fat, or heated (as when exposed to sunlight). BPA may also leach into some canned foods from can linings. BPA acts as an endocrine disrupter, a substance that mimics natural human hormones such as estrogen.[29]

Since both tap and bottled water are questionable sources, I recommend you consider filtering the water in your home. There are several types of filtration systems. Granular activated carbon or carbon block filters work best when there is a low water flow rate. They are usually rated by the size of the particles they are able to remove from the liquid. Ratings are generally expressed in microns, with 50 microns being the least effective and 0.5 microns the most effective for carbon-type filters.

Reverse osmosis (which produces substantial amounts of wastewater), gravity flow microfiltration units, and water-distilling systems remove the most contaminants—almost everything right down to the smallest molecule. The question that has been raised involves the health-promoting components of water—the minerals and other trace elements—that also may be removed by such systems. While there is no perfect solution, I believe the contaminants are of far more concern. This is why in the powerfoods section on p. 112 I provide recommendations for mineral supplementation to replace the important minerals and other trace elements that may be filtered out. More information on water quality is available on the LOC website.   ⓘ

Making the Transition

On the LOC website you can find a seven-day plan for transi- ⓘ
tioning from a diet heavy in animal foods, sugar, and chemicals to low-fat, plant-based eating. Follow the suggestions day by day and at the end of the week you'll find that you've made a quantum leap from your current diet to a LOC plan.

The Daily Food Quantity Recommendation table on p. 104 contains four calorie levels. If you weigh less than 120 pounds, use the 1,200–1,400 calorie level. If you weigh 120 to 144 pounds, use the 1,500–1,700 calorie level. If you weigh 145 to 189 pounds, use the 1,800–2,000 calorie level. And if you weigh more than 190 pounds, use the 2,400–2,500+ calorie level.

In addition to making the right choices about what you eat, you also need to pay attention to how much you eat. Most of each meal should consist of vegetables, whole grains, and plant-based proteins.

Caloric recommendations for weight loss, weight gain, and specific conditions or treatments are given in Chapter 6. Whatever the total recommended, complex carbohydrates (from whole grains, vegetables, and fruit) should provide about half of your daily calories. About 1½ cups of starchy vegetables or 2 slices of bread can be counted as the equivalent of a cup of cooked grain. At each meal and snack you should consume some grains or starchy vegetables (see list) or 1 or 2 slices of whole-grain bread.

I encourage my patients to eat at least a dozen servings of vegetables and fruits each day (2½–4 cups a day). Yes, twelve! I realize this sounds difficult if not unrealistic, so later I'll explain how you can make this easy by getting several of these servings from concentrated sources such as green drinks, vegetable juice, dehydrated vegetable or fruit powders, and vegetable extracts.

Adequate protein can usually be gotten in two protein-containing meals a day (usually lunch and dinner) plus snacks. However, if you are consuming more than 2,400 calories a day, you may want to consider three protein-containing meals a day. A protein serving consists of approximately ½ cup cooked beans *or* ½ cup soy foods such as tofu or tempeh *or* 2 eggs *or* 4 egg whites *or* 4 ounces of fish (a piece the size of your palm). Be sure to eat a variety of protein foods over the course of a week.

Some foods are fine in reasonable quantities, but too much may contribute to a decline in your condition: I am talking about fats, salt and sodium-containing items such as soy sauce, sweets, and (if you really overdo it) even fruits. Look at these food groups as accents for your meal.

While you do not want to zero out fat, you should consume no more than 2 to 5 teaspoons of oil a day unless you are very active and must eat well over 2,500 calories per day. Include at least 1 teaspoon daily of high-quality (the kind you will find in the refrigerated section of health food stores) cod liver oil (the kind with vitamins A and D removed), which is packed with omega-3s; if you don't like the taste, taking 5 grams of fish oil in capsule form is fine. Fish oil supplements made from fish caught in the northern Arctic Ocean are likely to be the most healthful. They tend to have high levels of the most important omega-3 fatty acids, and no detectable heavy metals, pesticides, or other contaminants. Enterically-coated fish oil supplements contain a special outer layer that prevents the "burpiness" of many fish oil supplements; these may be easier to take. For more information on fish oil and where to find high-quality formulations, see our website.

Fruit contains sugars, so it can satisfy a craving for something sweet. But be careful, since the high sugar content of fruit can make you gain weight and cause your blood sugar to fluctuate. I recommend for most patients no more than 1–3 pieces or five ½-cup servings a day. To further reduce the impact of fruit on blood sugar levels, choose whole fruits over fruit juices or other more processed fruit products, because the fiber in whole fruits helps slow down digestion and keep your blood sugar more stable.[30] If you have fruit juice, limit the amount (about ½ cup counts as a fruit serving) or dilute it with water. Also, spread fruit intake out throughout the day, rather than having a lot at once. If you eat fruit with a meal or snack containing protein or fat, you will digest it more slowly, also tempering the rise in blood sugar levels.

As I've noted, I recommend sweeteners that are less likely to lead to the spikes in blood sugar that refined sugars cause. Agave has a very low glycemic index (discussed in Chapter 18) and has a more concentrated sweet taste than conventional sweeteners, so it is less caloric. Barley malt and rice syrup contain sugars that are absorbed more slowly. However, you should remember that even these sweeteners should be used in limited amounts, especially by people who should lose weight or keep their weight stable, since consistently overdoing even "healthy" sweets and desserts can boost your caloric intake with surprising ease!

DAILY FOOD QUANTITY RECOMMENDATIONS FOR CORE DIET

1,200–1,400 Calories	1,500–1,700 Calories	1,800–2,000 Calories	2,400–2,500+ Calories	Trade-Off Approximations
Whole grains				
2 cups	2½ cups	3 cups	4 cups	I cup cooked grain = I½ cups starchy vegetable = 2 slices bread = I½ cups dry cereal
Vegetables				
2½ cups	3 cups	3½ cups	4 cups	½ cup cooked = 4 oz vegetable juice = I cup raw veg. = 3 cups raw lettuce
Protein				
5½ servings	5½ servings	6 servings	7 servings	I serving = ½ cup cooked legumes = ½ cup tofu or tempeh = 3 oz seitan = 4 oz fish = 4 egg whites or 2 whole eggs
Dairy alternatives, calcium-fortified				
I cup	I½ cups	2 cups	2½ cups	I cup soy, oat, rice, or multigrain low-fat beverage = I oz nondairy cheese

1,200–1,400 Calories	1,500–1,700 Calories	1,800–2,000 Calories	2,400–2,500+ Calories	Trade-Off Approximations
Fruit				
1 serving	1½ servings	2 servings	3 servings	1 serving = 1 piece of fruit = ½ cup fresh or frozen = ¼ cup dried fruit = 4 teaspoons fruit spread = 8 oz diluted juice (½ water and ½ juice)
Fat				
2 tsp	3 tsp	4 tsp	5 tsp	1 teaspoon oil = 1 tablespoon chopped nuts or ground flaxseed = 1½ teaspoons tree nut butter = 1 teaspoon peanut or soy nut butter = ¼ avocado = 6 large olives

See the LOC website for a description of how our food quantity recommendations were calculated; they were developed with the assistance of registered dietitians at the center.

I consider these recommendations to be a core regimen for all adults: patients, family members, and caregivers. For someone who is generally healthy, of course, you can be more relaxed with the guidelines.

However, for cancer patients in the throes of clinical disease, active treatment, or uncontrolled weight loss, it is critical to make sure you get enough food of the right kinds. If you find it difficult to consume the volume of food recommended above you can easily improve your intake by using an appropriate protein-calorie shake. I will detail how to go about this in Chapter 6.

► **At Home**

It is important to enjoy eating, so put in some time and effort to create wholesome and delicious meals. After you cook and eat this way for a few months, planning healthful meals will become a habit—a good habit!

- **Locate a health food store** or health section in your supermarket. Be on the lookout for local farmers' markets where you can purchase high-quality produce, particularly organic. If some of the nonperishable staple food items are hard to find, (i) check the suppliers guide on the LOC website.

- **Stock your natural pantry.** Use the start-up shopping list (i) on the LOC website to get your kitchen up to speed. Have a cupboard-cleaning party to get rid of foods that undermine your health.

- **Learn to use seasonings.** Many spices and herbs have antioxidant properties in addition to making food taste better. You can experiment by buying different individual varieties or preblended seasonings.

(i) • **Purchase appealing cookbooks.** On the LOC website, you will find a list of cookbooks our dietitians at the center find particularly useful. Don't be afraid to try cookbooks that use ½-star foods, since you can substitute ingredients—halibut in place of beef, soy milk in place of milk, or agave or rice syrup in place of sugar or honey.

- **Enlist the support of family members.** Whenever someone changes his or her diet, the rest of the family may experience some stress. Explain why you have chosen to adopt the LOC program. Ask your loved ones for their understanding. Ask them to eat as much of the healing diet as they can, especially when eating with you. This is a powerful expression of love, support, and encouragement. Also ask them not to criticize your dietary choices especially before they have read this book; it does you no good to hear negative comments. Your loved ones want you to get well; tell them this is one way you can do so.

- **If you are feeling ill.** Try to get members of your A-Team to shop or make appropriate meals for you for a few weeks until you feel better. If you are hospitalized, ask them to bring you fresh meals that are in keeping with your diet. Hospital foods rarely follow the LOC guidelines, and they can be so unappealing that it's no surprise 40 percent of hospitalized patients are malnourished.

▶ **Away from Home**

- **At work.** Bring meals from home. In the box below I offer plenty of healthful ideas for meals on the go.

- **At restaurants.** Carry a copy of the food-group lists above, and try to stick to three- or two-star choices, ordering one-star foods only in a pinch. Try to pick restaurants that generally have healthier choices, such as vegetarian, Asian, seafood, natural, and Middle Eastern. When ordering, look for choices such as a veggie burger, grilled fish, vegetable-based soup, pasta with low-fat marinara sauce, steamed vegetables, stir-fried veggies with rice, salads, hummus, or a fruit plate. Request little or no oil, or see if the restaurant can use olive oil. Order small portions, a half portion, or split an entrée with a friend. Eat slowly.

- **Social occasions.** If your host or hostess is planning a meal that resembles the standard American diet rather than the Life Over Cancer diet, you might want to explain your medical situation and ask if you could bring a dish that all could share. Most people are happy to accommodate those who have had to change their eating habits because of medical conditions. Or eat a substantial snack at home and just nibble on healthier items at the party. Instead of alcohol, have water with lemon or, if you prefer, nurse a glass of wine or beer throughout the event.

- **If you slip up.** Don't beat yourself up! Just get back on track and keep going.

Use these quick-start meal and snack ideas to get going.
(i) *There are additional ideas on the LOC website.*

Breakfast Ideas

- Whole-grain bread or toast, bagels, English muffins, French toast, mochi, muffins, pancakes, pita bread, or waffles, with toppings such as:
  - Mock butter/margarine spreads such as Spectrum Spread or olive oil
  - Fresh fruit such as berries or sliced bananas
  - Fruit spread
  - Nut or seed butters such as almond or peanut butter
  - Bean spreads such as hummus
  - Nondairy cream cheese or cheese alternatives
  - Cream cheese alternative with capers and diced onions on a bagel
  - Syrup such as agave or brown rice syrup
  - Vegetables such as sliced tomatoes, onions, garlic, avocado

- Kashi Breakfast Pilaf, cooked whole grains (oatmeal, brown rice, barley, quinoa, grits, etc.), or cold whole-grain cereals (muesli, Barbara's O's, shredded wheat), with toppings such as:
  - Milk alternative such as soy, oat, rice, or almond
  - Fruit, fresh or dried
  - Nuts or seeds
  - Spices such as cinnamon or cardamom
  - Sweetener such as stevia or agave syrup

- Eggs and egg dishes (made from omega-3 eggs if you use yolks) such as an omelet with peppers, onions, and tomatoes
- Scrambled tofu with seasonings and vegetables
- Energy bars such as Multigrain Cereal Bars by Nature's Choice (good for when you are on the go)
- Fresh fruit
- Healthy leftovers from other meals

Soup Ideas

- Split pea
- Lentil
- Black bean
- Vegetable
- Miso
- French onion with herbed croutons
- Corn chowder
- Vegetarian chili
- Butternut squash
- Sweet potato
- Creamy asparagus

Salad Ideas

- Fresh mixed greens
- Blanched vegetables
- Coleslaw
- Carrot-daikon
- Tossed green salad with chickpeas and fresh vegetables
- Tabouli (bulgur salad)
- Fruit salad
- Italian quinoa salad
- Grilled tuna salad

Sandwich Ideas

- Broiled fish
- Tuna salad made with a canola oil or vegan-based mayonnaise
- Toasted soy cheese
- Grilled vegetables with hummus
- Almond butter or peanut butter and fruit spread
- Tempeh Reuben
- Falafel in pita with tahini
- Millet-chickpea patties
- Tofurkey slices
- Soy-based deli-style slices
- Roasted tempeh and grilled vegetable sub
- Veggie burger on whole-grain bun

Entrée Ideas

- Grilled tuna salad
- Grilled, baked, oven-poached, or steamed cold-water fish
- Sweet-and-sour salmon with peapods
- Couscous with vegetables and seitan
- Udon noodles with carrot-basil sauce
- Veggie pizza with soy cheese
- Bean burrito with salsa and guacamole
- Stir-fried rice, vegetables, and tofu
- Vegetarian egg rolls
- Enchilada with black beans
- Pasta with broccoli and sun-dried tomatoes
- Lentil-stuffed cabbage rolls
- Gingered salmon steaks
- Pasta or rice with peanut sauce
- Vegetable lasagna
- Buckwheat noodle stir-fry
- Seitan potpie
- Vegetable fajitas
- Wild rice pilaf with vegetables
- Tofu fettuccini
- Seitan Stroganoff on pasta
- Whole-wheat pasta marinara

Snack Ideas

- Whole-wheat crackers
- Almonds or soy nuts
- Whole-grain pretzels
- Rice cakes with fruit spread
- Whole-grain bagel chips (low-fat or fat-free)
- Low-fat whole-grain muffins
- Hummus with raw vegetables
- Popcorn (air-popped or Bearitos)
- Soy Delicious (nondairy frozen dessert)
- Barbara's cereal bars
- Black bean dip with baked tortilla chips
- Raw veggies and tempeh dip
- Low-fat cookies (no sugar)
- Baba ghanoush (eggplant/tahini spread) with pita bread
- Applesauce with cinnamon
- Quesadillas with soy cheese
- Sunflower or pumpkin seeds

To get you started, let me offer a sample 1,800- to 2,000-calorie one-day meal plan; you can find others on the LOC website, along with recipes.

Breakfast	Lunch	Snack #1	Dinner	Snack #2
Grains				
½ cup oatmeal or 1 slice whole grain toast	1 cup brown rice	¼ pita bread, toasted	1 cup quinoa or wild rice	
Veggies				
Omelet: ¼ cup spinach ¼ cup shiitake mushrooms	1½ cups tossed salad with romaine lettuce and ½ cup sliced veggies	½ cup fresh carrot sticks	1 cup steamed broccoli	
Protein				
Omelet: 4 egg whites or 2 egg whites and 1 whole egg	1 cup lentil soup or 1 cup 3-bean chili	⅓ cup lowfat hummus or other bean dip	4 oz roasted salmon with garlic and shoyu	
Fruit				
2 teaspoons fruit spread	2 teaspoons dried tart cherries on salad			½ cup mixed berries
Fat				
1 teaspoon olive oil	1 tablespoon vinaigrette dressing (⅓ oil, ⅔ vinegar)		1 teaspoon olive oil	1 tablespoon chopped walnuts
Dairy Alternatives				
1 oz nondairy cheese				½ cup nondairy frozen dessert

If you adopt the meal recommendations above, you will be well on your way toward depriving your cancer of the nutrients that it needs. The next step is to emphasize your intake of the "Healthy Dozen" powerfoods. These are (mostly) plant foods that contain powerful anti-cancer compounds that I consider essential to your recovery. We advise our patients to get as many of them as possible, but at least one choice from each of the healthy dozen every day.

Since it can be a challenge to get all these anti-cancer compounds from food alone, you may find it easiest to get half or more of your powerfoods in concentrates, mixtures of concentrated juices, or extracts of these foods. To do this, I recommend that you find an organic powerfood concentrate (often called a "green drink") that you enjoy and make it a part of your diet. These "green drinks" are widely available in health food stores. Some cancer patients do make their own vegetable juices, but it is hard to get the diversity of foods you need at home. At the LOC website, you can find mail-order and online sources for a variety of powerfood concentrates that we feel are of high quality.

Here are the Healthy Dozen:

1. **Carotenoids** are red, yellow, and orange plant pigments such as those in carrots, tomatoes, pumpkin, and winter squash. Carotenoids have important anti-cancer properties. For instance, lycopene, which makes tomatoes red, has the ability to inhibit the cancer-promoting growth factor IGF-1.[31] In addition to eating whole foods containing carotenoids, the center recommends the freeze-dried juice of the carotenoid vegetables, which gives you the equivalent of several servings in one glass.[32]

2. **Cruciferous vegetables** are rich in glucosinolates, a veritable treasure trove of anti-cancer compounds. These vegetables include cabbage, broccoli, brussels sprouts, collards, and kale. Among the glucosinolates are indole-3-carbinol, which increases

the activity of enzymes that make estrogen less effective, thereby blocking the growth and progression of hormone-responsive cancers of the breast and endometrium.[33,34] The sulforaphane in broccoli also targets breast cancer: at least six studies have demonstrated that women with breast cancer who consume high amounts of sulforaphane-containing vegetables have significantly better survival rates, lower recurrence rates, or both.[35] Since cooking glucosinolates breaks them down, I recommend eating them raw whenever possible or, even easier, taking them in powerfood extracts. By taking extracts that concentrate the phytochemicals of cruciferous vegetables, you can get the equivalent of several servings in one drink.

3. **Allium family** vegetables are rich in organosulfides such as allicin, which help the body remove toxic compounds, including carcinogens,[36] enhance immune function,[37] reduce blood clotting,[38] and lower blood pressure.[39] They include fresh garlic, high-allicin garlic supplement, aged or pickled garlic, onions, leeks, scallions, and chives. To increase the activity of the organosulfides in fresh garlic, crush the cloves and let them sit for ten minutes before using.

4. **Roots and rhizomes** concentrate many biologically active phytochemicals that squelch free radicals and reduce the body's inflammatory cascade. They include ginger, turmeric,[40] burdock, beetroot, daikon, and Spanish black radish.

5. **Leafy greens** are nutritional powerhouses, containing compounds that have strong antioxidant activity.[41] Good sources are parsley leaf, watercress, dandelion greens, chard, and turnip or beet greens.

6. **Fruits** are rich in flavonoids that can enhance the efficacy of chemotherapy. The ellagic acid in raspberry, cranberry, pomegranate, and strawberry extracts, for instance, has been shown to

act synergistically with chemotherapy for advanced prostate cancer: a 2005 study found statistically better treatment responses and less treatment-related toxicity for patients receiving ellagic acid along with chemotherapy than for those undergoing chemotherapy alone.[42] While more research is needed on the clinical application of this finding, one explanation for the improved response is that ellagic acid inhibits NF-kappa-B, a molecule that fuels malignant growth and allows cancer cells to resist chemotherapy drugs.[43] Ellagic acid has also been shown to trigger apoptosis in many types of cancer cells and to curb tumors of the lung, liver, skin, and esophagus in the lab.[44] Good sources of flavonoids include blueberries, raspberries, strawberries, cranberries, pomegranates, tart cherries, apples and apple skins, and Concord grapes.[45]

7. **Sprouted seeds and cereal grasses** contain powerful compounds including antioxidants, a number of enzymes, and chlorophyll.[46] It is often easier to obtain these compounds in the form of juices. Excellent choices are broccoli sprouts, alfalfa sprouts, kale sprouts, sunflower seed greens, wheatgrass juice, barley grass juice, oat grass juice, cabbage sprouts, and cauliflower sprouts. Broccoli sprouts are particularly important as a source of the cancer-inhibiting phytochemical sulphoraphane.

8. **Medicinal mushrooms** contain compounds that can enhance the effectiveness of chemo while reducing side effects such as nausea, vomiting, and loss of appetite, as well as suppress metastasis and increase levels of natural killer cells.[47] One type of mushroom compounds, beta-glucans, has been shown to boost the cancer-fighting powers of the immune system's cytotoxic T cells.[48] Again, it is difficult to obtain clinically meaningful quantities of the mushroom phytochemicals from even the healthiest diet, which is why I recommend getting them in the form of extracts. Look for those containing maitake (*Grifola frondosa*), agaricus (*Agaricus blazei*), shiitake (*Lentinula* [or *Lentinus*] *edodes*), reishi (*Ganoderma lucidum*), turkey tails (*Trametes* [or *Coriolus*] *versicolor*), and caterpillar fungus or cordyceps (*Cordyceps sinensis*).

9. **Probiotics and prebiotics.** Probiotics are a live form of "good bacteria" in your intestinal tract that produce natural antibiotics to keep the "bad" or pathogenic bugs in check, thus preventing diarrhea and infections. They also bolster digestion and produce some B vitamins in the small intestine, where they can be absorbed.[49] Some may improve your quality of life during cancer treatment and recovery by fortifying the immune system and preventing urinary tract infections and inflammatory bowel disease.[50] Some probiotics even reduce the growth of colon tumors and bladder cancer: randomized trials showed significant reductions in colon cancer biomarkers and in bladder cancer recurrences in patients given probiotics.[51] Prebiotics are the foods that encourage and sustain the growth of these bacteria. You can buy these supplements in the refrigerator section of health food stores. Look for acidophilus powder that contains *Lactobacillus bifidus, L. plantarum, L. casei, L. delbreuckii,* or *L. bulgaricus.*

10. **Essential fatty acids.** In the section on fats I explained the need to balance omega-6 and omega-3 fatty acids. You can do this by cutting down on omega-6s (in corn oil, soybean oil, safflower oil, and baked goods), which I definitely recommend. You can also balance these fats by eating fatty fish a few times a week. But since even eating fish every day will not likely allow you to reach ratios of 1:1 or 1:2 omega-6s to omega-3s, a better strategy is to use supplements, either as fish oil capsules or in specially formulated foods. Fish oil contains both eicosapentaenoic acid (EPA) and docosahexaenoic acid (DHA), both of which have anti-cancer activity. I recommend fish oil that is molecularly distilled to remove heavy metals and as much omega-6 fatty acids as possible, while concentrating the omega-3s; the one I use has a high (over 10:1) ratio of omega-3s to omega-6s. Since the source, the freshness, the level of contaminants, and the method of processing are all extremely important, choose your fish oil carefully from the list on the LOC (i) website. We recommend oil from fish caught in the Arctic Circle and processed under low-oxygen conditions. There are also plant forms of omega-3s. While fish oil is generally a more potent anti-inflammatory, the plant omega-3s can also be useful.

Black currant oil contains gamma-linolenic acid (GLA),[52] and ground flaxseeds contain alpha-linolenic acid (ALA),[53] both of which can help reduce inflammation and thus make your internal biochemistry more hostile to cancer cells.[54]

11. Sea vegetables and algae are an excellent source of minerals,[55] amino acids, and cancer-fighting phytochemicals. Fucoidan, for instance, found in kombu and other seaweeds, can inhibit tumor growth, angiogenesis, and metastasis.[56] Seaweed phytochemicals can boost the activity and the number of important cancer-fighting immune cells called T-cells and natural killer (NK) cells.[57] It is important to pick sea vegetables from a reputable source that grows them in clear, clean waters, since they can soak up heavy metals.[58] Good choices are chlorella, spirulina, kelp granules or powder, dulse, and mekabu.

12. Vitamins, minerals, and other cofactors. While healthy people, or those in long-term remission, may be able to do without vitamin and mineral supplements if they eat right, those with more advanced cancers or those who are undergoing chemotherapy or other cancer treatments need a basic vitamin-mineral supplement. It is important to take one that has been specifically designed for cancer patients, who have unique needs and concerns. For instance, high-dose vitamin B_{12} may fuel the progression of some cancers, such as prostate cancer.[59] Some cancer cells have been shown to overexpress the receptor for vitamin B_{12}, so excess in the bloodstream can accelerate the growth of some cancers. Also, some cancers have receptors for vitamin B_1 or folate, which some chemotherapy drugs target.[60] That is why it is important to follow the recommendations below, into which I have built the cautions I have gleaned from the scientific literature over the years. If you receive one of these antifolate chemo drugs, your doctor will give you specific instructions about supplementing with B vitamins and folate to prevent adverse side effects. For similar reasons, as long as a deficiency does not occur, take little or no iron or copper in supplements: iron has strong oxidizing properties (which can promote cancer growth),[61] and copper promotes angiogenesis,[62] which feeds metastatic tumors.

Don't worry, since you should generally get adequate amounts from your diet. To obtain sufficient quantities of such important health-promoting nutrients as vitamin D, vitamin E, zinc, selenium, and magnesium, I recommend either concentrated food sources or a formula that includes the following nutrients:

Vitamins

- 2,000–4,000 mg vitamin C

- 3 mg vitamin B_1

- 20 mg vitamin B_2

- 100 mg vitamin B_3

- 100 mg vitamin B_5

- 20 mg vitamin B_6

- 150 mcg vitamin B_9 (folate)

- 20 mcg vitamin B_{12}

- 25,000 IU vitamin A (naturally occurring form, from cod liver oil; if you have liver dysfunction, stay under 10,000 IU)

- 1,000 IU vitamin D (naturally occurring form, from cod liver oil)

- 1,000 mg vitamin E (the naturally occurring family of mixed tocopherols standardized with 400 IU of alpha-tocopherol)

- 250 mg ascorbyl palmitate (fat-soluble form of vitamin C)

Bioavailable Minerals
(amounts reflect the elemental mineral content)

- 1,000 mg (for men)/1,500 mg (for women) calcium ascorbate

- 400 mg magnesium ascorbate or glycinate

- 75 mg zinc ascorbate or glycinate (if you have prostate cancer, take only 10 mg)

- 400 mcg selenium (selenomethionine)

- 100–200 mcg chromium picolinate

- 150 mcg iodine

- 1–2 mg manganese

- 75 mcg molybdenum

- 1–3 mg boron

- 100–200 mcg vanadium

I hope you will come to view diet as an integral part of your healing toolbox. The information in this chapter will help you get started modifying your diet in a way that eliminates foods that feed cancer and includes those that slow the growth and spread of tumors, act synergistically with chemotherapy drugs, and reduce chemo's side effects. Now let's turn to some situations in which you'll want to modify the basic Life Over Cancer diet.

CHAPTER 6

INDIVIDUALIZING YOUR DIET

There are some situations in which you will need to deviate from the Life Over Cancer core diet in terms of caloric intake, supplement use, or other details. These include cachexia, certain treatment situations or side effects, and remission. In this chapter I'll help you identify whether you would benefit from modifications to the core diet and how to use diet to manage the side effects of treatment.

Steve: Too Late to Benefit

Steve Rogers was diagnosed at age forty-nine with pancreatic cancer and liver metastasis. Several oncologists had told Steve that his prognosis was poor and his options were limited. After considerable thought, Steve opted against conventional treatment and instead began searching for alternative therapies. After learning of some pancreatic cancer patients who had fared well on a macrobiotic diet, he decided to try it himself. Soon after, he learned about our center and how I had made modifications to the macrobiotic diet to make it more medically and nutritionally sound for patients with cancer.

Steve came for his first visit in 2003. He told me he had followed a typical American diet most of his life, often indulging in pastries and ice cream. But on the diet he had adopted, a typical day's total intake looked like this: oatmeal with skim milk, a half turkey sandwich on sourdough wheat bread, seitan with steamed vegetables and brown rice, a few peanuts, an apple, wheat crackers, green tea, and water. After totaling his food intake, I found myself alarmed at the dangerously low level of calories and protein he was getting. Pancreatic cancer can cause rapid weight loss, making a diet higher in protein and calories from healthful foods (not sugar and unhealthful fats) a must.

Steve was already lean, carrying 180 pounds on his six-foot frame. Soon after his first visit, he told me he had decided to go on a strict macrobiotic diet to better combat his cancer. In spite of my pleas that he maintain a more balanced nutritional program, which would supply him with the protein and calories he needed, he started an overly rigid regimen in the hope of starving his disease. This is an all-too-common mind-set in the world of alternative medicine. Over the next five months, Steve lost fifty pounds, mostly muscle. Along with the continual weight loss came marked fatigue and weakness so severe he was no longer able to climb stairs. Soon his weight was down to 112 pounds— and his disease kept progressing.

At this point, along with the help of his wife, Steve finally allowed me to adjust his diet. I upped his calorie intake and advised him to consume more fish, eggs, soy, legumes, and other high-protein foods. In the first week, Steve gained eight pounds and experienced an immediate surge in energy. He could once again perform most of the normal activities of daily living. Steve was now willing to consider tumor-killing treatments, but he was still too weak and nutritionally depleted to receive treatments. Had he embraced a sounder nutritional plan sooner, we might have been able to get him to a point where he was strong enough to be treated. Instead, without more aggressive therapies, his disease progressed rapidly, and he passed away shortly afterward.

As Steve's tragic story shows, proper nutrition is critical for cancer patients with cachexia, the involuntary weight loss that is accompanied by muscle wasting, fatigue, impaired immune function, and diminished physical and mental function. Steve had what could be called a "catabolic cancer," one that is prone to catabolize (break down) normal tissue. Catabolic cancers include lung cancer and cancers of the gastrointestinal system, including the pancreas. Cachexia, in which people sometimes experience an unwanted loss of five to ten pounds in a month, has long been recognized as a hallmark of advanced cancer, and nutritional solutions for it have been sought by both alternative and conventional medical practitioners. But the approaches of these two groups can differ radically. A number of alternative practitioners, as in Steve's case, misguidedly take aim at the cancer and try to "starve the tumor" by denying it the calories it needs, but this denies the rest of the body the calories needed for normal functioning while doing little to eliminate the tumor (caloric restriction alone has little to no effect on a malignant tumor). Most mainstream oncologists, after doing what they can to eradicate the tumor, advise the cachectic patient to eat as many calories as possible, whatever the source, including and even emphasizing saturated and omega-6 fats, sugar, and red meat in the form of milk shakes, mayonnaise, margarine, ice cream, and supplement drinks based on milk products, sugar, and omega-6 fats.

Both approaches miss what has turned out to be the underlying cause of cachexia: out-of-control inflammation caused by substances secreted by the tumor and imbalances in the patient's internal environment. To help address cachexia in a scientifically sound way, the LOC program offers what I call **High-Intensity Nutritional Support.** It is much higher in calories than the core diet described in Chapter 5. Because you may be shedding five to ten pounds a month, you need to stabilize and reverse this loss. High-Intensity Nutritional Support also contains foods from the core diet that, based on laboratory studies, should help control the underlying inflammation.

Cachexia is not the only situation in which you may need more calories. During cancer treatment, even if you are not losing weight to cachexia, your body will be under extra nutritional stress, and both your caloric and your protein needs may be higher. Nutritionists have long recognized that during times of physical stress (and chemotherapy, radiation, and surgery certainly count as stress), the body's need for energy and protein increases. Protein is especially crucial, since during cancer treatment you are likely to experience tissue breakdown and stress on both your immune system and your liver's chemical detoxification system; all of these can be stabilized and reversed by boosting your protein consumption. And since chemo and radiation can kill your appetite and cause nausea and vomiting, you are at risk of undernutrition while undergoing treatment. For our patients with these problems, I formulated the **Treatment Support** diet, in which protein and calories are increased, but not quite as much as in the High-Intensity Nutritional Support diet for patients with cachexia.

I also recommend the Treatment Support diet for patients with advanced cancers whose levels of blood proteins, especially albumin, are mildly low, between 3.1 and 3.5 g/dL, which is correlated with an increased risk of mortality.[1] (Patients with moderately low albumin, 2.6 to 3.0 g/dL, would fare better with the High-Intensity Nutritional Support diet, whereas levels under 2.6 g/dL should be treated as a marked decline and require immediate and aggressive intervention.) Although this problem can often be remedied, many patients' malnutrition goes unrecognized, and most hospitals don't even try.[2] As a result, malnutrition worsens, leading to a severely depressed immune system with runaway cancer and infections. You should feel comfortable monitoring your own levels and regularly asking your doctor if your levels of albumin or blood protein are dropping. If you are also experiencing weight loss or muscle wasting, I recommend the High-Intensity Nutritional Support diet.

Breast cancer patients undergoing treatment, though, should be cautious about using the Treatment Support diet. If you are receiving chemotherapy for the first time, either right before surgery (neoadjuvant) or after surgery (adjuvant), and especially if you are overweight, you may want to increase your protein consumption but not your caloric intake. Because your metabolic rate may actually fall during chemotherapy, and because you may not be keeping up your usual fitness program, you may well gain weight during chemo.[3] That can increase your chances for recurrence or worsen your prognosis. If, however, your doctor feels you are experiencing mildly abnormal weight loss, or you have metastatic breast cancer and are on at least your second round of chemo, you should consider the Treatment Support diet. More serious weight and muscle loss would still warrant the High-Intensity Nutritional Support diet.

There are also special **Symptom Management Tips** for when you suffer the side effects of cancer treatment, such as nausea and vomiting, constipation, diarrhea, mouth sores, and appetite loss. And finally, I provide a **Remission Support** diet for when your goal is to keep your cancer from returning; think of it as a supercharged cancer prevention diet. Especially during the first years of remission, your dietary needs are markedly different from when you are undergoing treatment. This Remission Support diet is centered on avoiding weight gain and also on including foods strongly associated with cancer prevention, since a major aim during this period is to prevent a few stray cancer cells from ganging up on you and becoming an active tumor.

Gladys: Diet Made the Difference

When Gladys was diagnosed with inoperable metastatic pancreatic cancer in June 1993, she was treated at a clinic at the M. D. Anderson Cancer Center in Houston with intensive chemotherapy and radiation for six and a half weeks. But the treatments did not eradicate her cancer, and her doctors said there was nothing more that could be done. Her cancer and the treatment had caused Gladys to lose a tremendous amount of weight. Malnourished and weak, she was told she had four to six weeks to live. A short while later, after her son saw me interviewed on television, Gladys came to our Evanston clinic in February 1994.

At the center, our dietitians started her on the High-Intensity Nutritional Support diet to aggressively treat her malnutrition and weight loss, since she faced a real risk of dying of malnutrition or infection (uncontrolled weight loss can suppress the immune system). Gladys soon began to feel stronger and move around more. Now that she no longer faced life-threatening malnutrition, we shifted her onto the core diet in the last chapter as part of a full integrative program. By November 1994, Gladys' scans showed no tumor. As I write, she remains alive and well and, since she is more than a decade past her initial diagnosis, is now able to relax the core diet and sprinkle it with a few more one-star "celebration" foods.

Use the table below to determine whether you need the High-Intensity Nutritional Support diet, the Treatment Support diet, a diet tailored to treatment side effects, or the Remission Support diet. If you have any questions or concerns, I strongly encourage you to get a phone or face-to-face consultation with a dietitian from our center or one with experience working with patients utilizing an integrative cancer treatment approach.

WHAT SPECIAL DIET DO YOU NEED?

Condition	Diet
Cachexia/muscle wasting/weight loss. If you are not trying to lose weight yet are still dropping more than two pounds in one week or five pounds in one month, or if you have an albumin level under 3.0 g/dL consult your physician, an integrative cancer specialist, or an integratively minded dietitian.	**High-Intensity Nutritional Support**

Depleted albumin. If you have advanced cancer or are going through chemotherapy, ask for your most recent total protein and albumin levels. If these have not been measured, ask that they be ordered at the next blood draw. If your serum albumin level has dropped below 3.6 g/dL (but is not below 3.0), seek expert medical and nutritional consultation immediately.	**Treatment Support**
Catabolic cancer. If your weight is stable but you have pancreatic, ovarian, stomach, colon, or lung cancer, your goal is to maintain muscle mass, especially during conventional treatment. (With excessive or rapid weight loss, or muscle weakness, consider the High-Intensity Nutritional Support approach.) If you are overweight, you may lose some weight initially with this plan.	**Treatment Support**
Cancer treatment. If you are undergoing rigorous treatment to shrink your tumor, having difficulty tolerating treatment and have difficulty maintaining weight, or have long periods of diminished appetite, shifting from the core diet to the Treatment Support diet may be enough. (With a further decline in weight, appetite, and albumin, the High-Intensity Nutritional Support diet may be needed.) Exceptions are patients with minimal weight loss who are receiving hormonal blockers for breast cancer, hormonal therapies for prostate cancer, other medications that are given for prolonged periods, or breast cancer patients receiving chemo for the first time: you can stick to the core diet, but watch your appetite and weight.[4] (See page 104.)	**Treatment Support**

Treatment side effects. Among the side effects that can be ameliorated through diet are reduced appetite, nausea and vomiting, diarrhea, constipation, taste changes or loss, sore mouth or throat, dry mouth, and thick saliva.	**Symptom Management Tips**
Remission. If you have been in complete remission for at least a year and are not undergoing major treatment (that is, have been off conventional therapy for six to twelve months), your goal is to develop a lifelong healthful eating style that is realistic for you.	**Remission Support**

High-Intensity Nutritional Support for Cachexia

If you have struggled with being overweight, cancer-related weight loss may seem like a positive thing, especially since in some cancers being overweight is associated with a worse prognosis. But unintentional, uncontrolled weight loss can quickly turn into a nightmare as muscles waste away and the immune system falters, raising the risk of life-threatening infections. The more malnourished the patient, the more suppressed the immune system (in particular, the more depressed natural killer cell and interleukin-2 activity), resulting in heightened susceptibility to metastases, too.[5] Rapid weight loss alone is an independent risk factor for poor survival in people with cancer.[6] In general, the more rapid the weight loss, the worse the prognosis.

With the exception of AIDS patients, cancer patients have the highest prevalence of malnutrition of any hospitalized group, approximately 30 to 50 percent.[7] Worse, nearly half of all patients suffering from advanced-stage cancers die from malnutrition-related complications.[8] No wonder, then, that most doctors respond to cachexia out of a visceral sense of desperation. Loading up the patient with calories, no matter what their source, seems the only option. But calorie-loading diets by themselves do not control cachexia. This is because cachexia is not the result of a rapidly growing tumor with a high metabolic rate sucking calories from the rest of the body, as doctors used to think. Instead, it results from high levels of inflammatory biochemicals (cytokines) that are secreted by cancer cells and synthesized by other processes in the body.[9] These processes are part of the body's defense against the tumor (which is one reason cachexia may subside when a tumor shrinks or is eradicated). To combat cachexia, then, you need to lower the production of these inflammatory biochemicals. Although diet alone will rarely accomplish this (hence the role of the medical treatment, as well as fitness, mind-spirit, and supplement regimens aimed at reducing inflammation, as I'll discuss in the next sections), it can help. Most important, you need to stay away from foods that encourage the production of more inflammatory biochemicals.

The High-Intensity Nutritional Support diet therefore serves two purposes. Most important, it reduces inflammatory molecules through a high intake of omega-3 fats and antioxidants and avoidance of inflammatory omega-6s and simple sugars.[10] In addition, it emphasizes healthful calories, supplements, and medications to rein in the inflammatory process, including polyphenols such as those found in tea, olive oil, and pomegranates. When needed, it also includes appetite-stimulating drugs.[11] Chapter 15 will explore in more detail what you can do to combat inflammation, but the anti-inflammatory High-Intensity Nutritional Support diet is something you can start on right away.

To build up your muscles and make up for the lost weight, your diet will need to be high in protein (about as high as athletes in training get) and calories. But the source of calories is crucial. Although you should stick to foods in the core diet, as listed in the previous chapter, you may eat more one-star foods, since the two- and three-stars are less dense sources of protein and calories. In particular, the High-Intensity Nutritional Support diet includes more dried fruits, whole eggs, oils, seeds, and nuts and more liberal use of animal foods such as fattier fish, organic chicken breasts, and the like. This is far more than

I recommend for someone in remission who is following the core diet. However, the core diet's advice about fat quality holds for the High-Intensity Nutritional Support diet as well: you need to avoid pro-inflammatory fats such as saturated fats and omega-6s and instead consume more omega-3s and omega-9s.

To get going with the High-Intensity Nutritional Support diet, first find your caloric requirement in the table below.

CALORIC RECOMMENDATIONS FOR CACHEXIA

| Height | | Estimated Daily Requirements |
Women	Men	Calories
Up to 5'3"	Up to 5'1"	1,800–2,000
5'3" up to 5'8"	5'1" up to 5'5"	2,100–2,300
5'8" up to 6'1"	5'5" up to 5'10"	2,400–2,600
Over 6'1"	Over 5'10"	2600+

If you are in the middle of two height ranges, aim for the lower calorie level; if you are at the lower end of the height range, or the higher level if you are at the upper end. Similarly, if you have a small frame, you should eat somewhat less than the recommended calories, whereas if you have a large frame, you should eat somewhat more. For a quick estimate of your frame size, wrap your left middle finger and thumb around your right wrist. If your finger and thumb don't meet, you have a large frame. If they just meet, you have a medium frame. If they overlap, you have a small frame. If you are in the 2,600+ calorie level, and if your appetite allows or demands, you may add one or two more servings to each food category listed in the table below for the first five inches over 6'1" (women) or 5'10" (men), and an additional one or two servings if more than five inches over.

Now use the table to find the corresponding number of daily

food servings for each calorie level for grains, vegetables, fruits, and other foods. Notice that protein servings in this diet are supplemented with protein powders. Whey, soy, egg white, and rice protein supplements are widely available; they are an easy and healthful way to boost protein intake. Protein powders can also be used in the meal replacement shake described on page 131. Be sure to eat a variety of proteins each day, especially if you use rice protein powder, which is an incomplete protein.

DAILY QUANTITY OF FOOD RECOMMENDED FOR HIGH-INTENSITY NUTRITIONAL SUPPORT

1,800–2,000 Calories	2,100–2,300 Calories	2,400–2,600 Calories	2,600+ Calories	Trade-Off Approximations
Whole Grains				
2½ cups	2½ cups	3 cups	3½ cups	1 cup cooked grain = 1½ cups starchy vegetable = 2 slices bread = 1½ cups dry cereal
Vegetables				
3 cups	3½ cups	4 cups	4 cups	½ cup cooked = 4 oz vegetable juice = 1 cup raw veg. = 3 cups raw lettuce
Protein				
5 servings + 3 tbsp protein powder	5½ servings + 3 tbsp protein powder	6 servings + 6 tbsp protein powder	6½ servings + 6 tbsp protein powder	1 serving = ½ cup cooked legumes = ½ cup tofu or tempeh = 3 oz seitan = 4 oz fish = 4 egg whites or 2 whole eggs

1,800–2,000 Calories	2,100–2,300 Calories	2,400–2,600 Calories	2,600+ Calories	Trade-Off Approximations
Dairy Alternatives, soy, calcium-fortified*				
2 cups	2½ cups	3 cups	3 cups	I cup soy, oat, rice, or multigrain low-fat beverage = I oz nondairy cheese
Fruit				
2 servings	2 servings	3 servings	4 servings	I serving equals: I piece of fruit = ½ cup fresh or frozen = ¼ cup dried = 4 teaspoons fruit spread = 8 oz diluted juice (½ water and ½ juice)
Fat				
5 tsp	6 tsp	7 tsp	8 tsp	I teaspoon oil = I tablespoon chopped nuts or ground flax = I½ teaspoon tree nut butter = I teaspoon peanut or soy nut butter = ¼ avocado = 6 large olives

*Note: these beverages can be used to make meal replacement shakes that can help you consume the correct volume of food for the day.

If you think the diet above asks you to eat a lot, you're right. In fact, it may be more than you feel up to. In this case, our dietitians at the center would recommend a protein-calorie supplement in the form of a homemade "shake" drink to reduce the volume of food you need to eat. Unlike most commercial nutritional supplements ("enterals") recommended to cachectic patients, which are high in sugar, unhealthful fats, and growth-promoting dairy proteins, the formula we give our patients has a very different composition. It includes high-quality protein, a low-glycemic-index sweetener, and easily absorbed fats that are high in omega-3s. The ingredients can be purchased at health food stores.

LIFE OVER CANCER MEAL REPLACEMENT SHAKE

Yield: I shake

1½ cups rice, soy, or oat beverage

6 tbsp protein powder (cold-processed whey, egg white powder, or soy protein isolate; breast cancer patients may choose to substitute more whey)[12]

2 g chlorella, or to taste (optional)

2 g free-form USP L-glutamine (optional; if omitted, take in a capsule)

2 g L-leucine (optional; if omitted, take in a capsule)

6 g medium-chain triglyceride oil[13] (if you use the shakes for an extended period, you can substitute almond or hazelnut oil)

8–12 grams high-quality, high-potency fish oil (optional; this can be taken as fish oil capsules instead)

I small banana

I tbsp agave

Combine all ingredients in a blender and blend well. Chill.

The formula counts as 3 servings protein, 2 cups grain, 2 servings fruit, 1½ cups dairy alternative, and 2 tsp. fat (for 580 calories). Replacing each of two meals with this shake will provide up to half of your daily calorie needs. See the LOC website for other shake recipes. If you are allergic to one type of protein powder, substitute another that you can tolerate. (i)

If you need to build or maintain muscle and albumin, I recommend eating egg whites, Egg Beaters, and cold-water fish, and including protein shakes for most of your daily protein, in order to keep the volume of food you need to eat tolerable. Supplementing with various probiotics such as those containing

Lactobacillus bacteria, available at health food stores, can improve digestion and increase absorption. Also add prebiotics, which can also be purchased at health food stores, and encourage and sustain the growth of these probiotic bacteria. We include herbal adaptogens such as schisandra and ashwaganda in the formulations we use with our patients in the clinic, since these may help the body deal with stress; you can find them at health food stores.[14]

Although the High-Intensity Nutritional Support diet is appropriate for patients suffering from weight loss for any reason, you can modify it depending on your situation. If your unintentional weight loss is due to cachexia (a doctor or dietitian should be able to determine this through a clinical workup and laboratory testing), you can consume more fat servings than recommended above.

Our dietitians are available for professional consultations if you have a significant problem, or you may look on our website to find other integrative physicians and registered dietitians.

The Treatment Support Diet

The Treatment Support diet is appropriate if you have no weight issue or unexplained weight loss but have mildly low serum albumin, are dealing with a catabolic cancer but have not yet experienced weight loss, or are undergoing treatments such as radiation, surgery, or chemotherapy (not hormonal therapy for breast or prostate cancer). These cases necessitate more protein and slightly more calories than the core diet provides for your body weight and size but less than the High-Intensity Nutritional Support diet. Comparing it to the core diet volume in the last chapter, you will notice that I have increased the volume of protein servings and slightly reduced the volume of grain to more easily meet your nutritional needs.

As its name implies, the Treatment Support diet is formulated to maximize the benefits of therapy—surgery, radiation, or chemotherapy—by providing the basic protein, fats, carbs, and calories you need to soldier on. If you are overwhelmed by treatment-related toxicity, or have to stop or delay treatment because you are too weak or are experiencing debilitating side effects, you are obviously not going to benefit from treatment. In fact, according to a 2005 study published in the *Journal of Clinical Oncology,* failure to complete chemotherapy led to shorter survival in women with early-stage breast cancer.[15] But even if you are strong enough to undergo treatment, you may not reap the full benefits if you are malnourished: in many cancers, losing as little as 5 percent of body weight (due to something as seemingly innocuous as developing an aversion to food, as many cancer patients do) can substantially reduce your response to cancer therapy.[16] One reason for decreased responsiveness to treatment may be inflammatory cytokines, which inhibit the killing of cancer cells and so work at cross-purposes with radiation and chemo.[17] On the other hand, research has found that omega-3s (especially docosahexaenoic acid, or DHA) appear to sensitize cancer cells to the effects of chemo.[18]

Another aim of this diet is to restore important blood albumin levels, which can plummet, especially in cases of advanced cancer. Albumin serves as a major transporter of drugs, hormones, fatty acids, and metabolites. Besides placing a patient at greater risk of infections and poor treatment tolerance, low albumin levels are associated with poor prognosis in cases of lung cancer, head and neck cancers, gynecological cancers, colon cancer, and other cancers of the digestive tract.[19] As noted in an earlier table, however, breast cancer patients who are taking adjuvant chemotherapy, who have a tendency to gain weight, do not need the extra protein and calories of the Treatment Support diet.[20] They can follow the core diet in the previous chapter. Only if you are having difficulty tolerating treatment or have long periods of low appetite should you try the Treatment Support diet. Breast cancer patients on their second (or later) round of chemo, or whose doctors feel they are losing weight abnormally, can also use the Treatment Support diet.

First, find the daily nutritional requirements for your height:

CALORIE RECOMMENDATIONS FOR TREATMENT SUPPORT

Height		Estimated Daily Requirements
Women	**Men**	**Calories**
Up to 5'3"	Up to 5'1"	1,500–1,700
5'3" up to 5'8"	5'1" up to 5'5"	1,800–2,000
5'8" up to 6'1"	5'5" up to 5'10"	2,100–2,300
Over 6'1"	Over 5'10"	2,400+

If you are in the middle of two height ranges, aim for the lower calorie level; if you are at the lower end of the height range, the higher level if you are at the upper end. Similarly, if you have a small frame, you should eat somewhat less than the recommended calories, whereas if you have a large frame, you should eat somewhat more. For a quick estimate of your frame size, wrap your left middle finger and thumb around your right wrist. If your finger and thumb don't meet, you have a large frame. If they just meet, you have a medium frame. If they overlap, you have a small frame. If you are in the 2,400+ calorie level, and if your appetite allows or demands, you may add one or two more servings to each food category (listed in the following table) for the first five inches over 6'1" (women) or 5'10" (men), and an additional one or two servings if more than five inches over.

DAILY QUANTITY OF FOOD RECOMMENDED FOR TREATMENT SUPPORT

1,500–1,700 Calories	1,800–2,000 Calories	2,100–2,300 Calories	2,400+ Calories	Trade-Off Approximations
Whole Grains				
2 cups	2½ cups	3 cups	4 cups	I cup cooked grain = I½ cups starchy vegetable = 2 slices bread = I½ cups dry cereal
Vegetables				
3 cups	3 cups	3½ cups	4 cups	½ cup cooked = 4 oz vegetable juice = I cup raw veg. = 3 cups raw lettuce
Protein				
5 servings	5½ servings	6 servings	6½ servings	I serving = ½ cup cooked legumes = ½ cup tofu or tempeh = 3 oz seitan = 4 oz fish = 4 egg whites or 2 whole eggs
Dairy Alternatives, calcium-fortified				
I cup	I½ cups	2 cups	2½ cups	I cup soy, oat, rice, or multigrain low-fat beverage = I oz nondairy cheese

1,500–1,700 Calories	1,800–2,000 Calories	2,100–2,300 Calories	2,400+ Calories	Trade-Off Approximations
Fruit				
1½ servings	2 servings	2½ servings	3 servings	I serving = I piece of fruit = ½ cup fresh or frozen = ¼ cup dried = 4 teaspoons fruit spread = 8 oz diluted juice (½ water and ½ juice)
Fat				
5 tsp	6 tsp	7 tsp	8 tsp	I teaspoon oil = I tablespoon chopped nuts or ground flaxseed = 1½ teaspoon tree nut butters = I teaspoon peanut or soy nut butter = ¼ avocado = 6 large olives

Be sure to eat a variety of protein foods each day. You may use the protein-boosting drink below to help meet your increased protein requirement if needed. However, if you are not eating well, you may need the meal replacement shake on page 131.

PROTEIN-BOOSTING DRINK

Yield: I drink

I cup rice, soy, or oat beverage

3 tbsp protein powder (cold-processed whey, egg white powder, glutamine, or soy protein isolate; breast cancer patients may choose to substitute more whey). Be sure to include the glutamine regularly.

2 tbsp brown rice syrup
Fruit for flavor (optional; if used, count as I fruit serving)
Put all ingredients in a blender, blend, and chill.

The protein-boosting shake has 310 calories, 22 grams of protein, and replaces I dairy serving, 1½ protein servings, and 2 fruit servings (the brown rice
syrup in the recipe substitutes for fruit).

To reach the recommended intake of the powerfoods described in Chapter 5, you may also find it helpful to use the
powerfood concentrates (green drinks) suggested there.

Symptom Management Tips

Undergoing treatment for cancer, not to mention having the disease itself, can cause a number of side effects ranging from unpleasant to debilitating to dangerous. Below are listed some
common side effects and advice on how to combat them.

▶ **Loss of Appetite**
Chemo can kill not only your cancer cells but also your appetite. First, be sure that nausea and vomiting are not the underlying problem; if so, they must be addressed first (see below).
Otherwise, consider when your appetite is at its best. For many
patients, it is at breakfast time. If so, try to get most of your
nutrients and calories for the day then. Just be sure to follow the
meal with mild exercise for proper digestion and metabolism.

I also recommend healthful sources of carbohydrates to raise
energy levels between meals. Dried fruits are great for this; even
people who are not hungry can usually manage to chew and
swallow some raisins, prunes, or dried apricots. To avoid the
glucose spike (hyperglycemia) that can feed cancer cells, combine the dried fruits with a protein such as some roasted seeds
or nuts, a nut butter or soy product, or small amounts of fish or
whey protein. Some patients who have no appetite can manage
to drink the meal replacement shake given above.

Exercise can also stimulate appetite. Try it. If it does, exercise shortly before mealtime. If it has the opposite effect, wait an hour or more after exercising before you try to eat.

I urge all our patients and their loved ones to attend cooking classes to make food more appealing. They learn to make meals more appetizing and more inviting to the eye, nose, and mouth by using garnishes and plenty of color. If you learn to think creatively about cooking and food selections—adorning boring-looking rice or cauliflower with red and green peppers, chives, and the like—you may find you have more desire to eat.

Pain and pain medications can interfere with appetite. Get treatment for pain, and if you're taking pain meds, schedule your meal or snack at least thirty minutes after you take the medicine.

In intractable cases of appetite loss, you may need pharmacological appetite stimulants such as Megace, Oxandrin, or Marinol. But you can accomplish a lot on your own.

Tips for Low Appetite

1. Eat small amounts frequently throughout the day. Rather than regular-size meals, have a snack every two to four hours, even if you don't feel hungry. Snack before bed unless this disrupts your sleep.
2. Keep ready-to-eat snacks such as nuts, dried or fresh fruit, crackers with nondairy cheese or nut butters, pretzels, vegetable juice, and appropriate nutritional supplement drinks handy. Carry snacks when you go out, and keep easy-to-prepare foods available so you are not deterred by the idea of food prep and cooking. Consider preparing food in quantity and refrigerating or freezing it for later. If family members or friends offer to help, take them up on it. Nothing increases appetite like someone else doing the cooking!
3. Try to make every bite or sip count by choosing foods that are rich in calories, protein, and other nutrients and limiting low-calorie foods that fill you up (such as broth or lettuce). Eat more fruit, fat, and sweeteners,

but in the healthier forms (for example, olive oil, nuts, and avocados as fats; agave, rice syrup, and barley malt as sweeteners).

4. Make eating more enjoyable by creating a pleasant, relaxed mealtime atmosphere. Try setting the table with pretty dishes and flowers, or playing music. Experiment with eating in different surroundings. Eat with others, or while watching a good television program.

5. During meals, limit the amount of liquid you drink, since drinking may make you feel full.

6. Try softer, cool, or frozen foods such as a shake, a frozen juice bar, or pureed frozen fruit.

7. If you don't feel like eating solid foods, try juice, soup, and shakes.

8. Herbal teas such as fennel or anise, mixed with verbena or mint, may stimulate appetite.

9. Since stressors can interfere with normal appetite, seek assistance for relaxation strategies that can help relieve tension.

▶ **Nausea and Vomiting**

Nausea and vomiting are all too familiar to many chemotherapy and radiation patients. Cisplatin, cyclophosphamide, doxorubicin, and dacarbazine are particularly notorious for causing nausea and vomiting, although these can also be symptoms of tumors themselves. Merely thinking about chemo can make you nauseated, an effect called "anticipatory nausea." Whatever the causes, nausea and vomiting can now be tamed by antiemetic drugs such as Aloxi (palonosetron) and Emend (aprepitant). Your doctor may, however, start you out on an older antiemetic, such as Reglan (metoclopramide) or Zofran (ondansetron), which may be effective for you.

Complementary therapies can also combat nausea. In one study, ginger was about as effective as the antiemetic drug metoclopramide but not as effective as ondansetron. Many of my patients have used ginger, as a tea or supplement (500 mg every four hours), successfully.[21] Ginger should not be taken when your platelet count is low due to chemotherapy, since it may have anticoagulant effects. Aromatherapy with peppermint oil may also tame nausea; you can carry a small bottle of peppermint oil with you throughout the day and sniff it occasionally, something some of our patients find helpful.[22] Mild exercise such as walking or using an exercise bike for ten to thirty minutes can also help.[23]

Acupuncture, acupressure, and acupuncture point electrical stimulation can also relieve nausea.[24] Stimulating a point on the underside of the wrist called the P6 point, even by drumming it with the fingers of the other hand, seems to be quite effective. Ask someone experienced in acupressure how to do this, or go to our website, www.lifeovercancer.com, for instructions. You can also buy a wristband with a small button that presses on P6; often used for seasickness, it is sold under the name Sea-Band.

These remedies for nausea should control vomiting, too, but because vomiting can lead to electrolyte imbalances and land you in the hospital with dehydration, you need to do all you can to stay hydrated. Try sucking on ice chips, sprinkled with a little salt and fruit juice or rice syrup, to keep your electrolytes balanced. Try to drink 8 cups of water a day. You can also try electrolyte-restoring drinks based on fruit juices and natural products, such as those at www.knudsenjuices.com or www.ceralyte.com. Once the vomiting is controlled, go back to normal foods slowly, starting out with 1 tablespoon of clear liquids at a time, then ¼ cup, moving on to plain, easily digested starchy foods.

Tips for Nausea and Vomiting

1. Eat small amounts of food frequently throughout the day; feelings of nausea may be intensified if you get very hungry.
2. Choose foods that appeal to you and that you feel you can tolerate. Your tastes may change from day to day and hour to hour.
3. Try dry toast or cereal, plain crackers, pretzels, rice cakes, pita bread, plain rice, cold pasta salad, potatoes, hot cereal, applesauce, canned fruit, fruit-juice-sweetened sorbets or

ices, tofu, egg whites or omega-3 whole eggs, and cooked vegetables.

4. Foods that are served cold or at room temperature may be easier for you. Avoid foods with strong odors as well as smelly cooking areas, smoke, perfume, and warm stuffy rooms.

5. Avoid fatty, fried, spicy, and overly sweet foods.

6. If there is a bad taste in your mouth, rinse your mouth before or after meals, or suck on a hard candy made with two-star or three-star sweeteners (such as Sweet Rice Candy made by Mitoku).

7. Don't go overboard with your favorite foods, or you may begin to associate them with feeling queasy.

8. Try eating a small amount of grated or finely chopped fresh ginger (if your blood platelets are less than 60,000 cells per microliter, check with a medical professional first), or a teaspoon of gomasio (a seasoning made from crushed sesame seeds and salt), or try sucking on the pit of a umeboshi plum. Gomasio and umeboshi plums are available in the macrobiotic section of health food stores. Herbal teas (such as ginger, alfalfa, chamomile, fennel, and slippery elm), oranges, or tangerines may also help.

9. Eat slowly and try to relax. Distractions may help keep your mind off nausea while you are eating. Try listening to music, books on tape, the radio, or looking out a window.

10. Avoid stress, noisy environments, and commotion, and limit conversation if the effort of talking worsens the nausea. Stress reduction strategies may be useful if stress worsens or triggers your nausea.

▶ **Diarrhea**

You can develop diarrhea as a result of chemotherapy; radiation to the abdomen or pelvis; intestinal infections; some antibiotics, antinausea medications, and other drugs; gastrointestinal graft-versus-host disease following bone-marrow transplantation; lactose intolerance resulting from chemotherapy effects on the digestive tract; blockage of the intestinal tract by a tumor, hard stools, or scarring from surgery or radiation; or surgery that has removed part of the stomach, small intestine, or colon. And people with cancer can develop diarrhea for the same reasons healthy people do: food allergies, inflammatory processes, or poor absorption of fats or carbohydrates.

Diarrhea is not merely unpleasant. It can lead to dehydration, enervation, and/or nutrient malabsorption because the partly digested food is moving too rapidly for the intestines to absorb nutrients. For this reason you need to be especially vigilant about maintaining your fluid intake when you have diarrhea (drink lots of filtered water). You also need to maintain your electrolyte balance, and you can do so by eating fish, bananas, and potatoes, all good sources of potassium.

To reduce your chances of developing diarrhea, and to get rid of it as soon as you can, avoid foods that speed up peristalsis (the rhythmic contractions of the intestine that propel food through the gut). These include gas-producing foods such as beans and bean products; greasy or fatty foods; spicy foods; acidic foods such as citrus or tomatoes; caffeinated foods and beverages; and raw fruits and vegetables. High-fiber foods such as brown rice or whole-grain bread should be eaten in moderation—about one or two and a half cups a day rather than the two to three and a half recommended in the Treatment Support diet or the two to four of the core diet—and in ground form rather than as whole grains. If diarrhea forces you to restrict your normal consumption of vegetables, you can still get their benefits from a green food concentrate. Diarrhea-fighting foods include rice porridge, tapioca, barley broth, miso (a Japanese soup base made from soybeans), potato-based vegetable soup, and carob-powder tea. And of course there are antidiarrheal medications such as Imodium and Lomotil. (Caution: too much of an antidiarrheal drug can cause constipation.)

If your diarrhea is especially severe or persistent, you may need to consume only water or dilute juice for two or three days, paying close attention to weight loss. Once the diarrhea has abated, slowly reintroduce easily digested, hypoallergenic foods such as vegetable broths, grated apples, steamed carrots, and rice or barley cooked in twice the usual amount of water so that it becomes a thin porridge. Ginger tea and umeboshi plum tea, sold in health food stores, may be helpful, as may miso combined with a potassium-rich vegetable broth made from carrot, spinach, celery, and parsley.

Supplements that might be helpful include glutamine (3 grams, three times a day), quercetin (250–500 mg two to four times daily), or powdered carob (½–1 teaspoon every hour, mixed in applesauce or half a banana). Chemotherapy can deplete lactose, the enzyme that digests milk; if you are consuming dairy products, cut back on or eliminate them. If diarrhea began when you started taking an antibiotic, use a supplement of *Lactobacillus acidophilus* (1–2 billion organisms per day).

Tips for Diarrhea

1. Sip small amounts of clear liquids often throughout the day to prevent dehydration. Clear liquids include water, broth, green tea, herbal tea, clear fruit juices (but avoid large amounts unless diluted with water), and kanten (a seaweed-based gelatin substitute available in health food stores) made with fruit juice. Choose room-temperature liquids, since very hot or very cold drinks may stimulate bowel movements.

2. Eat small, frequent meals and snacks throughout the day. Avoid large amounts of food at one time.

3. Avoid greasy, fried, very spicy, or very sweet foods; caffeine; carbonated beverages (unless open for at least ten minutes beforehand); and chewing gum. Also avoid fruit juices such as apple, cherry, or prune juice, which often contain large amounts of sorbitol, a stool softener.

4. You may need to temporarily cut back on fiber by limiting or avoiding whole-wheat products and bran; raw vegetables and gas-forming vegetables such as beans, broccoli, cauliflower, and cabbage; fruits with seeds, unpeeled fruit, dried fruit, juices with pulp; and legumes, nuts (except smooth nut butters), and seeds.

5. Foods that seldom exacerbate diarrhea, and sometimes alleviate it, include white rice, cream of rice cereal, and

refined white flour products such as white bread and noodles; eggs (not fried); smooth natural unhydrogenated almond butter; fish (baked or broiled); low-fiber vegetables such as acorn squash, peeled summer squash, peeled cucumber, peeled potato, peeled zucchini, and mushrooms; and low-fiber fruit such as applesauce, grapes, peeled peaches, bananas, mandarin oranges, tangerines, melons, mango, and plums. Bananas and applesauce are especially good choices because they contain pectin, a water-soluble fiber that can produce a firmer stool.

6. Try to choose foods high in potassium and sodium for electrolyte balance. High-potassium choices include bananas, baked or boiled potatoes without the skin, avocados, carrot juice, tomato juice or vegetable juice cocktail, and orange juice (diluted with water and without pulp). Foods high in sodium include miso, crackers, and pretzels.

7. Try two or three cups a day of ume-kuzu tea until normal bowel movements resume. To make the tea, dissolve 1 teaspoon of kuzu root chunks or powder in 1 cup of cold water. Simmer over low heat, stirring in 1 teaspoon of umeboshi paste and 1 teaspoon of shoyu or tamari (traditional Japanese soy sauce varieties). These ingredients are all available at health food stores. Note: I have seen better results in patients with this traditional tea consumed in Asia for many centuries than with most any medications.

8. Contact your doctor if your diarrhea is severe or bloody or if it lasts for more than two days or if light-headedness and dehydration are worsening.

▶ **Constipation**

There is considerable debate among health professionals about how infrequent bowel movements have to be to qualify as constipation. A normal number of bowel movements can range from three per day to one every three days. A good yardstick is whether you are having a bowel movement less frequently than you used to. Since constipation can be extremely dangerous—a fecal impaction, in which feces collect in the lower colon or rectum, or a partial or complete obstruction resulting from a tumor can be fatal if not treated—if you have not had a bowel movement in three days despite eating normally, you should contact your physician.

For cancer patients, constipation can be a side effect of chemotherapy or narcotic pain medications. It can also result from a low-fiber diet, lack of physical activity, low fluid intake resulting in dehydration, intestinal blockage due to a tumor or scarring from surgery, other medications, chronic overuse of laxatives, spinal cord compression that interferes with bowel movement, and hypercalcemia (an abnormal buildup of calcium in the blood).

To relieve constipation, avoid dairy products, salty foods, sugar, coffee, chocolate, caffeine, cheese, fried foods, spicy foods, tea, alcohol, white-flour products, and other refined and processed foods. Drink six to eight glasses of water daily. Increase your fiber intake from whole grains, legumes, and a wide variety of fruits and vegetables; you might also consider a fiber supplement, such as one of the psyllium-based supplements available at drugstores, as a temporary measure. Foods that can relieve constipation include those high in sodium, such as seafood; prunes soaked in water; flaxseed (1 tbsp ground on cereal or mixed with half a glass of water or dilute juice); whey protein; seeds such as sesame and sunflower; sprouts or sprouted seeds, such as alfalfa and broccoli sprouts; fruits such as raw apples, grapefruit, pears, cherries, persimmons, berries, pomegranates, currants, and figs; and vegetables such as asparagus, bok choy, burdock root, cauliflower, cabbage, sauerkraut, Jerusalem artichokes, radishes, spinach, and sweet potatoes. As always, if dietary changes do not relieve your constipation within two or three days, see your doctor.

Tips for Constipation

1. Drink plenty of fluids, 8 to 12 cups daily. Warm or hot beverages or prune juice may stimulate bowel movements. Avoid caffeinated beverages.
2. Gradually increase your intake of high-fiber foods such as beans, whole grains, vegetables, and fruits. Aim for 25

to 35 g of fiber a day (you can find fiber content on nutrition labels). Some particularly high-fiber foods include ground flaxseed (add 1 to 2 tbsp to breakfast cereal, juice, or other foods, ideally buying whole seeds and grinding them as needed), Uncle Sam's Laxative Cereal (½ to ¾ cup with nondairy milk), wheat bran (1 heaping tbsp on breakfast cereal or mixed into other food), or psyllium-husk products that do not contain sugar or artificial ingredients.

3. Walking or other regular exercise can relieve constipation. Even five or ten minutes of walking can help, but a half hour or more is ideal.

4. Check with your doctor about using a stool softener, such as citrate of magnesia or Dulcolax, which draws water back into the colon and stimulates the colon muscles. Stimulant herbal laxatives do the same thing but can be habit-forming and tend to weaken bowel tone, so avoid using them for more than two days. But for a day or two, you might try Senokot granules or tablets (a vegetable-based laxative that contains senna), cascara sagrada (one or two capsules with a large glass of water an hour before bedtime), or whole aloe leaf capsules or liquid. These are all available at most pharmacies or health food stores.

5. Check with your doctor if the problem persists in case there is an underlying disorder that needs to be addressed.

► **Taste Changes or Lack of Taste**
About half of all patients report changes in their sense of taste during and after chemotherapy. The cause is probably damage to the sensitive cells of the tongue from chemo, though the association of nausea or vomiting with particular foods may make you lose your taste for them. It is thus a good idea to limit food intake and avoid your favorite foods for two hours before chemotherapy and three after. Chemo tends to make people more sensitive to bitter tastes and less sensitive to sweet tastes, and can also produce a metallic taste. There is some evidence

that deficiencies in zinc, nickel, niacin, and vitamin A might be related to taste changes, so a good multivitamin and mineral supplement tailored for the needs of cancer patients would be useful during chemotherapy (follow the recommendations in the powerfoods section in Chapter 5).

Radiation therapy to the head and neck can also cause taste and smell changes. These usually start to clear up about two months after therapy but in some cases last for a year or longer. There are no medications to help with such taste changes once they have occurred, though having a dentist make sure that you do not have a mouth infection is a good idea.

Tips for Taste Changes or Lack of Taste

1. Food may taste better if served cold or at room temperature instead of hot.
2. Foods that are well tolerated include fresh fruits and vegetables; fruit smoothies and fruit sorbet (made with healthful sweeteners); fruit-juice ice pops (which you can make at home); pasta; dairy alternatives; tofu; eggs, preferably omega-3 rich if you are using whole eggs.
3. Choose strongly flavored foods. Use sauces, herbs, and spices, and condiments such as mustard for more taste.
4. Add tart ingredients to help cover any metallic taste, unless you have mouth or throat sores. For instance, add orange juice, lime juice, lemon juice, or orange marmalade to sauces, salsa, stir-fried or cooked vegetables, salad dressing, or fruit salad; add vinegar, lemon juice, or pickles to dressings for bean, potato, pasta, tuna, egg, or coleslaw salads; add lemon juice to soup, broth, or guacamole.
5. Try adding something sweet, such as applesauce or fruit preserves, to protein foods.
6. Select foods that smell appetizing. Avoid foods with strong odors.
7. Before eating, rinse your mouth with tea, club soda, salted water, or fruit juice to clear your taste buds.

8. Drink fluids with your meal to rinse away any bad taste.
9. Eat fresh fruit to get rid of a bad taste in your mouth between meals, or suck on hard candy made with two-star or three-star sweeteners (such as Sweet Rice Candy made by Mitoku).
10. If a metallic taste persists, avoid using metal utensils. Substitute plastic utensils, porcelain soup spoons, or chopsticks. Similarly, avoid metal cooking utensils; aluminum, copper, and cast-iron cookware; and metal dishes. Instead use plastic, rubber, or wooden cooking utensils, and stainless-steel or glass cookware.
11. Avoid strong smells by using an exhaust fan when cooking, grilling outside, or using precooked foods. Also avoid cigarette smoke.

▶ **Sore Mouth or Throat (Mucositis)**
Mucositis is an inflammation of the mucous membranes causing a painful or dry mouth, mouth sores, burning, peeling, or swelling of the tongue. In cancer patients mucositis is typically a result of chemotherapy or radiation. As many as 40 percent of those getting standard chemotherapy will develop mucositis, as will 70 to 90 percent of patients undergoing bone marrow transplants.[25] Severe mucositis can result in increased infection rates, increased need for intravenous nutrition and opiate medications, and an increased risk of mortality.

Relieving moderate to severe mucositis usually requires pain medicine, starting with acetaminophen and moving on, if necessary, to stronger pain medications. Since eating will likely be painful, you can use a special mouthwash that a pharmacist can prepare, which includes lidocaine, hydrocortisone, and other medications. Used half an hour before eating, it will numb the mouth. A prescription gel called Gelclair adheres to the inside of the mouth; it contains an extract of licorice, an herb traditionally used for mouth sores and digestive system inflammations. If you use lidocaine, avoid very hot foods and do not take large bites, since this might cause gagging if your mouth is numb. Hypnosis is also a possibility for pain control.

If you develop mucositis, it is especially important to practice good oral hygiene (using a soft toothbrush) and good hydration. Avoid alcohol-based mouthwashes, substituting aloe vera juice as a swish-and-swallow mouthwash.

Researchers have reported seeing terrific results treating mucositis with glutamine, an amino acid.[26] They mix water with 20 grams of glutamine and have patients carry a bottle of this all day when they are receiving treatment and one day after treatment ends so they can swish and swallow. They recommend that this be done approximately every hour. Indeed, this can also prevent mucositis in the first place, so you might consider it before you begin chemo or radiation therapy.

Tips for Mucositis

1. Try soft, moist, nonirritating foods such as bananas, applesauce, melons, other soft or canned fruits, or baked fruit; fruit nectars (such as peach, pear, and apricot) rather than acidic juices; kanten (a juice dessert made with a seaweed-based gelatin alternative); soups; oatmeal or other cooked cereals; pasta; soft cooked grains; pureed or mashed foods such as squash; tofu; scrambled eggs; soft cooked beans; and organic baby foods.
2. Cook foods until they are soft and tender. Reduce spices.
3. Cut foods into small pieces, or use a food processor or blender to puree them if necessary.
4. Add sauce or gravy to food to make it easier to swallow.
5. Try cold foods such as shakes, fruit-juice ice pops, frozen berries or grapes, and nondairy frozen desserts. Sucking on ice chips may also provide some relief.
6. Drink through a straw to bypass mouth sores.
7. If swallowing is hard, tilting your head back or moving it forward may help.
8. Maintain good mouth care. Rinse your mouth often with water to remove food and bacteria and promote healing. If your teeth and gums are sore, your dentist may be able to recommend a special product for cleaning your teeth.
9. For relief, try swishing with and then swallowing 1 ounce of aloe vera gel two or three times per day, swabbing

mouth sores with a Q-tip saturated with vitamin E three times per day, sucking slippery elm throat lozenges, or drinking slippery elm or marshmallow root tea.

10. For severe discomfort, request pain medication. Ask about anesthetic lozenges and sprays that can numb your mouth and throat long enough for you to eat.

▶ **Dry Mouth**

Both chemotherapy and radiation can cause dry mouth. With chemotherapy, the symptom is usually temporary, but with radiation, it can last longer, especially if the salivary glands received a direct hit. If your mouth feels dry, check with your doctor, because some medications, including certain antidepressants, diuretics, and pain medications, can cause it. In addition, you may have a mouth infection or be dehydrated. There are no medications for dry mouth, but food tips can improve your symptoms.

Tips for Dry Mouth

1. Add sauces, gravies, broth, and dressings to foods.
2. Suck on ice chips, fruit-juice ice pops, or hard candy made with two-star or three-star sweeteners (such as Sweet Rice Candy made by Mitoku) to keep the mouth moist.
3. Add citric acid in your diet to stimulate saliva production. Citric acid is present in oranges, orange juice, lemon, and lemonade. (But if you also have mucositis, acidic beverages or foods are not advised.)
4. Drink liquids with your meals.
5. Avoid plain meats, bread products, crackers, or dry cake.
6. Avoid very hot foods or beverages.
7. Avoid alcohol.
8. Practice good mouth care.
9. Ask your nurse or doctor about commercial saliva substitutes such as Salivart, Mouth-Kote, or Saliva Substitute.

▶ **Thick Saliva**

Thick saliva, which is related to dry mouth, is also common in patients who receive radiation to the head and neck, especially the salivary glands. Salivary glands may take a long time to recover, and may never do so. This makes adapting to this condition through diet modification a good investment.

Tips for Thick Saliva

1. Drink sparkling water or hot tea with lemon, or try papaya juice. If you also have mucositis, avoid acidic beverages and foods.
2. Try sucking on lemon drops made with two-star or three-star sweeteners.
3. Eat a lighter breakfast if you have a buildup of mucus in the morning, and bigger meals in the afternoon and evening.
4. Rinse frequently with a saline solution (1 quart water with ¾ tsp teaspoon salt and 1 tsp–1 tbsp baking soda).
5. Drink lots of fluids.
6. Eat soft, tender foods such as cooked fish, noodles, thinned cereals, and pureed fruits and vegetables diluted to a very thin consistency.
7. Eat small, frequent meals.
8. Drink diluted juices and vegetable, miso, or fish broth-based soups.
9. Switch to a liquid diet if the problem is severe.
10. Don't eat bread products, gelled desserts, oily foods, hot cereals, thick cream soups or nectars, hot spices, tomato products, or foods that require much chewing.

Remission Support Diet

The key to maintaining your remission long-term is chemoprevention—the scientific concept of preventing and reversing malignant cell transformation by changing your internal biochemistry through food, supplements, or medications. Nutrients and pharmaceuticals may play a role not only in prevention but also in reducing the long-term risk of tumor recurrence as well as second cancers (those that begin in a different location from the original cancer). I believe the likelihood of attaining long-term freedom from cancer, or remission maintenance, is greatly enhanced by implementing the core diet with the modifications of the Remission Support diet. Although the guidelines for preventing cancer in the first place can be extended to the prevention of recurrences, sustaining a remission argues for a more aggressive approach:

- **Eat solely (or mostly) plant foods.** A plant-based diet is the best for those in remission; however, deep-sea fish caught from clean waters is fine.
- **Eat on the leaner side.** Try not to overeat. If you are of normal weight, simply eat about 100–200 fewer calories than are recommended for your weight level in the core diet program, as given on page 104. This would mean cutting out about ⅓ cup of whole grains and ½ cup of beans from your daily diet. If you are overweight and trying to lose weight, cut out 200 to 300 calories per day (⅔ cup grains and up to 1 cup beans), and increase your exercise time to account for another 250 calories (a forty-minute brisk walk).
- **Control your total fat intake.** Limit fat to 2 tsp a day.
- **Consume a high proportion of omega-3s and some omega-9s.** Cut way back on omega-6s.
- **Bulk up on high-fiber and phytochemical-rich whole grains, vegetables, and fruits.**
- **Moderate protein intake.** Reduce protein servings by one or two a day.
- **Incorporate foods that have shown chemoprevention activity at every meal.** These include cruciferous vegetables (broccoli, cabbage, cauliflower, brussels sprouts, bok choy, mustard greens, watercress, and kale; these contain sulforaphane and indole-3-carbinol, which help convert unhealthy estrogens

into healthy ones),[27] cherries (with anthocyanins, potent natural anti-inflammatories),[28] tomatoes (whose lycopene is a powerful antioxidant and anti-inflammatory),[29] garlic (whose organosulfides improve blood flow characteristics and stimulate the immune system),[30] salmon (whose omega-3s reduce inflammation and may improve response to chemotherapy),[31] turmeric (whose curcuminoids exhibit anti-inflammatory activity, as well as protect against DNA-damaging free radicals),[32] soy in the form of miso, tofu, and tempeh (because its phytoestrogens may reduce your risk of developing colon cancer or prostate cancer),[33] green tea (whose catechins may prevent and fight breast and prostate cancers),[34] flaxseed (whose good fats and cancer-fighting lignans reduce angiogenesis),[35] fruit such as pomegranate, strawberries, cranberries, and raspberries (which contain ellagic acid, which inhibits cancer cell growth),[36] and grapes (whose resveratrol acts as a chemopreventive for some forms of skin cancer and can inhibit proliferation of several cancers).[37]

Should you simply take a pill containing ellagic acid for chemoprevention instead of changing your diet? Randomized trials on individual phytochemicals—antioxidants such as beta-carotene and vitamin E—indicate no cancer preventive effect. In retrospect, the futility of trying to overcome years of junk-food diets with a single phytochemical should be obvious. More research on cancer chemoprevention is definitely needed, but researchers now realize that they must study whole foods and whole diets rather than isolated compounds.[38] Supplements can be enormously useful, and randomized studies indicate that single phytochemicals can be used for specific treatment objectives. But for cancer chemoprevention, you need the entire panoply of phytochemicals that come in whole plants, and not just an isolated active chemical. I emphasize with patients the use of supplements based on whole plant extracts and complex mixtures. Preventing cancer—and its recurrence—also requires a sound overall diet that replaces cancer-promoting omega-6 fats and sugary sweets with salmon, green tea, and colorful fruits.

CHAPTER 7

THE PHYSICAL CARE PLAN: THE CASE FOR FITNESS

What if I told you that by just conditioning your body with appropriate activity during the day and attaining deep, restorative sleep at night, you could improve your odds of surviving cancer and reduce the chance of suffering debilitating side effects of treatment? And that establishing new, healthier patterns of body alignment and movement could reduce pain and enhance your ability to heal?

Not so long ago, advising cancer patients to get fit was unheard of. I recall vividly during medical training in the 1970s being taught that cancer patients should rest and reduce their physical activity after treatment, and that message has clearly reached laypeople, too: my patients often seem surprised when I urge them to work out and tell them that a 2006 *Journal of Clinical Oncology* study, for instance, showed that exercise is linked to survival and decreased recurrence even in stage III colon cancer patients.[1] Yet once they get over their incredulity, their response is always the same: "Exercise," they tell me, "helps me feel more vital, more peaceful, and more hopeful."

Despite the conventional wisdom of the past, my own clinical experience with patients in my care, along with recent research, has repeatedly confirmed the therapeutic benefits of exercise for people with cancer. Even walking at a moderate pace for three to five hours a week is correlated with a 50 percent decline in mortality from breast cancer.[2] If walking were a drug, pharmaceutical companies would be in a frenzy to patent it. Moreover, numerous studies show that inactivity can result in frailty, fatigue, and the loss of critical lean muscle; it can disrupt sleep cycles and impair tolerance and response to cancer treatment. My patients have shown me time and again that exercise is among the most powerful ways to break the vicious cycle of decreased activity, impaired sleep, low mood, and increased fatigue that strikes so many people with advanced cancer.[3] More than that, exercise can mitigate some of the taxing symptoms and life-threatening complications of cancer and can even reduce some of the side effects of cancer treatment. Physical activity can be—indeed, must be—a key part of your recovery.

I'll go further: exercise may be crucial to your very survival. A sedentary lifestyle is a bad idea no matter what your health, but it is a really bad idea for cancer patients. For one thing, malignant cells secrete inflammatory biochemicals that promote the breakdown of skeletal muscles, amplifying the muscle-degrading effects of inactivity.[4] Loss of muscle is dangerous because muscle provides a buffer against protein losses from more vital tissues—the visceral proteins that constitute your glands and organs and which are crucial for, among other things, a healthy immune system. As the skeletal muscle protein reserves become depleted by chronic exposure to inflammatory molecules, visceral proteins begin to go as well. So while you may think that advanced cancer earns you a dispensation from exercise, the opposite is true: in such patients the lack of physical activity will lead to even greater muscle wasting and an immune system so compromised that you place yourself at real risk of pneumonia and other potentially fatal infections.[5]

Unfortunately, this new understanding has not changed most clinical practice. Because of lingering misconceptions about exercise and cancer, few oncologists will recommend physical activity as part of your treatment. The most common rationale is that bed rest will help you save your energy, whereas exercise will deplete it. This is what I was taught in the 1970s, and the idea has persisted to this day: studies show that a large percentage of cancer patients exercise less after their diagnosis.[6]

Don't worry—I am not going to recommend that you start training for a triathlon. Overdoing exercise, especially without adequate preparation, can damage tissue and increase oxidative stress and inflammation, both of which encourage the survival and spread of malignant cells.[7] Overdoing it can also leave you exhausted, unable to cope with the demands of cancer treatment.

You may be surprised to learn that fitness is not only about activity and exercise. Just as crucial is proper rest. If you or someone you know has cancer, I do not need to tell you that the disease and treatments bring on deep, lasting fatigue. This fatigue can be ruinous to your quality of life, of course. But chronic exhaustion can also worsen your prognosis: if you are always feeling enervated, you are unlikely to summon the energy to exercise. The importance of proper rest extends beyond giving you the energy and stamina to keep fit, however. Banishing the anxious, sleepless nights (followed by lethargic days) that so many cancer patients suffer, and replacing them with restful sleep and healthful activity at the right times of the day-night cycle, is correlated with dramatically prolonged survival for people with metastatic cancer, as demonstrated by a study published in the journal *Clinical Cancer Research* in 2000.[8] The study compared patients with metastatic colorectal cancer, some of whom had abnormal sleep-activity rhythms and some of whom had normal and (as we now know) healthful rhythms. The former tossed and turned all night, got up and wandered around, napped excessively, and were generally sedentary during the daytime—a pattern scientists describe as "disturbed circadian rhythms." These patients were five times more likely to die within two years of their diagnosis than comparable patients with normal circadian rhythms. One possible explanation: patients with disrupted circadian rhythms have higher levels of cancer-promoting biochemicals called cytokines than patients with similar tumors but normal circadian rhythms, according to a 2005 study.[9]

Survival wasn't the only difference. As anyone who has suffered insomnia will appreciate, patients with disturbed circadian rhythms also reported a poorer quality of life.[10] How miserable can abnormal circadian rhythms make a cancer patient feel? If one patient experiences few side effects of chemotherapy but has abnormal sleep-activity cycles and another has debilitating side effects but normal circadian rhythms, the former will report a worse quality of life than the latter. Disturbed sleep-activity rhythms appear to exacerbate chemo-related symptoms as well as patients' perception of them, while healthful sleep-activity rhythms may diminish them.

Studies such as these pointed me to one conclusion: the most effective approach to fitness takes in the entire daily cycle of rest and activity. The Block Center fitness program therefore targets your rest patterns as well as your activity patterns over the course of a full 24-hour day. It reflects decades of experience as well as the growing number of studies testifying to the importance of physical activity for cancer patients—those undergoing treatment as well as those in remission. I will sketch out some of that evidence here; you can find details of the studies supporting the advice at www.lifeovercancer.com. There, for instance, you will find a summary and a link to a 1998 randomized controlled trial—the gold standard in biomedical research—in which cancer patients who underwent aerobic training experienced a 25 percent reduction in diarrhea (a common side effect of radiation), a 28 percent reduction in pain, a 15 percent reduction in low white blood cell counts, and a 12 percent reduction in hospital stays, as well as significantly less fatigue and emotional distress than their sedentary counterparts.[11]

Of course I am concerned about whether your tumor is shrinking. But I have seen too many patients felled by smaller, seemingly minor symptoms such as fatigue, anxiety, depression, bowel irregularities, and disturbed sleep patterns, that can—if untreated—cascade into major complications, impacting not only your quality of life but your ability to tolerate treatments, respond to treatments, and go into remission. That's why circadian fitness is as important as diet and mind-spirit interventions in making your biochemical environment as hostile as possible to tumors and metastases.

Why Fitness?

My own epiphany about the importance of exercise for cancer patients came when I was fifteen and my grandmother's breast cancer returned twenty-five years after a radical mastectomy and chemotherapy had beaten it into remission. I visited her almost daily for two weeks. In those days, it was customary for patients receiving chemotherapy to be confined to a hospital bed. To my astonishment, her body began to shrink. Either the members of her medical team hadn't noticed or they didn't care; maybe they figured there was nothing they could do. As my grandmother dutifully followed her doctors' orders to rest and conserve her energy, with each passing day she wasted away before my eyes. She died in that bed a few weeks later.

It would be some years before I fully grasped the importance of what I had observed and just how harmful bed rest—what I call "excessive rest syndrome"—can be for a cancer patient. At the most basic level, inactivity accelerates muscle wasting, resulting in less endurance and less physical activity, which in turn leads to ongoing muscle loss. This is especially pernicious for cancer patients, who can lose over 80 percent of their muscle mass. Losing muscle is bad for several reasons, starting with the simple fact that you need your muscles to move and perform the activities of daily life.[12] But muscle also serves as the primary reservoir for glutamine, an amino acid that powers the anti-cancer immune defenses. Muscle loss means glutamine loss and thus a decline in your cancer-fighting arsenal.[13] In addition, the longer you remain inactive, the less efficient your body's energy-generating capacities will be: physical inactivity promotes a vicious cycle in which diminished blood circulation and lack of oxygen (as well as other nutrients) result in less energy and more fatigue.[14] This reinforces the tendency to remain sedentary. In time, the fatigue and inertia become so overwhelming that the mere thought of exercise is exhausting.

The rationale for physical activity is not only that inactivity is harmful. It is that activity is beneficial, with numerous studies showing that it is associated with decreased death rates from cancers of the colon, lung, prostate, testicles, breast, ovaries, and uterus.[15] How? According to new research, exercise counters cancer-fueling molecules called growth factors, oxidative stress, the immune system, and how the body responds to inflammation.

• Growth factors include estrogen, insulin, and a compound related to insulin called insulin-like growth factor 1 (IGF-1) that promote breast, lung, prostate, and other solid tumors. Exercise can reduce the levels of these growth-stimulating factors. It lowers excessive IGF-1 production and increases the levels of blood proteins that bind it, making less of it available to promote tumor growth.[16] Exercise also reduces insulin resistance, thereby lowering your blood levels of insulin, also a growth factor.[17] Regular exercise also reduces estrogen production in women, depriving estrogen-sensitive cancers of the breast, ovaries, and endometrium of the fuel they feed on.[18]

• *Oxidative stress* refers to the surplus of free radicals, which are reactive molecules that promote cancer. Exercise seems to boost enzymes that curb free radicals, resulting in lower levels of them.[19] One caveat: if you exercise irregularly, infrequently, or too strenuously, especially if you are in poor shape to begin with, you may increase your levels of oxidative stress and thus weaken your anti-cancer defenses.[20] What you want is regular but not overly strenuous exercise, which is what the Life Over Cancer fitness plan offers.

• The immune system includes natural killer (NK) cells, which stem the spread of cancer cells from the primary tumor.[21] Exercise can increase your population of these cells, probably because it halts and reverses the loss of glutamine, the amino acid that is stored in muscle cells and that stimulates the cancer-killing cells.[22] Exercise also boosts production of anti-cancer compounds from immune cells called macrophages.[23]

• Inflammation drives cancer, but exercise increases the activity of anti-inflammatory molecules and thus can slow the progression of cancer.[24] Inflammation is also a critical part of the muscle-wasting syndrome called cachexia; exercise appears to moderate it, although more specific research is needed.[25]

In addition to reducing the levels of cancer-promoting molecules, exercise can improve your response to chemotherapy and reduce the number of times you need to interrupt or delay treatment due to fatigue or other debilitating side effects, such as a plunge in white blood cell count.[26] Treatment interruptions and discontinuations reduce the efficacy of chemo, with the result that your tumor will not shrink as much or as quickly. In some cases, avoiding such interruptions can be the difference between success and failure. In one study, for instance, colon cancer patients over sixty-five who dropped out of their chemo regimens before five months survived only half as long as patients who completed five to seven months of treatment.[27]

How can exercise improve your ability to stick it out? Clinicians refer to something called *performance status,* which is basically your ability to function physically. Performance status is highly predictive of prognosis—in fact, it may be the single best predictor of survival—in most types of cancer.[28] Aerobic exercise can substantially improve your performance status.[29] It can also reduce common symptoms and complications of cancer that can impede your chances of getting the most out of treatment. Among them:

• **Anxiety and depression.** Exercise reduces both anxiety and depression in people with cancer, in a direct dose-response way.[30] That is, the more regularly you exercise, the less anxious and depressed you will be. Part of this effect comes from the fact that exercise improves your sleep quality, energy levels, ability to function in daily life, and inner resilience, all of which improve your mood.[31] But exercise also raises levels of molecules that act directly on the brain to decrease anxiety and improve mood.[32]

• **Sleep.** Fifty percent of cancer patients have insomnia, which—as even people without cancer know—severely reduces your quality of life. In cancer patients, though, the effects can be more dire. Fitful sleep at night tends to mean inactivity during the day. In contrast, exercise can enhance the quality of sleep.[33] The effect is not limited to any specific form of exercise: it has been seen in studies of the ancient Eastern practice of tai chi and Tibetan yoga as well as plain old aerobic conditioning and strength training.[34] Regular sleep is correlated with dramatically prolonged survival for people with metastatic disease who are receiving certain chemotherapy regimens.[35]

• **Fatigue.** Eighty percent of cancer patients report suffering from fatigue, which is not surprising.[36] Radiation therapy is notorious for causing fatigue.[37] The emotional toll the disease takes can leave you wrung out, and poor sleep can leave you feeling as if you are never more than half awake.[38] Exercise seems to decrease fatigue, especially during the crucial period when you are undergoing chemotherapy. Just half an hour daily of aerobic exercise can decrease fatigue as chemotherapy goes on (the opposite of what usually happens).[39] Even gentle forms of exercise, such as tai chi, can markedly improve energy levels and quality of life.[40] An advantage of tai chi, which my wife and professional partner, Penny, has practiced for nearly thirty years, is that it's just about impossible to overdo it: the practice involves slow, graceful, continuous movements that produce a state of relaxed alertness. Indeed, we have incorporated movements from tai chi and other Asian fitness traditions, such as qi gong, into a system we teach at the Block Center, the Block Be Fit program.

• **Embolisms.** Because chemotherapy and inactivity both raise the risk of clots, patients with cancer have a higher than normal risk of developing pulmonary embolisms and other dangerous blood clots, which can break loose from where they formed—the leg, say—and travel to the lungs with fatal results. Exercise, however, can reduce blood viscosity and blood cell (platelet) aggregation, lowering the chances of clots.[41] What seems to happen is that exercise increases circulation and makes the blood more fluid. Also, improved blood circulation delivers more oxygen and nutrients to tissues. Malignancies spread more slowly in oxygen-rich conditions.

• **Nausea and loss of appetite.** A big reason cancer patients are at risk of cachexia is that they have no desire to eat, because of the inflammatory effects of cancer or the nausea caused by chemo. Exercise can decrease nausea and increase appetite.[42] When one of my patients, Karin, was undergoing several cycles of strong chemotherapy for advanced colon cancer, she suffered from nausea for several days after each treatment and as a result stopped taking her morning walk—understandable, but precisely the wrong thing to do when hit with chemo-induced nausea. We worked out a plan of aerobics, including fifteen minutes of low-intensity walking whenever nausea hit. To her delight, Karin found that the walking, along with relaxation and visualization, suppressed the nausea. She subsequently began each chemo visit with twenty minutes on a treadmill at the Block Center. By overcoming the nausea, Karin was able to avoid debilitating weight loss during her long treatment, a significant risk for patients with advanced colon cancer.

• **Compromised digestion.** Conventional cancer treatments can block or limit the absorption of key micronutrients, particularly trace elements. Exercise improves absorption, which is definitely what you want. The most healthful diet in the world will not do you much good if your digestive system doesn't absorb what you swallow.

• **Constipation.** Many patients develop constipation as a result of chemo. Physical activity appears to decrease bowel transit time, or how long it takes waste products to move through the intestinal tract, by increasing peristalsis, the rhythmic contractions of the bowel.[43]

Individualizing Exercise

Let me address one point you may hear from your doctor about exercise and fitness: namely, that it is harmful for a cancer patient to lose weight. Patients sometimes do lose weight on the Life Over Cancer program, often intentionally. But if you lose the right kind of weight, your prognosis is likely to improve. If you are obese, you have an increased risk of dying from almost all cancers, partly because obesity tends to raise levels of sex hormones and insulin, which promote tumor growth.[44] This is especially so for patients with breast or prostate cancer, who need to lose fat if they are overweight (excess fat increases the risk of having distant metastases) but at the same time conserve or even build muscle tissue.

Several years ago, a doctor who had encouraged one of his breast cancer patients to work with us called me in alarm to say that she had lost thirty pounds on our regimen. His concern was reasonable, if misplaced: although weight gain with breast cancer patients undergoing chemotherapy worsens prognosis, weight loss of the wrong type can be equally worrisome. Center staff faxed him the patient's body composition analysis, which showed that her weight loss had in fact been the right kind: she had lost excessive body fat while building up lean muscle. I explained to this concerned physician that by eating well and following our fitness program, she had changed her body composition and improved her prognosis.

This example underscores that, as with all components of the Life Over Cancer program, fitness must be individualized. If you are an overweight stage II breast cancer patient, you want to lose weight. If you have advanced pancreatic cancer, weight loss may be life-threatening, and may actually be a result of cachexia, since in this cancer an underlying inflammatory state often drives this wasting syndrome. In addition to determining whether a patient needs to lose weight, gain weight, or keep weight stable, individualizing fitness also means determining which type of exercise is most motivating or best suited to a patient's physical capacities. This includes determining whether muscle rebuilding is needed and more important than focusing on regaining cardiac fitness. Although in this chapter I've mostly treated exercise generically, in fact it is important to match the right exercise—walking, running, weight lifting, tai chi, favorite sports—to the right patient. I explain how to do that in Chapter 9, but first let's look at the ingredients of the Life Over Cancer fitness program.

CHAPTER 8

THE LIFE OVER CANCER
CORE FITNESS PLAN

The Block fitness program is designed around the circadian cycle. It therefore has two phases: the rest phase and the activity phase. Although you might assume that any program with *fitness* in its name emphasizes activity over rest, in fact I regard them as equal contributors to fitness. That's because when you sleep more deeply at the right time, you have more energy to engage in whole-body conditioning; when you engage in conditioning during the day, you are likely to sleep better.[1] The two phases of the circadian fitness program are therefore mutually enhancing: healthful sleep will improve your ability to exercise, while exercise will improve the quality of your sleep. The result will be an improvement in your general well-being and the ability to keep up your usual activities. You will also preserve the energy you need for battling cancer. Thus the exercise program begins with taking a rest!

The Rest Phase

Restful, restorative sleep is the foundation for well-being, mental and physical. To get an idea of your level of sleep disruption, answer the following questions:

1. Do you go to bed and get up at different times each day?

2. Does it usually take you more than twenty minutes to get to sleep?

3. If you nap during the day, do your naps total more than twenty minutes?

4. Do you sleep less than seven hours a night?

5. Do you awaken more than two times during the night?

6. Do you feel unrefreshed when you awaken in the morning?

7. Is your exposure to sunlight limited (less than fifteen minutes) most days?

8. Do you exercise fewer than three times per week?

If you answered yes to:

1 to 3 questions: Your sleep patterns are not disrupted. Review the sleep hygiene program for preventive care.

4 to 6 questions: Implement the sleep hygiene program. Incorporate the recommendations in this chapter, and proceed with regular testing, continued monitoring, and reevaluation.

7 to 8 questions: Fully implement the sleep hygiene program and also seek out help from a medical professional with expertise in sleep disorders.

Sleep Hygiene: Lifestyle Strategies to Improve Sleep Quality

No, this is not a one-sentence section that recommends taking a prescription or herbal sleep medication. We actually do recommend sleep aids to patients going through a brief, particularly stressful period. But sleep medications, particularly prescription ones, are not very effective for long-term sleep problems: their efficacy drops with time, and they may have adverse side effects. Instead, research has found that lifestyle changes, such as when and where you sleep, are much more effective, especially in the long term, because sleep is essentially a conditioned psychological response that is most easily evoked with a routine and predictable environment. The idea, then, is to create that environment through behavioral changes known as "sleep hygiene."[2] Try them one by one until you find the combination that works for you:

- **Improve your sleep space.** It is crucial to create the proper environment for sleep, so reserve the bedroom for sleep and intimacy only. You should not use your bedroom for work, and you should not have a TV there. Do not fall asleep watching television.
- **Avoid caffeine.** Even if you don't feel that caffeine affects your sleep, too much of it can keep you on edge. If you feel uneasy or jittery during the day, gradually eliminate caffeine. At least do not consume coffee, tea, colas, or other sources of caffeine after midday.
- **Regularize your daily schedule of sleep, work, physical activity, bedtime, and waking.** If you set 11:00 P.M. to 7:00 A.M. as your sleeping hours and stick to them, your body's circadian rhythms are more likely to normalize. If you move your bedtime by more than an hour or so, and if you sleep late (such as on weekends), you can count on a couple of nights of disturbed sleep as your body struggles to regain its rhythms.
- **Maintain a relaxing bedtime routine.** Find a soothing ritual, such as quiet music, meditation, or a warm bath with relaxing essential oils, a pinch of baking soda, or bath salts—or whatever works for you.
- **Sleep in complete darkness.** Use heavy curtains, blackout shades, or eye covers to keep out light.
- **Watch out for purposeful sleep deprivation.** Staying up late and waking up early to get more work done or watch more TV is epidemic in American society. If you have cancer, you need to avoid this bad sleep habit. Readjust your attitudes about work, call on your support network, or have someone tape your favorite late-night shows—but go to sleep!
- **Get at least a half hour of bright daylight exposure each day.** Bask in sunshine or take a brisk morning walk in good

weather. Sunshine signals the brain to stop producing the sleep hormone melatonin.[3] If you can't get out, use a light box first thing in the morning. (A light box contains full-spectrum lights. For more information on where to locate a light box, go to www.lifeovercancer.com.) This will keep your biological clock properly set. As a result, your production of melatonin—which is produced only at night in the normal circadian cycle and causes drowsiness—will be properly timed to enhance your sleep.

- **Engage in a balanced fitness program.** Combine relaxing and meditative practices such as yoga, tai chi, or qi gong with aerobic exercise appropriate for your condition. Moderate exercise is a great way to improve your sleep.
- **Exercise during the morning, late afternoon, or very early evening, at least five to six hours before bedtime.** That will synchronize your circadian rhythms. Avoid late-night vigorous exercise.
- **Avoid heavy meals close to bedtime.** This is especially true if nighttime heartburn keeps you awake.

The Activity Phase

The goal of the activity phase is to give you energy, vitality, and physical and physiological resilience. Resilience is the ability to quickly recover from exertion, trauma, and stress. For example, if a thirty-year-old and an eighty-year-old undergo surgery or chemotherapy, the eighty-year-old will probably take many months to recover, while the thirty-year-old will bounce back much faster. Internal fitness, and particularly cardiac recovery training, can give you that bounce-back ability and help you get through the physiological challenges of cancer and its treatment. This kind of fitness is characterized by a low heart rate at rest, the ability to quickly increase heart rate to its maximum, rapid recovery of normal heart rate after exertion. Muscle strength and flexibility are also crucial.[4] To help you achieve this, the Life Over Cancer fitness program uses the principle of *complementary opposition*—the idea that to develop fitness you need opposing but complementary components. That's why the program comprises rest and its opposite, activity. Similarly, it includes weight training, which shortens muscles, as well as flexibility training, which lengthens them.

The ideal fitness program if you have been largely sedentary consists of regular, short bouts of low-to-moderate exercise that increases in intensity and duration as your fitness improves. Even brief periods of aerobic activity are often sufficient to reduce fatigue and improve your mood, daily functioning, and quality of life. This is especially relevant to people with cancer, since surgery, radiation, chemo, and their side effects—to say nothing of the disease itself—can limit your ability to exercise. But let me be clear: it takes real commitment, especially if you are debilitated or used to being sedentary. The trick is to individualize an exercise regimen to your needs and capabilities.

Tom: Advanced Cancer and Fitness

While we were developing our fitness plans, Penny and I held regular weekend workshops called the Intensive Health Training Program. There, we instructed patients and their A-Teams in the use of diet, exercise, and supplements to fight their cancers. I've never forgotten a patient who came for an office visit shortly before one of these workshops. Tom had advanced gallbladder cancer. His family wheeled him into my consulting room on a stretcher. The whites of his eyes were yellow, his skin was green from the tumor obstruction and backup of bile into his blood, and he was so debilitated and weak it was hard for him to sit up. I took one look at Tom and knew he did not have the strength to participate in the full intensive weekend training program. But I felt he could participate in our less arduous Block Be Fit program, which we held twice each day of the workshop. At first, Tom couldn't do much at all. He stayed seated as my staff and I showed him exercises and movements he could perform while reclining. But he made continual small gains, first sitting, and then standing. By the last morning of the three-day workshop, he not only spent most of the day sitting up but was able to stand and perform an entire low-intensity exercise routine with the weekend group. In the final fitness session, to everyone's astonishment, Tom was able to complete the entire thirty-minute exercise program.

Tom's example shows how incremental increases in fitness can help you break "excessive rest syndrome" and improve performance even when you are fighting advanced cancer. Tom went on to become more active and survived more than a year after the workshop. Thanks to Tom and patients like him, I never assume that even a late-stage patient is unable to benefit from internal fitness.

The activity phase of the fitness program starts with the exercise fundamentals: good postural alignment, engagement of your core abdominal muscles, and proper breathing. These provide significant benefits and, once learned, take so little effort I hope they become second nature to you. Once the fundamentals are in place, you can begin *whole-body conditioning*. This includes lengthening your muscles by improving flexibility, strengthening muscles through resistance or weight training, increasing endurance through aerobic exercise, and practicing recovery exercise through interval training. The program should give you the resilience to derive the greatest benefit from your cancer therapy, and minimize the side effects of the disease and its treatments. You will also sleep better, have more energy, and get through your treatments more easily. I will explain the benefits of each component—in the hope of motivating you!—and then the types of exercise that can help you achieve it.

Exercise Fundamentals

▶ **Postural Alignment**
Why: Most of us have posture problems, ranging from the common post-pregnancy swayback to the hunched-over posture of

desk workers. Cancer patients may develop posture problems as a result of unconsciously "protecting" an area that has gone through surgery, or because of persistent involuntary muscle contractions or pain. Unfortunately, this typically leads to more muscle imbalances and pain.

If you are starting (or continuing) a fitness program, poor posture can make you more susceptible to injuries and keep you from getting the most benefit from an exercise. Improper alignment can also block energy flow as well as vascular and lymph circulation. It is therefore important to practice better body alignment daily: work on your posture whether you are doing a vigorous aerobic routine or standing in line at the grocery store. You'll feel taller, stronger, under control, and empowered.

Benefits

- Prevents injury during exercise

- Relieves or prevents muscle pain in back, neck, and other areas

- Improves your self-image and self-presentation

- Relieves pressure on internal organs

- Balances the muscular system

- Serves as a basis for good breathing patterns

- Improves vitality and energy

- Prevents vascular and lymphatic circulatory blockages

How: You do not have to practice good postural alignment or any other exercise fundamental at a specific time. In fact, it's better if you practice whenever you remember to, multiple times over the course of a day, so it becomes a habit. For instance, set up your work space so you can sit with good posture, especially if you work at a computer all day.

In excellent postural alignment, heels are together and toes are turned slightly outward. Your buttocks are slightly tightened and tucked under, to open the lower spine and mid-back. Your spine has a natural curve, so don't try to stand ramrod-straight; just keep your spine erect and your chest lifted. This will elongate and stretch your upper spine and neck, helping with the alignment of the chest. Your shoulders should be down and slightly back, as if you were holding a ball between your shoulder blades (but don't scrunch your shoulders back). Keep your head pulled up, with your chin pointed slightly down. Start all of your exercises and fitness techniques with good postural alignment; it will protect you from injury (especially backache) and help engage core muscles.

Pilates and yoga can help you with posture. A massage therapist or physical therapist can also help; you may also want to consult with a chiropractor.

▶ Engage Core Abdominal Muscles

Why: Abdominal muscles tighten slightly when you achieve good posture because they play a key role in supporting the body. Without them, good posture is impossible. These core muscles provide dynamic stability during exercise as well as everyday movements, and help prevent injury during exercise.[5] Too often, though, these muscles are weak from years of bad posture and neglect, or from disease. Breast cancer patients, for instance, appear to easily lose muscle from their lower trunk, the location of core muscle groups; patients with colon or other abdominal cancers suffer from disruptions to the core muscles.[6] Besides your abs, core muscles include those from the pelvis to the rib cage and surrounding the internal organs. Engaging these muscles actually massages these organs. Because initial work on the core muscles does not require much exertion, it can be a first step in self-care for cancer patients who are debilitated from treatment or disease and who feel that any exercise is beyond them, opening a door to improved quality of life and rehabilitation.

Benefits

- Improves balance and stability

- Supports good posture and alignment

- Helps with daily activities involving lifting and turning

- "Massages" the internal organs and supports digestion

- Helps with better coordination

- Prevents or alleviates back pain

- Increases confidence and functionality after abdominal surgery

---

How: You don't need to do crunches or endless sit-ups, which are likely to be counterproductive, since they bulk up the abdominal muscles rather than engage the core muscles in a way that promotes good postural alignment and other benefits. Instead, exercise systems such as Pilates and yoga are much better suited to this. (In fact, the fitness system Joseph Pilates so brilliantly designed for developing core muscles and establishing optimal alignment was initially for disabled and bedridden patients.)

Here's an exercise we teach at the Block Cancer Center that will make you aware of and engage a broad range of core muscles. It uses the muscles of the pelvic floor, which many women will be familiar with from Kegel exercises. These are the muscles you use to stop the flow of urine. Lie on your back with your knees bent and your feet flat, about hip width apart, arms by your sides. Breathe in so your rib cage expands and your spine lengthens. When you breathe out, engage your pelvic floor muscles by imagining you are trying to stop urination. When you breathe in, release these muscles. Do this three times. Next, assume the same position and breathe in, but when you breathe out think about engaging muscles deep in your core, around your abdominal organs. Eliminate the space between your lower back and the floor by pressing your lower back flat against the floor. Do this three times. Don't let your buttock muscles do this work, and don't just suck in your gut. This isn't as easy as it sounds; it takes some thinking and body awareness, but will make you more sensitive to the core muscles.

▶ **Proper Breathing**
Why: Most of us are shallow "chest breathers," taking small, frequent breaths that fill only the top of the lungs. This type of breathing is insufficient to support aerobic exercise, and results in suboptimal oxygenation of the blood. Proper breathing for vigorous activity fills the entire lung, all the way to the bottom, but without expanding your belly. It can be slow and relaxing when you are still, faster and more vigorous when you exercise. Exhale fully so you expel old air.

Benefits

- Helps oxygenate the blood, necessary for energy

- Engages abdominal muscles, which stabilize your torso

- Allows entry of new air rich in oxygen

- Offers better lung capacity and circulation

- Provides better body awareness

- Improves muscle lengthening and flexibility

How: While resting, move your diaphragm (located at the very top of your abdomen) downward and the sides of your chest outward, while your abdominal muscles keep your navel pulled up and in toward the spine. When you engage your diaphragm this way, you will feel the back and sides of your chest expand, and the breath will go all the way to the bottom of your lungs. Don't let your shoulders hunch up; that will keep the top of your chest from expanding fully. Pace your breathing to the intensity of your activity; don't overbreathe if you are doing mild activity, or you will become light-headed. Many of my patients learn proper breathing with minimal training, but Pilates is terrific for teaching it. As with postural alignment, proper breathing is not something you should practice only during some period you set aside for it. It should become second nature, something you do while walking, reading, driving, shopping . . . living!

Whole-Body Conditioning

▶ **Muscle Lengthening**
Why: Combined with proper alignment of your skeletal structure through good posture, lengthening your muscles will bring increased flexibility, greater range of motion without pain or discomfort, reduced likelihood of injuries, faster and fuller recovery from trauma, and a greater sense of comfort in your body. In addition, the same regimen that lengthens muscles also helps stretch the fascia, which are connective tissues that surround the muscles. Fascia tightened by overuse and inadequate stretching can cause myofascial pain that impedes exercise and the activities of daily living such as cooking, doing laundry, and working. If you find that pain makes it hard to exercise, you may benefit from massage focused on the fascia or on "trigger points" associated with myofascial pain.[7]

Benefits

- Improves relaxation and sleep

- Reduces tension, improves circulation and lymph flow

- Diminishes stress on other body parts

- Reduces risk of muscular injury and pain

- Improves muscular and joint flexibility

- Improves range of motion

- Increases comfort in body

How: Any activities that encourage joint flexibility, stretching, and alignment can lengthen muscles, including Pilates, yoga, and tai chi. Do lengthening/flexibility exercises every day, ideally for at least fifteen minutes straight. If you are not well enough to do this, try it three times a day for five minutes each time. As your fitness improves you should increase both the duration and the intensity of your stretching workout.

Select stretches that lengthen the muscles you use the most in your fitness routine (many training tapes include proper stretches for the exercise they feature). Yoga is an excellent system for learning a variety of stretches, as are tai chi, Pilates, qi gong, and the Block Be Fit program taught at our center. Be cautious, though, as some programs—such as more advanced yoga or Pilates—may be over-strenuous if you are just beginning. With proper alignment and breathing, you can lengthen your muscles with minimal movement, especially when you use what I call complementary opposition. For instance, you can lengthen your neck by reaching the crown of your head toward the sky, but even better is bringing your shoulder blades together and down toward the floor at the same time.

▶ Muscle Strengthening
Why: With more lean muscle mass, you will enhance immune function and be better able to carry out the activities of daily living as well as engage in exercise, sports, and leisure activities.[8] You can strengthen muscles with isometrics, calisthenics, weights, or the weight-bearing exercise known as resistance training. The goal is not to bulk up but to gain strength so your quality of life improves.

Benefits

- Increases lean muscle mass

- Improves musculoskeletal strength

- Increases the ability to perform your activities of daily living

- Improves sensory nervous system response

- Improves immune system (glutamine reservoir in skeletal muscle)

- Improves albumin levels

- Improves bone density and reduces the risk of osteoporosis[9]

How: You have a number of options here, from push-ups and calisthenics to isometrics, strenuous yoga, weight lifting, and resistance training. Whatever you choose, remember two things. First, it is important to train a variety of muscle groups, so include exercises for your back, arms, legs, and abdomen on different days to allow each group to properly recover from its workout. Second, warm up with aerobic exercise such as walking, jogging, or just gently moving your arms and legs as well as lengthening or stretching. (Winding down with stretching and lengthening, to keep muscle tension at bay, is just as important as warming up with them.) Start each new exercise with good alignment, engagement of core muscles, and proper breathing.

A comprehensive program will include eight to ten different exercises, each performed several times before you move on to the next. The number of repetitions depends on your condition. Since your goal is building internal fitness, it is more important to perform correctly and build the number of reps than to use ever-heavier weights. To start, select a weight that will let you do three to five reps with minimal fatigue. When this becomes too easy, add reps a few at a time, to eight to ten, and eventually increase the weight. If you are inexperienced in weight training, obtain some instruction first so you get the most out of it and avoid injury. The LOC website lists a number of books and tapes that have been very helpful to our patients. You can also work with a trainer or physical therapist, who can design a routine that best fits your condition and needs. If you go this route, try to find someone with experience in caring for cancer patients and the knowledge to individualize care.

Be sure to breathe with each movement. Exhale on the part

that causes you the greatest exertion, and inhale during the part that is least difficult. Our physical therapy staff encourages patients to exhale loudly through pursed lips, while inhaling slowly through the nose. Slower breathing is generally calming, while shorter, faster breathing is more energizing.

If you don't need assistance, do strengthening exercises at least fifteen minutes daily. If you are bedridden, you may need a therapist to help you move your limbs. No matter how debilitated you are, there are exercises for you: Thera-Band resistance bands (stretchy bands color-coded for levels of resistance), stability balls, small exercise balls, and resistance cords. Many of these assisted exercises can be performed lying down, utilizing the resistance provided by your own limbs or your helper or physical therapist.

► Cardiorespiratory Endurance Conditioning (Aerobic)

Why: Cardiorespiratory fitness describes the capacity of the lungs to exchange oxygen and carbon dioxide with the blood without undue fatigue, shortness of breath, or pain. One component of cardiorespiratory fitness is cardiorespiratory endurance, which is the ability to engage in physical activity for prolonged periods—and, in the case of cancer patients, to endure the battle against disease and withstand the rigors of treatments. The most immediate benefit of cardiorespiratory endurance is better cardiorespiratory functioning, which brings better oxygenation of your body's tissues. This is beneficial to everyone, but particularly to cancer patients: as I will explain in greater detail in Chapter 14, a low-oxygen environment supports the growth and spread of malignant cells, but a highly oxygenated environment deters both.[10] Another benefit of cardiorespiratory endurance to cancer patients is less likelihood of nausea while you are undergoing chemotherapy, and even improved immune function, which may reduce your risk of recurrence or improve your reach for remission.[11] In addition, improved heart and lung function may lower your risk of developing potentially fatal blood clots.[12]

Benefits

- Improves cardiorespiratory function

- Increases oxygenation of tissues, creating a less hospitable environment for cancer

- Improves peripheral circulation

- Improves movement of lymphatic fluids

- Reduces risk of deep vein thrombosis and emboli

- Improves rest

- Decreases nausea and vomiting during chemo

- Improves immune function

How: First, a note of caution. Ask your doctor whether you should have an EKG, a MUGA scan, or another test before starting endurance training, especially if you have had a difficult time with chemotherapy or other treatments. You may need to begin with interval training (below) or shorter periods of endurance training. Also consult with your doctor if you have taken any heart-damaging chemotherapy drugs (such as Adriamycin or Herceptin), have bone metastases, lymphedema, surgical adhesions, or neuropathy, or are taking hormonal or other drugs that help maintain your remission. All of these increase your risk of injury, and your doctor may recommend ways to avoid that.

Cardiorespiratory fitness is best achieved through aerobic exercise, which is continuous exercise that uses the large muscle groups and increases oxygen consumption. We find that simple walking is terrific endurance training, especially if you pick up your pace enough to feel mildly winded. But your aerobic options are almost limitless, so pick the activity that most appeals to you: walking, running, biking, stair-climbing, swimming, basketball, and tennis are just the tip of the iceberg. You can use a treadmill, stationary bike, or rebounder (a mini-trampoline). You can stand in one place doing high knee lifts, jumping jacks, or "conducting" (moving your arms to your favorite music). Aim for thirty minutes each day. If you are in fairly good shape, you should be able to do this all at once. If you are out of condition, have recently had surgery, or are a total neophyte when it comes to endurance exercise, try fifteen minutes twice daily, or as little as three to five minutes four to six times daily to start with. Breaking up sessions can restore stamina.

If you run out of ideas or get bored, aerobics classes or tapes are a good option. Unless you are experienced, don't do aerobic exercise outside in the bitter cold (it can be hard on your respiratory function), and be aware of the possibility of heatstroke or heat fatigue if you are working out in hot weather. Stay hydrated with an electrolyte-containing drink, ideally a natural fruit-juice-based one rather than a sugar-based drink.

I will cover special cases more in the following chapter, but let me mention here that an important consideration in endurance training is whether you need to prevent muscle loss or to lose excess fat. If you are losing weight or muscle involuntarily, probably because you have cachexia or a cancer of the gastrointestinal system or lungs—or have poor caloric intake—you should reduce endurance training and instead work on regaining lean muscle through the muscle-strengthening exercises described above. If, on the other hand, you have breast or prostate cancer and are overweight, your extra fat is encouraging the growth of your cancer; endurance exercises are a great way to burn calories, and increasing your proportion of lean muscle through strength training promotes weight loss because lean muscle burns calories at a higher rate than fat tissue. As a rule, if you need to lose weight, try for forty-five minutes a day or more of endurance exercise rather than thirty minutes.

Cardiac Recovery Conditioning (Interval Training)
Why: During cancer treatment, you will undergo repeated stressful events both emotionally and physically, such as

surgery and chemotherapy. One of the few ways to improve your recovery capacity is by placing yourself in a physically stressful situation, over and over, and then training your body to tackle the stress and return to its healthy baseline—for instance, returning your heart rate to normal after strenuous physical activity. This recovery time is a good index of health: a healthy heart will slow down by more than twelve beats per minute after a workout until it reaches a healthy resting rate, but an unhealthy heart will slow down only ten beats per minute or less.[13] Excessively slow heart recovery rates are associated with an approximate *doubling* of the risk of dying of heart failure,[14] according to several studies, and even from other, unrelated diseases.[15] Since heart damage is a side effect of some chemotherapy drugs, cardiac recovery conditioning is arguably even more important for cancer patients than for the general population.

Benefits

• Reduces risk of death from all causes

• Increases ability to recover from the trauma of chemo, surgery, and radiation

• Reduces fatigue

• Increases vitality and resilience

• Increases capacity to perform work

• Improves recovery of cardiac system

How: The most effective route to a healthy cardiac recovery capacity is interval training, alternating periods of aerobic activity and rest. Even if you are extremely debilitated, you can exercise gently for a few minutes, then rest for a few minutes. Interval exercise will also help increase your heart rate variability, or how much your heart rate varies from moment to moment. Perhaps surprisingly, a metronome-like regularity is not really healthy, since it reflects a heart that is less resilient and less able to cope with the changing demands. The lower your heart rate variability, the higher your risk of death from cancer, heart disease, obesity, diabetes, AIDS, multiple sclerosis, and Parkinson's disease.[16]

As long as you are in reasonably good condition, you can do recovery training with any of the exercises used for endurance training. In recovery training, you perform an aerobic workout for one to five minutes to get your heart beating much faster than usual, followed by five to ten minutes of rest. A period of activity followed by a rest is called a "set." I recommend doing five sets each day, preferably consecutively. Calculate your maximum target heart rate by first subtracting your age from 220 (for a fifty-year-old, 170 beats per minute). Your initial target rate is 50 to 60 percent of the maximum. You can gradually increase this percentage as you become more fit, but do not attempt more than 80 percent of maximum without medical consultation. Take your pulse or wear a monitor to determine your heart rate. Assess your heart rate immediately after you stop exercising, and again after resting for one minute. A decrease of 12 beats per minute or more (for instance, 102 beats to 90 beats) is optimal.

Recovery training has the virtue of being easily adaptable for patients who are in poor physical condition and who cannot undertake a regular endurance program. Patients with cachexia and those who are bedridden fall into this group. If you are bedridden, try to sit up or be propped up, and try "conducting" with your arms. If you have cachexia, for which exercise appears to be one of the few effective treatments, try to exercise for even thirty seconds, and then rest for five to ten minutes. Aim for five to eight repetitions, and try to do two of these sessions a day. Thirty seconds may seem ridiculous, but I have worked with markedly debilitated patients who saw remarkable results even with very short but frequent workouts.

Let me recap the chief benefits—the *why*—of each component of the fitness program:

I've mentioned many different types of exercise for each of

BENEFITS OF A WHOLE-BODY FITNESS PROGRAM	
Postural alignment	Reduces pain, exertion
Engage core muscles	Stabilizes and establishes balance, avoids injury, improves small muscle viability
Proper breathing	Improves vitality, quiets agitation, reduces anxiety, supports exercise
Muscle lengthening	Maintains blood and lymph circulation, improves relaxation and sleep
Muscle strengthening	Improves functional capacity and immune activity
Cardiorespiratory endurance	Improves stamina
Cardiorespiratory recovery	Bounces back from strenuous treatments

the components of whole-body fitness. As you've probably noticed, each exercise can be used for one or more. Here is a summary:

While the standard thirty minutes per day of exercise is an acceptable minimum, our recommendation for optimal whole body conditioning is sixty minutes a day. You can certainly break this into several shorter sessions if that better fits your schedule or your clinical needs. A quarter of your workout time should be spent in lengthening, a quarter in strengthening, and half in aerobics. That works out to a minimum of thirty minutes in endurance and/or recovery training, fifteen minutes strengthening, and fifteen minutes lengthening. This is a maintenance level. To improve your present condition, you may need to

TYPES OF EXERCISE AND THEIR BENEFITS

	Lengthening	Strengthening	Endurance	Recovery
Block Be Fit	X	X	½ X	½ X
Pilates	X	X	½ X	½ X
Meditative yoga	X	X		
Aerobic yoga	X	X	X	
Qi gong	X	X	½ X	
Jumping jacks		½ X	X	X
Push-ups and calisthenics		X	X	X
Weight training		X		
Thera-bands	½ X	X		
Treadmill			X	X
Stationary bike		½ X	X	X
Rebounder			X	X
Track		½ X	X	X
Stair-climbing		X	X	X
Walking			X	X
Swimming	X	X	X	½ X

spend more time. At the Block Center, we may even have a debilitated patient engage in training for as much as two hours per day broken up over several short sessions. I cannot tell you how many hospitalized patients I have motivated to work out in bed, beginning with only thirty seconds at a time once an hour, who were eventually able to get up and walk again.

This may sound counterintuitive, but as you get older I want you to spend *more* time, not less, on whole-body conditioning. The thirty-minute minimum is fine at age forty. Starting at fifty, you should work toward an hour a day. By seventy, a longer period is optimal if you can manage it, due to more rapid deconditioning. This may sound a bit overwhelming, but we decondition more rapidly as we get older, particularly if we have an illness or are undergoing treatments. Remember that many of the "exercises" lend themselves to multitasking, such as walking vigorously while you do errands, practicing muscle lengthening while you watch television, or doing recovery training by using a treadmill while reading a book. That said, keep in mind that these times are goals. If you cannot carve out an hour or more each day, just exercise as much as you can. You can incorporate additional activity into your day by making some simple changes in your routine. For example, use the stairs rather than the elevator or escalator. Park your car a distance from the door and walk the extra distance. While I have espoused the value of exercise since the early 1980s, leading experts in cancer and exercise such as Melinda Irwin, from Yale University School of Medicine, are now, as of 2008, urging the same. Exercise will become a "targeted therapy, similar to chemotherapy or hormonal therapy." Irwin said any regular physical activity—the equivalent of a thirty-minute walk five times a week—will do.[17] I agree, although I encourage you to commit to the more extensive program I outline above. Note that if you schedule exercise for the same times each day, you are more likely to stick to your program. And try to exercise outside in the sun sometimes, especially if you have sleep problems.[18] You may find that you feel so good afterward you do want to spend more time at it!

Greg: Developing Good Fitness Habits

In January 1998 Greg Gibson, a forty-three-year-old accountant, began feeling lethargic. At work, he opted for the elevator over the stairs, even though his office was on the second floor. Even household chores became a challenge. Eventually Greg got a CT scan, which showed massive swelling and inflammation in the lymph nodes throughout his abdomen and upper chest. He had lymphoma. The news left Greg and his wife quite depressed. "The statistics they presented were so dismal," his wife, Sharon, recalls. "They told us he had a 30 percent chance of survival with chemotherapy." Greg felt that his world had turned upside down. His shock and sadness quickly turned to desperation.

After combing the Internet and skimming through books on alternative cancer care, Greg opted for an alternative clinic in New York. There, the physician administered high-dose vitamin C and hydrogen peroxide. But Greg's disease did not improve. A staff member at the clinic advised him to visit us.

In the fall of 1998, Greg came to our clinic and, after an extensive workup, agreed to begin a full integrative program. We counseled him to undergo nine cycles of a chemotherapy protocol that included four drugs, classically known as CHOP. He completed this in June 1999. As Greg underwent treatment, we helped him make major changes in how he lived. Greg was a big meat-eater, so we put him on a modified version of the Treatment Support diet in Chapter 6, with emphasis on lowering his intake of animal protein while increasing his consumption of whole grains, legumes, and vegetables. We encouraged him to eat powerfoods. Greg adopted the diet enthusiastically and adhered to it faithfully.

On his first visit I told Greg that while rest is important, excessive bed rest is not something I encourage. "The more you exercise and improve your aerobic fitness," I told him, "the better you will sleep, the better your energy levels will be, and the better you're going to handle your treatments and illness." I discussed with Greg and Sharon research showing that lymphoma patients who engaged in aerobic fitness training experience much less fatigue and fewer toxic side effects from high-dose chemotherapy. Other studies of lymphoma patients have shown that exercise can lead to substantial improvements in overall well-being, as well as significant reductions in anxiety, depression, and hospitalization.[19] "Perhaps most important, improving your aerobic capacity after a cancer diagnosis reprograms your metabolism," I told Greg, "shifting it in a direction that's unfavorable to the cancer itself." Exercise can also boost the activity of the immune system's natural killer cells. In other words, the more physically active you are, the better your chances of controlling your disease.[20]

Greg leaped into our fitness program, taking up bike riding, aerobic workouts, and strength building through resistance training. The Block Center staff trained him in both yoga and qi gong while he received chemotherapy. He did experience nausea, mouth sores, and some fatigue during the treatments, but these effects were quite mild. Acupuncture helped with the nausea, and the regular aerobic workouts were essential in helping him overcome fatigue.

At first, Greg's family seemed shocked that he was able to continue exercising, even during chemo. "I was walking, biking, and practicing yoga every day, regardless of which part of the cycle I was in during treatments," Greg recalls. "I feel sure that working out helped me to tolerate my treatments. I just felt stronger every time I exercised. I couldn't have envisioned before treatment that I would be taking fitness classes with the other patients, even while we were all receiving chemotherapy infusions." Being functional made a huge difference: Greg says he felt more "normal" and less like the stereotypical patient with an advanced malignancy. Since he completed chemotherapy with us in 1999, his CT scans have remained clear of cancer. As I write this, Greg is alive and well.

Contraindications and Precautions

Cancer patients who are experiencing side effects from treatment or complications of disease may need to put off whole body conditioning work for a day or more. The table below lists the special circumstances that can affect how and whether you can exercise.

EXERCISE CONTRAINDICATIONS

- After prolonged periods of bed rest or stress, which are common if you have cancer, discuss with your physician and consider a baseline EKG before starting an exercise program.

- If you have had heart-damaging chemotherapy drugs, get rechecked with a MUGA scan (the kind used to monitor your heart during chemo) to reassess your heart's contractile strength before restarting a strenuous exercise program.

• If you have blood clots (thrombosis), heart rate irregularities, high blood pressure, emphysema, lung cancer, or asthma, have your exercise program approved by your physician and physical therapist.

• If you have an infection or fever, are taking medications to promote growth of red blood cells or white blood cells, take hormone-suppressive medications (e.g., Lupron for prostate cancer), or have abdominal bloating, diarrhea, anorexia, or vomiting (more than three times a day), you may need to temporarily stop or modify your exercise program.

• If you are taking pain medication (e.g., Hydrocodone), it may not be safe for you to exercise on a treadmill, bike, or rebounder. Walking is the better choice, possibly with some support from a friend. If you develop blurred vision or become disoriented, dizzy, or confused, do not exercise, and seek medical evaluation.

• If you become overly fatigued while exercising, stop and rest. If you become pale or have blue lips or fingernails during exercise, or if you experience joint pain, dizziness, sudden shortness of breath, sudden nausea, chest pain or tightness, or pain down the left arm, the neck, or the back, stop exercising immediately. If the symptoms recur or persist, call your physician or go to an emergency room immediately.

• If you are experiencing neuropathy, poor general health, cachexia, bone cancer or bone metastases, lymphedema, swelling, inflammation, or lack of vitality, look at the next chapter on individualization for clinical problems. If your problem is not covered, please call or e-mail us to arrange for a professional consultation (see the LOC website), or consult with your doctor or physical therapist.

• If you have significant difficulty with any functional mobility (getting in/out of bed and/or chairs, walking, climbing stairs); deficits in your strength, range of motion, balance, posture; or severe problems with fatigue and/or pain, see a physical therapist before beginning an exercise program. Have your doctor write you a prescription with the words "evaluate and treat," along with the corresponding cancer diagnosis, any complications which would impact a physical therapist's evaluation, and any specific areas to be treated.

• If you have a primary bone cancer or bone metastases, you need to avoid physical activity that places stress or impact on affected areas, because bones weakened by cancer are more likely to fracture when stressed, which is definitely something you do not want to add to your problems. You might want to seek expert advice in putting together a personalized program, something I will explore in the next chapter.

• If you are a recent (within the last eight weeks) surgical or radiotherapy patient, you may be weak, may have new scar tissue, or may have seen changes in balance or coordination. To avoid injury, practice only range-of-motion/flexibility exercises, and use only very light (1- to 3-pound) hand weights during convalescence and recovery. Consult with your surgeon about any limitations; surgical patients should have preapproval from their surgeon prior to beginning a weight/resistance program. If radiation or surgery is radical, modified radical, or extensive, get specific rehabilitation guidelines from your surgeon, radiation oncologist, or physical therapist.

Assuming that none of the clinical contraindications apply to you, and that you are able to undertake a self-directed exercise program, there are still several precautions that you should be aware of:

1. Avoid exhaustion! Don't overdo exercise, particularly early on. You may get discouraged or harm yourself. Moderate exercise is most helpful for most people.

2. If you used to exercise regularly but haven't in a while, be patient and go easy on yourself. There is every reason to believe you can regain your previous conditioning, or close to it, even with cancer. Our physical therapy staff at the Block Center has seen many patients, even those in wheelchairs or bedridden, recover so well that they can play tennis again or, in one case, climb a Colorado mountain!

3. Be aware that your sleep needs may change. Initially you may require more, but as you become more conditioned you may sleep more soundly and require less.

4. Let family and friends know that you appreciate their encouragement, but pushing you to the point of guilt and resentment if you fall short of the Jane Fonda ideal is counterproductive. With many patients, our center therapists find that the best role for a spouse to play is that of providing support and nurturing, while mild pushing is left to others. After all, you don't want the mere sight of your spouse to make you think, "I didn't exercise enough today!"

5. You may need to change your diet to fit your new activity level. If you are trying to regain lean muscle, follow the recommendations on page 131 in Chapter 6.

6. Try hard not to skip your day's exercise. Adjust your daily choice of exercises based on how you are feeling (especially around treatment days), but do not go cold turkey even if you feel weak, nauseated, or in pain. It takes only two weeks of bed rest to lose significant muscle mass and strength, and days of a sedentary lifestyle will set you back. Train and regain slowly.

Setting Up Your Conditioning Program

If you belong to a gym, health club, or fitness center, you will have easy access to exercise equipment and trainers. If you do not, or if you prefer to work out at home anyway, see about getting a treadmill, stationary bike, rebounder, step (for step aerobics), exercise balls, mat (for yoga), or graduated set of hand, wrist, and ankle weights ranging from 1 pound up to 5 or 10 pounds. If you're not ready to commit to purchasing a set of weights, you can start out by using a 15-ounce can of food as a hand weight. If you are willing to put in the time and effort, Pilates training and equipment can be of immense value. Seeing a physical therapist or illness-sensitive trainer, even episodically, can have great benefits in developing a program suited to your needs.

If you are bedridden, you will be likely to need the assistance of a helper or physical therapist. But being confined to bed is no excuse for abandoning your fitness goals. You just need to make some adjustments. You may need such devices as stability balls, small exercise balls, resistance cords, or the Theraband resistance bands mentioned in the section on muscle strengthening. (A physical therapist or trainer can help you find these; the LOC website also lists sources.) Instead of lifting weights, you should use the resistance provided by the weight of your own limbs, isometric exercises, or resistance applied by the helper or physical therapist. If you can sit up but not walk, there are exercises you can do in a chair, such as biceps curls, "walking" while seated in a chair, and standing up and sitting down.

CHAPTER 9

INDIVIDUALIZING YOUR FITNESS PROGRAM

In the preceding chapter I mentioned a few situations, such as bone cancer, being bedridden, or having just had surgery, in which the standard Life Over Cancer fitness program—specifically the four components of the whole-body conditioning program (muscle strengthening, muscle lengthening, cardiovascular endurance, and cardiovascular recovery)—need to be modified. (The exercise fundamentals—postural alignment, core-muscle engagement, and proper breathing—can be done by anyone without restriction.) In this chapter I will describe specific modifications dictated by specific clinical situations. In some cases the fitness regimen also includes recommendations on individualized diets, as described in Chapter 6.

Bill: A Remarkable Comeback

Bill Dufty was a longtime family friend and the coauthor of Billie Holiday's autobiography *Lady Sings the Blues*. In the 1970s, Bill became deeply interested in a healthful diet and lifestyle. In 1976 he married the actress Gloria Swanson, who was a passionate advocate of natural foods. After experiencing firsthand the benefits of a macrobiotic diet, Bill wrote the best-selling book *Sugar Blues,* which detailed the health hazards of sugar. In his mid-seventies, Bill developed metastatic prostate cancer and, in 1990, came to see me in our clinic. From the beginning, he resisted the idea of conventional therapy. But in time we started and were successful with various medical integrative strategies beyond the impressive diet he already followed. Unfortunately, as time moved forward his disease advanced and spread to his bones; as his bone pain worsened and his condition declined, he finally elected to give chemotherapy a chance.

To Bill's surprise, the chemotherapy drug Taxotere substantially improved his quality of life, reversing the growth of the tumors that were causing him pain and incapacitating him. Nevertheless, by this time Bill was in his early eighties, the continued treatment and advancing medical problems left him with serious muscle weakness and fatigue, and he soon found himself needing a wheelchair. This was a terrible blow to Bill, who had always cherished his mobility and independence. He became extremely gaunt and weak. "I hate to look in the mirror these days," he told our physical therapist on arriving at the clinic. "I look like a prisoner of war. Where did I go?"

Despite his despair, Bill was able to stage a remarkable comeback. He had diligently followed our core physical care program, but now it was time to make therapeutic modifications. When he arrived in the wheelchair for his chemotherapy session, our physical care team began emphasizing muscle-strength training and gentle aerobic training, including riding on a stationary bike for about twenty minutes per day. For pain management, I recommended massage, shiatsu, and acupuncture along with some natural anti-inflammatories. Within a month, Bill was able to get out of his wheelchair and, eventually, walk up to a mile daily. He regained his appetite and experienced a dramatic resurgence in his energy levels.

Bill survived for twelve years with bone metastases, eventually dying of his cancer at age eighty-six. By adhering to the modified fitness program, Bill was able to walk to the very end, something that contributed substantially to his zest for life. His ability to maintain a high level of physical and mental performance— his dizzying intellect never ceased to inspire and humble those fortunate enough to be in his presence—was remarkable even during treatment for advanced cancer. His story of rising from his wheelchair to reengage in living will always be, to me, one of the most powerful examples of life over cancer.

Custom-Fit Fitness

"Doc, my arm hurts when I do this."

"Well, don't do that!"

Individualizing a physical care program for a cancer patient is a little more complicated than this old chestnut, although it is not entirely off the mark: little good comes of a fitness approach that aggravates pain. But there's much more to tailoring an exercise program than avoiding pain. To begin with, you must be a full partner in determining what activities will work for you. If you hate swimming, it's going to do no good for me to insist that you swim twice a week. If you love tennis, it would be silly for me to insist that you switch to basketball. But tailoring to your needs goes beyond likes and dislikes. If your cancer has spread to your bones, particularly your spine, you have to avoid exercises that risk fracturing your already weak bones. Following hospitalization or a period where you have been bedridden, you must be extra careful when you resume, or start, a fitness program.

WHAT FITNESS REGIMEN DO YOU NEED?	
Condition	Fitness Regimen
Cachexia/muscle wasting/weight loss Inexplicably losing more than two pounds in one week or five pounds in one month, or debilitation after disease and treatment.	**Rebuilding Program** (including High-Intensity Nutritional Support)

Condition	Fitness Regimen
Catabolic cancer (cancer of the pancreas, ovary, stomach, colon, or lung) without significant weight loss.	**Treatment Support** (including Treatment Support diet)
Cancer treatment to reduce the size of your tumor, including chemotherapy, radiation, or surgery. (If you are taking oral therapies like tamoxifen, Aromasin [exemestane], or Evista [raloxifene] for breast cancer, hormonal therapies for prostate cancer, oral molecular target therapies or other medications given long-term, or your first chemotherapy for early breast cancer, you can use the general program outlined in Chapter 8. Use Symptom Management tips later in this chapter if you are overweight).[1]	**Treatment Support** (including Treatment Support diet)
Treatment side effects including: • Gastrointestinal problem such as nausea, diarrhea, or constipation (see dietary tips in Chapter 6 as well) • Bone metastases • Balance problems (usually with brain metastasis) • Fatigue • Breathlessness • Overweight • Neuropathy • Heart failure (heart damage from cancer treatment drugs) • Lymphedema • Pain • Anxiety and depression • Osteoporosis	**Symptom Management**

Condition	Fitness Regimen
Crisis periods caused by complications of the disease or treatment: • Low albumin • Mucositis (mouth sores) • Diarrhea • Blood clots • Low blood count • Bleeding • Elevated blood calcium • Emotional crisis (e.g., learning that your disease has progressed or recurred)	**Crisis Care**
After conventional treatment	**Post-treatment Recommendations**

The Rebuilding Program

The Rebuilding Program is aimed at cancer patients with muscle-wasting cachexia, as well as those who have become severely debilitated during the course of disease and treatment. In these cases, you need to resist the siren call of bed rest and a sedentary lifestyle. It is arguably more important for you than for healthy people to exercise properly, since regular *moderate* physical activity may reduce your susceptibility to infections, minimize the protein losses that can cripple your immune system, restore or maintain your muscle mass, and even extend your survival.[2] To this end, I have worked with bedridden patients for more than two decades, teaching them how to get back their strength and conditioning.

The Rebuilding Program focuses on building muscle, reducing inflammation, and enhancing relaxation (because the stress hormone cortisol fuels muscle loss). For building and maintaining muscle, you need resistance training through gentle workouts with small weights (isometrics, light hand weights, or

Thera-Bands) or slow weight-bearing exercise such as qi gong and tai chi. Rather than overemphasizing regular aerobic endurance training, which might burn too many calories, substitute shorter periods of walking, "conducting" (mimicking a musical conductor with your arms), or "jarming" (jogging only with your arms). Include flexibility training—stretching—before and after strength training so that you do not experience excessive muscle tension and pain. Because exercise alone is not enough to overcome cachexia or deconditioning, combine this Rebuilding Program with the dietary recommendations in Chapter 6 and the program to reduce inflammation explained in Chapter 15.

EXERCISE FOR REBUILDING

Emphasize: Strength training with small weights, in short (five-minute) sessions as able, repeated several times each day

Emphasize: Flexibility training, using therapies such as yoga, basic/beginners Pilates, qi gong, or tai chi

Adjust: Endurance training, using gentle effort or shorter interval workouts as long as this does not risk worsening the cachexia, exhaustion, or further decline. Increase caloric intake as needed.

Continue: Recovery (interval) training

Cautions: Stop exercising during infections, fevers, gastrointestinal problems, or periods of excessive fatigue, and consult your doctor

Treatment Support Program

If you have cancer, at some point you will be undergoing treatment. That may seem obvious, but because treatment can profoundly change how you feel and function, it is important to tailor exercise to your physiological status while you are undergoing treatment, as we do at the Block Center.[3] To figure out what you're up for, see which performance level best describes you:

PERFORMANCE STATUS

Performance Level	Daily Functioning
Independent	Fully active and normal to somewhat restricted in strenuous activities; can do light or sedentary work (e.g., office work)
Minimally assisted	Ambulatory and able to care for personal needs, but unable to work; up and out of bed for more than 50 percent of the day
Moderately assisted	Limited ability to care for own needs; confined to bed or chair/wheelchair for more than 50 percent of the day
Maximally assisted	Incapable of self-care, fully disabled; confined to bed or chair/wheelchair

The lower your performance level, the less intense your fitness program should be, and the more physical assistance you will need with it. If you are performing at an independent level, you can use the core exercise plan in the previous chapter, easing up on treatment days as needed and working around your treatment side effects. If you are at a minimally assisted level, reduce the intensity of your exercise so you do not become exhausted. If you are functioning at the moderately assisted level, therapists, friends, or family members will need to give you physical support as you exercise, such as helping you mount and dismount a stationary bike. If you are at the maximally assisted level, you may need a therapist to help you move your limbs, and you may be restricted to isometric exercises, in which you alternately tense and relax your muscles.

You may fluctuate between performance levels, even day to day, usually due to side effects of treatment. If you drop from functioning independently to needing assistance, don't worry, and do not abandon the fitness program: recruit the member of your A-Team charged with giving you physical assistance, and plunge into the fitness routine that suits your capabilities. Base your choice of exercise on how you are feeling, and know that whatever you are able to do comfortably is the best program for you. Adjusting your exercise program in this way allows you to continue to reap its benefits throughout treatment and recovery.

▶ **Treatment Support for Chemotherapy**
If you are undergoing chemotherapy, you are likely to be under considerable physiological stress. When this occurs, I encourage my physical therapy staff to engage my patients more in recovery training, followed by endurance training only if they are able; the latter is less suitable for some chemotherapy patients. (However, if you need to control your weight—as is particularly important for breast cancer patients, in whom weight gain can impair long-term outcome—endurance training can better help you burn calories. Alternating endurance training during periods when you feel well with recovery training when you don't can maintain fitness and a healthy level of caloric expenditure.) Recovery training will be very beneficial, training your body to manage and recover from stresses—physical as well as emotional. The aerobic stimulation of recovery training should help with fatigue, depression, and quality of life, as well as the anti-inflammatory and antioxidant enzyme responses that make your internal biochemistry hostile to malignant cells.[4]

During chemo you can also practice strength training, using either weights or Thera-Bands, to maintain muscle mass, which is important in maintaining the competence of the immune system as well as your ability to engage in daily activities. As always with strength training, adjust to your performance level and practice flexibility training, as muscles should always be stretched before and after strength training. If you do not have as much time for exercising as you would like during chemo, you can shorten your flexibility training to basic stretches and emphasize recovery and endurance training. At the risk of repeating myself, let me emphasize that chemo is no excuse to become a couch potato: doing aerobic exercise can diminish treatment toxicity, and engaging in strength training can combat both the fatigue and the decline in lean muscle that often occurs with treatment.

Finally, please look at "Contraindications and Precautions" in Chapter 8, as some apply to chemotherapy, including the cautions about heart-damaging chemo drugs, infections, and acute gastrointestinal problems.

EXERCISE DURING CHEMOTHERAPY

Emphasize: Recovery training will help counter fatigue

Adjust: Strength training to your performance level

Emphasize: Endurance training (perhaps break into ten-to-fifteen-minute periods); if you feel able, however, it's fine to continue your endurance plan, which improves treatment tolerance

Continue: Flexibility training—basic stretches should always be used after strength training; helps counter malaise

Cautions: Heart-damaging chemo drugs, infections, or severe gastrointestinal reactions make exercise difficult if not inadvisable

---

► **Treatment Support for Surgery and Radiation**

At the center, we encourage patients who are undergoing radiation or who have done so in the previous eight weeks, as well as patients who have had surgery in the previous eight weeks, to practice muscle lengthening/flexibility exercises and mild, controlled movement exercises. Examples of the latter are tai chi, qi gong, or the Block Be Fit program. After checking with your surgeon, you should probably also do strength exercises; 1- to 3-pound hand weights are also appropriate during radiation treatment and convalescence from surgery. Even if you were functioning at the independent level before your operation, during recovery you should practice a moderately assisted level of strength training for several weeks in order to give scars time to form. If surgery is radical or extensive (including modified radical mastectomy), get specific rehabilitation guidelines from your surgeon or physical therapist to avoid injury and give tissues time to heal.[5] If your surgeon doesn't mention physical therapy or exercise, request a referral to a physical therapist and a prescription for physical therapy.

While undergoing radiation therapy, you should maintain recovery or endurance activities, or cut back if needed, but don't stop them. Try moderate walking instead, which decreased fatigue in a study of prostate cancer patients.[6] You can also engage in moderate walking after surgery; consult with your surgeon about when.

SURGERY AND RADIATION EXERCISE RECOMMENDATIONS

Emphasize: Muscle lengthening/flexibility (yoga, qi gong, Block Be Fit)

Adjust: Strength training, which should be done at the moderately assisted performance level with very light hand weights

Continue: Intensive recovery and endurance; moderately intensive exercise such as walking can be done as tolerated during radiation; you may need to lighten your aerobic program after surgery, but restart as soon as possible

Cautions: Consult with your surgeon or radiation oncologist before returning to your normal exercise routine; take care around incision sites

Symptom Management

There are various clinical conditions for which I suggest modifying exercise recommendations. Some result from cancer itself, and some are side effects of treatments. If you have any of these symptoms, you will need to adjust your fitness regimen to avoid injury. In some cases, though, modifying exercise may not be enough to deal with these problems. If your symptoms persist, you—like many of my patients—may find bodywork techniques to be highly effective. *Bodywork* refers to any of a wide variety of "hands-on" techniques, such as massage therapy, neuromuscular therapies, acupuncture and acupressure, electrical stimulation, shiatsu, and others. I include explanations of the major types of bodywork at the end of this chapter.

▶ **GI Problems: Nausea, Vomiting, Diarrhea, Constipation**
Many patients find that simple walking is a good preventive for nausea. Studies show that acupuncture can help relieve vomiting during chemotherapy, and acupressure can reduce nausea during and after chemotherapy.[7] It is not too difficult to learn and apply acupressure whenever needed, but you can also use acupressure wristbands. Commercially available wristbands that stimulate the P6 acupuncture point are often used for motion sickness. They have a small button on the inside that you position on the wrist acupressure point following package directions. Tiny acupuncture needles in the ear can also help prevent nausea and can be left in place for a few days. Electrical acupuncture point stimulation devices, such as the Acuscope and similar tools, can be helpful. We have found these to be quite effective with our patients in the clinic.

If you experience severe diarrhea, you may want to avoid endurance and recovery exercise. (Be certain to maintain your fluid intake during this time so you do not become dehydrated.) You may continue with low-intensity muscle strengthening and muscle lengthening, as well as "conducting." If your diarrhea persists, you should work with your doctor or a physical therapist to determine a manageable exercise program. Again, abandoning your fitness program, even during chemotherapy, will be likely to lead to deconditioning and the risk of greater toxicity, diminished quality of life, and lower odds of survival.

While exercise has long been prescribed for constipation, there is actually little research showing that increased exercise prevents or relieves constipation. It does appear to be a side effect of bed rest, however. If you are bedridden, you may be able to relieve constipation by getting even mildly active with exercises such as "conducting" or "jarming." Abdominal massage may also be useful, as may massaging the shoulders and neck, which stimulates acupuncture points that relate to the colon.[8]

▶ **Bone Metastases**

If cancer has spread to your bones, you need to avoid any kind of impact exercises, such as those in recovery and endurance training. Check with your doctor or radiologist to assess your vulnerability for fracture and how cautious you should be. If the cancer is in your leg, hip, or pelvis, try an exercise bike or swimming rather than walking or jogging.[9] If you do keep up your walking, go at a mild or moderate pace on an even surface as long as it doesn't hurt, at which point you should switch to an exercise bike or swimming. If cancer has spread to your spine, avoid bending or twisting it, as can happen in some sports or yoga poses, as well as high-impact exercise such as running. If it hurts to walk, try swimming or an exercise bike. If the cancer has spread to your ribs, be careful with exercises that involve twisting or bending.

▶ **Balance Problems**

Brain cancer, brain metastases, or weakness and fatigue can impair your balance. In this case, you may want to start out walking with a walker, or using a stationary bike with a friend spotting you. Or simply stand up and sit down repeatedly, using an armchair for support. Some videos offer exercises you can do while seated. You can also try to improve your balance through strengthening exercises that focus on the abdominal muscles. Yoga, Pilates, qi gong, and tai chi have poses and exercises that focus on balance.

▶ **Fatigue**

Fatigue is no reason to stop exercising. To the contrary: exercise is one of the best strategies for overcoming fatigue. Be cautious and get support if needed. Emphasize recovery training, choosing whichever aerobic exercise works best for you, and do it with the timing pattern suggested for moderately or maximally assisted patients at first. You can alternate this with endurance training by walking as little as ten minutes at a time. Strength exercises, beginning with very light weights, or just climbing stairs can help your muscles develop more resistance to fatigue.

▶ **Breathlessness**
If you have lung cancer, lung metastases, or fluid in the lungs, you may experience breathlessness. A physical therapist or nurse can teach you breath-control techniques, progressive muscle relaxation, and energy conservation, any of which may help.[10] Or try yoga or Pilates, each of which teaches methods of breathing that reduce anxiety, promote full utilization of lung capacity, and open the chest.

▶ **Overweight**
Do forty-five minutes a day of endurance or recovery training, all at once or divided into two to four daily sessions. Since excess weight puts extra strain on your joints, choose exercises that will not aggravate this strain, such as walking, swimming, or using a stationary bike rather than high-impact jumping or twisting. Strength training is important if you are overweight, since it builds muscle, which burns calories at a higher rate than fat.[11] A physical therapist or trainer can teach you safe strength training.

▶ **Neuropathy**
Several chemotherapy drugs can cause neuropathy, or tingling, numbness, and pain in the hands and feet. Severe neuropathy can make it difficult to walk or run and can lead to balance problems. You should therefore limit endurance exercises to those that do not cause pain or balance difficulties. If the neuropathy is mild, walking or climbing stairs is fine, but for more severe neuropathy switch to swimming or even walking in a pool (the water holds you up if you lose your balance). Be careful not to let your hands and feet get too cold; neuropathy can decrease the ability to sense heat and cold. You can also use an exercise bike, particularly a recumbent bike, or perform seated exercises. Gentle strength training may help the function of muscles in affected areas. At the Block Center, our physical

therapists use various techniques, including an infrared "cold laser" treatment, with neuropathy patients.[12]

▶ **Heart Failure**

Herceptin (trastuzumab), which has helped many breast cancer patients, can cause heart muscle injury or even failure, as can the chemotherapy drug Adriamycin (doxorubicin). Exercise is still beneficial, but you will need to make allowances. You need to exercise the muscles of the arms, legs, and trunk in ways that do not overstress your heart, such as by muscle strengthening and lengthening. Interval training with very short exercise cycles and longer rest cycles is also effective for patients with heart failure.[13] Pedaling a stationary bike for thirty seconds and resting for three minutes, or walking on a treadmill for sixty seconds and resting for an equal time, or up to five minutes, spares the heart from overexertion while improving fitness and increasing your exercise capacity. If you can get a referral to a cardiac rehabilitation center, the staff can help you design an appropriate exercise program. A physical therapist can also recommend exercise programs.

▶ **Lymphedema**

Surgery that removes lymph nodes, usually for breast cancer, can cause a debilitating condition called lymphedema, swelling due to altered flow of lymphatic fluid. Patients with other cancers can also develop lymphedema after radiation or surgery. It used to be thought that exercise aggravates lymphedema, but that is not so. To the contrary, muscle strengthening and lengthening (especially of the arms) as well as recovery and endurance training can help. Wear a compression sleeve during such exercises, to help prevent further swelling of the affected area due to the increased fluid load that exercise sometimes causes. If you have lymphedema in the legs, moderate walking or walking in a pool is fine. Specialized lymphedema massage may help.[14] A 2007 study showed that weight loss helped reduce lymphedema in breast cancer patients.[15]

▶ **Pain**

Massage, acupuncture, and acupressure can help alleviate pain, as can yoga, especially if the pain involves tension or imbalance in the muscles due to surgery, stress, or anxiety. Selected yoga and Pilates techniques, with coaching by a well-trained expert, can often provide relief.

▶ **Anxiety**

Yoga, massage, and other bodywork therapies can reduce anxiety, stress, fatigue, and depression.[16] Yoga teaches breathing techniques that can defuse anxiety. Many patients find that endurance and recovery exercises let them blow off steam, reduce anxiety, and improve sleep, itself a good way to combat anxiety.

▶ **Osteoporosis**

Aromatase inhibitors such as Arimidex (anastrozole), Femara (letrozole), and Aromasin (exemestane), given for breast cancer, decrease estrogen levels and so can increase the risk of osteoporosis. To counter that, breast cancer patients taking these drugs should emphasize weight-bearing exercise, such as walking or weight training, and include 1,200–1,500 mg a day of calcium and at least 400–800 IU daily of vitamin D.[17] Ask your doctor about bone density tests to check how you are doing. Prostate cancer patients taking hormonal drugs such as Lupron (leuprolide) and Zoladex (goserelin) face similar risks and should adopt the same exercise and diet or supplement regimen.

Crisis Care

If you suddenly develop an infection, a fever, or a severe gastrointestinal problem, you should consult your doctor. But once the situation resolves, you can do your daily exercise as a recovery program by breaking up your session into five to six short periods of two to five minutes each, with substantial rest periods in between, rather than a continuous half hour. If you can, try to get in five to fifteen minutes of strength training even during a crisis period, though do not push yourself to the point of exhaustion. Consult with your doctor to be sure there are no contraindications to such activity.

CRISIS CARE RECOMMENDATIONS

Continue: Strength training, in five-to-fifteen-minute sessions

Adjust: Recovery training, using timing and intensity appropriate to the moderately or maximally assisted levels as necessary

Emphasize: Flexibility training, but don't overstretch vulnerable areas affected by the crisis (e.g., a leg clot)

Adjust: Endurance training but don't push toward exhaustion

Cautions: Stop exercising during infections, fevers, gastrointestinal problems, or cases of excessive fatigue and consult your doctor; excessive fatigue should be evaluated to determine whether fitness and conditioning should be held off or pursued with caution. A physical therapy consult may be needed

After Conventional Treatment

As you may recall from Chapter 7, exercise can fight cancer in several ways, including controlling weight and body composition, reducing levels of growth factors, and increasing anti-inflammatory molecules. Once you have completed conventional treatment and are, I hope, in remission, you will be ready to go full speed ahead with circadian fitness. This will decrease your risk of recurrence and make exercise an integral part of your life. If you finished conventional treatment in a debilitated state, get your doctor's go-ahead before starting endurance training; an EKG or another test may be necessary. You can start with ten-to-fifteen-minute sessions, working toward at least thirty minutes. I do often recommend recovery training during such vulnerable periods. By pushing hard with intervals of aerobic training for only one to five minutes with five to ten minutes of rest in between, you can rebuild your vitality and overall condition more rapidly than by following an endurance plan (a longer period of milder aerobics). Check your performance level, as described above, to see whether you can graduate to a more challenging level.

This is also an excellent time to work on maintaining a healthy weight and losing excess fat. This is especially so for breast cancer patients, since being overweight and sedentary raises your risk of recurrence.[18] To lose weight, you should do endurance training for forty-five to sixty minutes each day, as long as you are able. This need not be done all at once; two or three shorter sessions are also useful. Strength training to maintain and increase muscle mass can help you lose weight, since muscle burns more calories than fat. Flexibility training is always important, so your muscles remain loose and you avoid injury. Rigid musculature can also reduce vitality. The first year after completing conventional treatment is when you should really commit to working on every aspect of circadian fitness.

POST-TREATMENT RECOMMENDATIONS

Emphasize: Endurance training, working toward ideal body weight (especially for breast and prostate cancer patients)

Emphasize: Finding an exercise program that is personally sustainable and gratifying; endurance and flexibility are excellent strategies to reduce recurrence risk

Continue: Recovery aerobics training, as needed

Caution: Ask your doctor if you should have an EKG before beginning or advancing your exercise program; make sure your instructors or trainers are properly certified; vary strength and endurance exercise to avoid overtraining and boredom

---

In the second year after conventional treatment, work out an exercise program that can help keep your cancer in check for the long term. If you are overweight or have trouble controlling your weight, keep up the endurance and strength components in particular. If you are over fifty, remember that strength training is crucial to combating the decline in muscle mass that accompanies aging. Since doing the same exercise routine month in and month out can be boring—and is a main reason people stop working out—try varying your routine by working with a trainer, taking classes, using exercise videos, or taking up a new routine.

Bodywork Techniques: A Summary

Several therapies classified as bodywork have provided much relief of pain and anxiety to cancer patients. You can consider them as another type of support to your physical care program. They may be especially helpful in symptom management.

▶ **Asian Systems**
In traditional Chinese medicine, chi (or qi), the vital energy of life, courses through the body in a set of channels, called meridians. These are conceptually similar to blood vessels but are not actual physical organs; you will not find them on Western anatomy charts. In Western terms, they may correspond to areas of variation in the body's electrical resistance. According to Chinese tradition, illness arises when the energy in these channels becomes blocked. Treating the illness therefore requires manipulating the meridians at particular points—the acupuncture points. Stimulation can be by needles or strong manual pressure, among other techniques. Shiatsu massage is particularly useful for stimulating the points, while qi gong and tai chi stimulate the flow of energy through the meridians. While these systems are difficult to understand from a Western viewpoint, many patients have found relief through traditional Chinese exercise and treatment systems.[19]

Another important medicine system is Ayurveda, the traditional medicine system of India. The bodywork system that evolved in Ayurveda is yoga, which we frequently recommend at the center both for flexibility training and as a mind-spirit tool, since it promotes meditation and relaxation. Several forms of yoga can be very strengthening. A system called Acu-Yoga combines yoga and acupressure techniques.

▶ **Pilates**
This system was developed nearly seventy years ago by Joseph H. Pilates. It focuses on building strength and flexibility and engaging both the body and the mind in fitness. It is the most effective system I have seen for building core muscles and developing the capacity for internal organ massage. Originally a fitness system for the weak and debilitated, it is ideal for recovering one's health. Pilates uses special apparatuses to build strength and develop sensitivity to the use of different muscle systems. By training the smaller abdominal and spinal muscles, the larger muscles can relax more. This can be helpful for reducing pain and spasms. From those who are bedridden to high-performance athletes, this program comes close to being a comprehensive and complete fitness program.

▶ **Meridian Stretching**
This system, also known as resistive stretching, redefines flexibility by addressing the strength of muscles throughout their full range of motion. It is based on two unique concepts. A muscle is strengthened by contracting through an entire stretch, and the strength is proportional to its degree of flexibility. By repeated strengthening through stretching, muscle fibers and entire sections of muscles are activated. Along with relieving tension, meridian stretching can cause body, mind, and emotional shifts, promoting overall health.

▶ **Aromatherapy**
Aromatherapy is the use of essential oils extracted from plants. These oils, the concentrated extracts of the plants' fragrance-bearing compounds, are typically applied in massage. They may affect the body through interaction with the skin or through inhalation, as in the use of pillows filled with lavender to promote sleep. Many cancer patients find some aromatherapy oils comforting and others energizing. But chemotherapy patients, who are often sensitive to smells, are sometimes disturbed by

aromatherapy oils. If you are undergoing chemo, you may need to experiment with different oils to see which you prefer.

▶ **Hydrotherapy**
Warm water can be relaxing, and taking baths may reduce pain. Immune-suppressed cancer patients need to be careful when using spas and other types of water therapies, however, since if poorly maintained they can harbor infectious organisms. If you are immune-suppressed from chemotherapy or radiation or are recovering from surgery, you should avoid spas, baths, or hot tubs open to the public or frequently used even by family and friends.

▶ **Massage**
A clinical massage therapist, rather than a massage therapist who specializes in relaxation-oriented massage at a spa, can show you basic types of self-massage to relieve muscle tension and pain. If you do self-massage, be sure to stay at least eight to twelve inches away from any tumor, because theoretically, direct massage to a tumor may encourage metastasis by stimulating growth signaling. (Massage in other areas of the body is not likely to promote metastasis and to date no research suggests a problem.) Deep therapeutic massage can help reduce pain and improve the well-being of bedridden patients in particular.

▶ **Saunas**
Saunas may provide some immune stimulation effects. Saunas raise the internal temperature of the body, as fevers do. Fevers trigger an activation of the immune system that may be relevant to helping suppress cancers, an effect used in hyperthermia as a cancer treatment.[20] Some studies have shown that artificially raising the temperature of the body results in activation of monocytes (immune cells)[21] or release of proteins associated with fevers (acute-phase proteins such as transferrin).[22] Saunas are used for promoting health in many countries; their effects include pain relief and relaxation. Research shows that they are generally safe for people accustomed to them, but there are concerns for people who have cardiovascular problems and those

who are unaccustomed to saunas, as well as those who have issues with potential infection and dehydration.[23] You should
also be cautious if you experience exhaustion or excessive
weakness. All users of saunas should make sure they are properly hydrated. While much research is needed, saunas may provide a heat-induced physiological change that may affect the
response to chemotherapy. Infrared saunas have been the subject of recent research in Japan showing health benefits in various conditions.[24] Compared to regular saunas they may better
increase core temperature and dendritic cell signaling to activate immune function.

► **Physical Therapy/Trainers**
A visit to a physical therapist is a must if you have severe problems with mobility, balance, range of motion, pain, or fatigue.
For that reason, we include physical therapy at our center, in order to provide consultations to people with these problems as
well as help other patients design exercise routines most suited
to their condition, needs, and schedule, training them in different exercises (even simple strength training should be done right
so you do not injure your muscles), and monitoring their
progress. A physical therapist who has specific skills in working
with patients who have more advanced cancers can design an
appropriate exercise regimen if you have a disability related to
cancer.

CHAPTER 10

MIND AND SPIRIT CARE: THE RATIONALE

Like an earthquake that strikes without warning, the simple words "You have cancer" can fracture your world and leave you dazed, confused, and even breathless from shock. Being stunned, terrified, incensed, incredulous, overwhelmed, bereft, or just plain numb—these are all normal reactions to receiving a diagnosis of cancer or to news that your cancer is progressing or that it has recurred. Don't let anyone tell you otherwise. Feeling depressed because of the profound changes that cancer makes in your life, worrying about treatments, or feeling angry about how your illness has upended your life are all very common among cancer patients—and all normal and understandable reactions. Indeed, surveys find that up to 50 percent of cancer patients experience symptoms of depression—and this does not include other forms of distress like anxiety.[1] But be reassured that you can feel joy and hope again. This chapter will give you tools that can enhance your inner resources, restore your emotional and psychological equilibrium, enable you to hang on to some measure of inner strength and serenity even when the going gets tough, and help you reengage in your life with vigor and vitality.

The feelings of depression, shock, and fear may seem to lie solely in the psychological or emotional realm, but the tools I offer in the next three chapters address something physiological as well: the stress response. Being diagnosed with cancer can trigger the same acute reactions as being accosted by an armed man in a dark alley. The muscles in your neck, shoulders, and back tighten. Your heart races. Your breathing becomes shallow and more rapid. This reinforces the message that there is indeed a reason to be on high alert. And the brain responds. It releases neurotransmitters (brain chemicals) through the hypothalamus-pituitary-adrenal axis that instructs the pituitary and adrenal glands to release a variety of stress hormones, called corticosteroids and catecholamines (whose cancer impact is explained in Chapter 19). These hormones are behind the fight-or-flight response, which is useful with transitory stressors such as that guy in the alley, but not so good when the source of the stress is an underlying illness that may be with you for years. In this case, the stress response begets chronic anxiety and distress, accompanied by a slew of biochemical changes that ultimately contribute to the cancer's ability to thrive in you. Among these stress-related shifts in biochemistry are excessively high levels of certain growth factors, free radicals, blood sugar, inflammatory cytokines, and immune-suppressive factors.

My wife, Penny, studied the perception of cancer among recently diagnosed patients for her University of Chicago dissertation.[2] Her analysis of in-depth interviews with twenty cancer patients revealed five common themes that can underlie the overwhelming reaction to a cancer diagnosis. (1) Patients feel stunned by what seems an invisible invasion by a hostile alien. (2) Cancer can activate a profound sense of uncertainty and vulnerability. (3) It triggers a keen awareness of death even if not imminent. (4) Former assumptions about life's predictability and normalcy seem permanently shattered. (5) Cancer represents not just a biological fact or diagnostic category but a challenging personal saga which unfolds as each patient enters the roller coaster of their cancer journey.

The Life Over Cancer mind-spirit strategies can help you manage disturbing emotions, reduce symptoms of depression and anxiety, and gain control over your stress hormones. Just as the brain triggers the stress hormone cascade, so the mind can turn it off. You *can* learn to relax and maintain equanimity. You *can* find a way to not just survive but enjoy life and experience peace and fulfillment.

This would be reason enough to master the mind-spirit strategies, but there are others. First, by reining in the growth factors, immune-suppressing biochemicals, and other compounds that chronic stress floods your body with, you can help improve your chances of beating cancer.[3] One, your mind-set will affect whether you pursue the best cancer treatments and stick with them; whether you are aggressive in gathering information on promising experimental, off-label, and integrative therapies; and whether you can maintain your commitment to cancer-fighting nutrition and fitness. Two, someone who feels hopeless or frantic is unlikely to pull this off. If you think, "There's nothing I can do," it can become a self-fulfilling prophecy. In that sense, your state of mind can be your own worst enemy. But it can also be your greatest ally. How you think, feel, react, and behave in response to having cancer affects your recovery.

However, let me note that if you try the techniques outlined in these chapters but still suffer from persistent depression or anxiety, please find professional assistance, especially if you have had past episodes of clinical depression or anxiety.

This chapter will look at the compelling scientific basis for the techniques we teach patients to manage and overcome stress. To start, let's dispel four myths that can impede your recovery from cancer.

Mind Myths

▶ **Myth #1: "Maintain a Positive Attitude"**
If you're like many cancer patients, well-meaning friends or family members have insisted that "you have to keep a positive attitude." Television talk shows, news programs, and magazines regularly deliver the same message. Yet this notion, which can feel like a moral imperative, is a distortion of the idea that the mind can influence cancer. While your mind can affect your recovery, reducing complex mind-body connections to the command to "think positive" is misleading and injurious.

For one thing, it's not scientifically accurate. Data do not support the simplistic notion that a positive attitude is a key to getting well. Instead, accepting the flux of emotions and learning how to manage them is healthier than trying to deny them. In one study of patients with a recurrence of breast cancer, for instance, scientists found that restricting the expression of difficult emotions was actually associated with *shorter* survival.[4]

Worse, perhaps, is that this misguided worship of a positive attitude can produce a blame-the-victim mentality. The flip side of "Be positive and you're more likely to extend your survival," of course, is that if you experience recurrences and other setbacks, then you might mistakenly assume it must be your fault for not maintaining a positive attitude. We have seen time and again how pernicious this is for patients. They mistakenly believe that if they let their optimism flag for one day, even though distress and depression are perfectly normal responses to cancer, they may doom themselves. This is factually incorrect: while your actions may help prolong your life or reduce your risk of recurrence, there are innumerable factors that are outside your control, including your genetic background and the inadequacies of conventional treatment. We don't always know why some people with cancer do better than others, and to blame your normal feelings for any setbacks (or for having cancer in the first place, or for "failing" chemotherapy as some people do) is wildly off the mark.[5]

Plus, hiding your emotions this way is the *opposite* of health-promoting. Squelching unpleasant thoughts and pasting on a smiley face means you do not work through emotional upset; you just try to ignore it. You can't develop effective tools for coping with stress unless you acknowledge emotional unrest. Contrary to popular belief, distress tends to grow rather than shrink when you try to deny its existence.[6] Further, if you smother negative emotions, you will inadvertently blunt positive ones. Emotional anesthesia is not selective.

The one kernel of truth in the "positive attitude" message is that hope and determination (quite different from forced positivity) may be healing. Genuine hope—the belief in the possible in the face of uncertainty, as Penny defines it—supports your resolve to get the best medical treatment and adopt psychological, nutritional, and fitness programs. It can also keep you on track when waning energy slows you down. Hopelessness, on the other hand, may augur shorter survival.[7]

Denise: Keeping the Lid On

A vibrant forty-year-old who was diagnosed with colon cancer, Denise was so nervous about acknowledging fear—as if doing so magnified her disease—that she outlawed the word and all its synonyms. If she so much as said she was afraid, she felt, then her condition must truly be fearsome; if she didn't, it couldn't be so ominous. She forbade her husband, two school-age children, and friends to voice any concern or worry. The result, as you might guess, was that everyone tiptoed around their true feelings and felt stiff and disconnected. Denise herself found "keeping the lid on," as she put it, exhausting. Never troubled before by insomnia, she now suffered restless nights, stuck in ruminations she could neither halt nor admit. The irony for Denise was that the more she insisted on banishing her fears, the larger they grew.

It took several months, numerous conversations, and two sessions on mind-spirit strategies before Denise was able to admit the futility of her obsession with maintaining a positive attitude. After counseling with our mind-spirit team, she and her husband sat down to a difficult but honest conversation about how they felt about Denise's cancer. The wall between them melted away.

▶ **Myth #2: "Statistics Say My Situation Is Hopeless"**
It's difficult enough to handle the news that you have cancer. But it's crushing to be told you have only a few months to live. As I said in Chapter 1, such statements are misleading and, coming from the lips of experts, injurious. I can't say this emphatically enough: it is wrongheaded, misguided, and worse for physicians to extrapolate from population data to an individual patient.

What is the basis for such statements? In studies of, say, a thousand patients with cancer X, some percentage—say, 35 percent—are alive after a year. This translates into the statement that *you,* an individual cancer patient, have a 35 percent chance of surviving one year. Or perhaps a study shows that the median survival with cancer X is eight months, which leads a doctor to tell you that you have eight months to live.

But statistics do not apply to any individual patient. A median means that half of patients live *longer* than eight months. And there is no way to tell who will be in which half—the half that lives longer than the median or the half that lives less than the median. Nor is there any way to tell who will be in the 35 percent who live longer than a year. I reiterate what I said in Chapter 1: such statistics have little relevance to you, a unique human being. It is not only cruel to tell someone she will die in six months, it is also factually unjustified.

Our center staff members have sat with many patients who have despaired after receiving the "you have less than a year" pronouncement. This statement can trigger a biology of death. Many acknowledged giving up after hearing such news and then choosing not to have treatments that may have improved and extended their life. In this way such pronouncements can be prophetic. If being told you have less than a year to live adversely shifts your biology, or makes you walk away from treatment, it's a good bet the doctor will turn out to be right. Yet a surprising number of patients who received such "death sentences" are alive and active years later. Especially if you adopt the full panoply of cancer-fighting dietary, fitness, medical, and mind-spirit strategies, *you may be one of the survivors.* If your doctor gives you a shocking prognosis—and many patients report this to me—you may need to tell him or her, "That is a population statistic, but you can't know how things will turn out for me." And then go ahead and commit yourself to a full Life Over Cancer program.

Consider one fascinating study of patients with metastatic cancers classified as "medically incurable." Some were highly involved in a program of self-healing practices; the others were not. The first group lived significantly longer than what an expert panel of oncologists had predicted. Although this was a small study of twenty-two patients, it suggests how important it is to look beyond the statistics and throw yourself into a comprehensive cancer-fighting regimen.[8]

▶ Myth #3: "Don't Delay, Decide Today"

Aside from saying yes or no to a very few emergency treatments or urgent surgical procedures, you will rarely have to make an instant, on-the-spot decision. Give yourself time to assemble and mull over information with your A-Team and consider additional opinions. It's hard to make critical decisions when stunned by the news of your diagnosis.

If you're being prodded by specialists to undergo a major procedure immediately, you may feel so agitated by their insistence that you can't focus. Consider taking time to calm, refocus, and reenergize yourself before you sit down to evaluate therapies and plan your strategy. Other than true emergencies, I have yet to see a patient for whom waiting a few extra days, a week, or even two or three before making an important decision jeopardized his or her chances of recovery and survival. However, if you have any bleeding, are experiencing shortness of breath, or have any of the other symptoms described in the list of medical emergencies in Chapter 21, your doctor is quite correct to urge immediate action, and you should heed his or her advice.

▶ Myth #4: "My Psychology Is Separate from My Medical Regimen"

Scientists who study mind-body medicine have in recent years put the brain into the equation—that is, they have worked out the intricate connections by which a thought or emotion in one region of the brain excites neuronal circuits that connect to the immune system, the gastrointestinal tract, and other parts of the body. Excessive and uncontrolled distress affects immune factors, stress hormones, and inflammation, all of which may affect the course of your cancer and of your recovery. Emotional distress can lead to a surge of inflammatory chemicals, which support the deadly process of metastasis. Unrelieved stress can also lead to elevated insulin levels, which can promote the growth of a number of tumor types.[9] (I address such biochemical aspects of stress in Chapter 19.) Please remember, though, that "staying positive" is not the best way to cope with the inevitable stress and distress of having cancer, and that despite their biological effects, your natural emotional reactions to disease are far from being the only reason that you may have experienced setbacks.

The assertion that *uncontrolled,* chronic emotional distress can contribute to cancer's growth and spread may sound simplistic in the case of advanced cancers, whose aggressiveness is probably the determining factor in progression. Nonetheless, every possible factor influencing the progression of cancer should be explored when you are fighting for your survival. I have seen time after time the difference it makes.

Mind-Spirit Care and Your Cancer

Mind-spirit techniques are one of the core therapies at our center, not a side note as in many other oncology practices. We feel these techniques are essential to helping our patients battle their cancer. The effect of your mind on your body can be helpful or hostile to cancer cells, help you tolerate treatments or make you more susceptible to its side effects, make you more responsive to chemotherapy or less. Learning to harness the extraordinary power of your mind and spirit can therefore be just the thing that gives you the survivor's edge. That's what the Life Over Cancer model is all about: chipping away at every vulnerability in the cancer with everything from conventional treatment to diet, tailored supplementation, fitness regimens, and mind-spirit techniques. After I have discussed what effects your mind can have on your disease and its course, I hope you will be sufficiently convinced to adopt the techniques I will introduce at the end of the chapter.

▶ **Cancer Growth**
Much as we might like it to happen, your mind and spirit will not directly attack malignancies. Wishing will not make it so.

But psychological factors can exert a potent *indirect* influence on the growth and spread of cancer because emotional states and coping style affect your internal biochemistry, even molecular factors, and the state of your immune system.[10] Plus, chronic, unrelieved distress can negatively alter the growth factor activity and cell signaling that are instrumental in metastasis.[11] The immune connection is captured in the tongue-twister *psychoneuroimmunology:* your psyche (mind) manifests itself in patterns of neuronal activity that affect your immune system.[12] The rapidly evolving field of mind-body science has discovered that our immune defenses and hormonal responses are partly regulated by the brain and the chemicals it produces. This is why breast cancer patients suffering from high levels of emotional stress experienced a 15 percent reduction in the activity of the immune system's natural killer (NK) cells, as one study showed, and why cancer patients who suffered unrelieved anxiety had significantly lower NK activity than patients who had tamed their anxiety.[13] NK cells act like a biological Pac-Man, gobbling up tumor cells in the bloodstream so they do not form metastases.[14] (I'll discuss NK cells more in Chapter 16.) You don't want these cells to be lying down on the job: decreased activity of natural killer cells is correlated with cancer spread and growth in tumor size. Lowering stress levels through social support, though, may improve NK function.[15] In a 1999 review of nineteen studies, high levels of social support—especially when the cancer patient viewed it as dependable and beneficial—were linked with a greater ability of natural killer cells to eliminate cancer cells.[16] Similarly, practicing progressive muscle relaxation (described later in this chapter) for one month increased the activity of natural killer cells by 30 percent.[17]

Stress has another direct effect on the progression of cancer. A substance called VEGF—vascular endothelial growth factor—stimulates the new blood vessels needed for tumors to grow and spread. Ovarian cancer patients who experienced more intense distress had higher VEGF levels than patients who felt they were coping better with their disease, thanks to high levels of social support according to a 2003 study. Stress, concluded the scientists, can "directly contribute to the progression of ovarian tumors."[18]

▶ **Treatment Side Effects**

Experts have estimated that approximately one-third of cancer patients bolt from chemotherapy prematurely because the physical and psychological distress makes the treatment unendurable.[19] Stopping chemo before you have a full course decreases your chance of going into remission.[20] Several other factors certainly influence whether you can stick with chemo, but I want to focus on one you can do something about.[21]

We usually think of controlling the side effects of drugs with more drugs, but mind-spirit techniques can be an effective and safe addition. Nausea and vomiting, among the most feared side effects of chemotherapy, are generally countered with drugs. But progressive muscle relaxation plus guided imagery has been shown to be more effective than antiemetics alone in controlling how often and for how long patients suffered severe nausea and vomiting.[22] Mind-spirit techniques can also control anticipatory nausea, in which you feel nauseated before you start receiving chemo.[23] That's not surprising, since anticipatory nausea originates in the mind, which learns to associate environmental cues such as the sight and smell of the chemo unit with feelings of nausea. Hypnosis, for instance, just about eliminated anticipatory nausea and vomiting in one group of patients in a 2000 study published in the journal *Oncology*. Systematic desensitization, a technique I will explain in Chapter 11, has also effectively curbed anticipatory nausea. Relaxation strategies and focused imagery had similar benefits.[24]

▶ **Quality of Life**

It is a sorry reality of modern cancer care that far too many patients silently endure serious impairment in their quality of living. Huge numbers of people are uncomfortable acknowledging their emotional unrest, and doctors are not very good at detecting it (or assume distress is inevitable with cancer and pay no attention to it).[25] For this reason, at the Block Center we use validated quality-of-life and well-being questionnaires to identify what each patient may be grappling with and how we can provide tools that match their needs. A number of mind-spirit strategies, both group and individual, can alleviate emotional issues triggered by cancer or its treatment. A combination of relaxation and imagery has reduced stress among breast cancer patients undergoing radiotherapy, and psychosocial programs have improved patients' ability to cope with unfamiliar and complex cancer issues, eased emotional distress and feelings of isolation, and enhanced physical functioning.[26] For instance, a ten-week stress management program using cognitive-behavioral techniques reduced the stress hormone cortisol and improved emotional well-being in women with early-stage breast cancer, according to a 2004 study.[27] A study first presented in 2007 found that quality of life, especially as it relates to social support, isolation, and help in coping with daily needs, significantly affected survival in lung cancer patients—a cogent reminder that your A-Team is powerful medicine in coping with cancer.[28]

▶ **Averting Serious Complications**
I still remember the astonished expression of a young woman who heard me say at a public lecture that "people don't generally die from cancer; they die from the consequences of cancer." Infectious disease, primarily pneumonia and sepsis, is a major cause of death among cancer patients. Emotional stress can make you more vulnerable to infectious diseases, particularly if you have received conventional treatments that compromise immune resistance to viral and bacterial pathogens.

The immune system can be compromised by acute threat, unrelenting personal difficulty, mild but persistent depression, and painful life disruptions.[29] Fortunately, certain mind-spirit techniques—structured relaxation practice, social support enhancement, and a process called Expressive Writing—can help restore some of the body's defenses.[30] Such practices can increase total lymphocytes and helper T cells, which guard against and fight infections.

Putting Together a Mind-Spirit Program

As this brief tour of the science shows, mind-spirit interventions have a lot to offer cancer patients. But how do you pick an intervention? Drawing on clinical experience, we have formulated the Life Over Cancer mind-spirit program based on what we call the five R's:

1. Recovering calm and creating emotional ease
2. Reestablishing balance
3. Reconnecting: support and social connectedness
4. Restoring control of symptom and side effect management
5. Revitalizing your life, bettering your circumstances

Each step is associated with particular problems cancer patients face, and each has specific mind-spirit interventions associated with it. I'll review these here, present the core program and basic techniques in Chapter 11, and discuss how to tailor the program to specific needs in Chapter 12.

▶ **Recovering Calm and Creating Emotional Ease**
The strategies for recovering calm are the most basic of all the mind-spirit methods. You will call on techniques such as relaxed abdominal breathing, progressive muscle relaxation, and comfort space imagery again and again as you deal with the ups and downs of cancer—helping you prepare for procedures like a repeat mammogram, helping you feel relaxed while you're lying on a table receiving radiation treatment and surrounded by intimidating machines, or helping you cope with the news of a possible cancer recurrence or tumor progression.[31] The techniques that help you recover calm can also counteract anticipatory nausea. In a 2005 study, for instance, breast cancer chemotherapy patients who were trained in progressive muscle relaxation with guided imagery had less anticipatory nausea and vomiting, less post-chemo nausea and vomiting, less anxiety, less depression, and less hostility than control patients.[32]

▶ **Reestablishing Balance**

A diagnosis of cancer brings almost daily emotional minefields. Every ache or pain makes you wonder, "Is this a sign of cancer spread?" The toll cancer takes on career and family life makes you worry that you won't make it financially and personally. The side effects of treatment make you wonder if it's worth the suffering. You may lie awake worrying that your cancer will recur or that your spouse might be repulsed by the aftermath of disfiguring surgery.

A number of techniques for regaining equilibrium can help you with these challenges. Using Expressive Writing, you can pour out your thoughts and emotions in complete privacy. Another technique will let you recognize "thought warps," self-defeating thinking that needlessly stirs painful feelings, and help you learn to reframe these thoughts so they reflect a more positive reality. Reimaging can transform frightening images, turning an impression of dangerous X-rays blasting you to an image of healing light. Examining your life systematically for sources of satisfaction and dissatisfaction can help you shift the balance toward the former.

The equilibrium techniques we teach patients are meant to complement something that many doctors (and society at large) disparage: denial. When you face a daunting diagnosis, it's human nature to try to escape implications. My patients say things like, "I feel fine, so it can't be all that serious," "It's just another lump, nothing to worry about," "The doctors think they got it all," and "Doctors do make mistakes. Maybe the diagnosis was wrong." Downplaying the gravity of bad news is one way we adapt, a natural strategy for holding it together in the face of adversity. And despite its bad press, adaptive denial can yield benefits initially, helping curb anxiety and making it possible for you to stay engaged in everyday activities and routines. Denial—at least as a stopgap measure that does not lead to avoiding needed treatment—is nothing to be shunned.

For instance, adaptive denial helps us generate "positive illusions."[33] A man with metastatic colon cancer once told me, "Since the PET scans indicate the tumors in my liver aren't actively growing, I think I'll just keep doing what I'm doing. If I do that, maybe I can stop them from ever growing again." This view about containing disease, with a treatment plan in place, is not completely implausible. Moreover, it's a positive way to frame a challenging situation, since patients are usually told that cancer that has spread to the liver has a poor prognosis. I was gratified that this individual chose *not* to focus on the statistics for his condition; people who do so often end up feeling overwhelmed with anxiety and succumbing to despair.

Let me offer you a more detailed example of healthy illusions. Barbara had suffered from fibroid tumors for many years. When she was diagnosed with ovarian cancer, she at first framed it as simply another fibroid that she had to eliminate. "I have gone through this before," she said. "I'm not going to freak about a tiny clump of strange cells. There are probably too few to amount to anything. Life goes on, you know? I've lived forty healthy years and I'm looking forward to another forty."

Barbara's denial of some hard truths about ovarian cancer— her ability to avoid catastrophic thinking—was a form of adaptive reasoning, also called cognitive reframing, that provided her with a desperately needed emotional buffer. Shielding herself from alarming information probably saved Barbara from lapsing into depression, which not only is destructive psychologically but can shift the body's biochemistry toward an immune-suppressive and tumor-promoting state. As long as you do not let the idea of having only "a few strange cells" keep you from making the changes in lifestyle and undergoing the aggressive medical and integrative treatments needed to battle cancer, there is nothing wrong—and a lot right—with adaptive denial. That's why our mind-spirit team confirms what I emphasize: that it's unfair to force recently diagnosed patients to confront the worst they may be facing. If you want to use adaptive denial as a temporary mechanism to cope with shock—saying things such as "I can't talk about this right now" or "I don't believe this is serious"—do so, while you regain the calm you need to sort out treatment options. I hope you can use the information here to ask loved ones or health care personnel to respect your pace in dealing with fears or despair. I do encourage you, though, not to hesitate to express and work through any distress you may feel when the time is right for you.

Positive illusions can help you manage the early onslaught and return to a new equilibrium. Once you achieve that equilibrium, I hope you will be able to move ahead to more productive methods, including those I describe in the next two chapters.

▶ **Reconnecting: Support and Social Connectedness**
Support groups are a fixture on the cancer landscape. Most hospitals offer them, a welcome change from the situation three decades ago, when cancer patients often did not even want to reveal their illness, much less discuss it with others. But do these groups merely provide feel-good experiences that help lower anxiety, or even cause more distress, or can they actually help transform the biological milieu that fosters healing? Can participating in a support group improve your chance of surviving cancer?

By my reading of the scientific literature, the answer is both a qualified yes and no.[34] When scientists assigned, at random, some cancer patients to support groups and not others, the results have been mixed. In five studies—of patients with breast cancer, malignant melanoma, lymphoma, leukemia, or gynecologic cancers—those who participated in group treatments lived significantly longer than similar patients who did not participate.[35] However, another five studies failed to show such a connection.[36]

But there is one telling observation in the five no-effect studies. In two of the five, the psychosocial treatments not only failed to improve survival but also failed to improve the patients' psychological well-being.[37] In another, the psychological benefits were only transient.[38] It seems clear to me that the psychological treatments offered in these support groups simply weren't powerful enough to make patients feel and cope better or, therefore, to substantially alter their internal biochemistry to one that is hostile to cancer. If the group does nothing but provide secure, safe hours for expressing sorrow, confusion, and other emotions, it is not likely to change psychological well-being; if it does not affect psychological well-being, it cannot affect the balance of stress hormones and thus the biochemical environment that encourages or discourages cancer; if it cannot affect the biochemical environment, it cannot affect survival. If, however, the support group trains patients in relaxation strategies, coping skills, more effective communication, and problem solving, it may do all of the above. Of the ten trials of support groups, only seven brought participants psychological benefits. Of those seven, five—71 percent—brought improved survival. The most recent support group study, published in 2008, used an intervention that did more than offer support and expression of feelings. It taught patients progressive muscle relaxation, ways to increase daily physical activity, healthy diet, ways to cope with treatment side effects, and communication skills. In this study, the intervention group had a 56 percent lower risk of dying from cancer after eleven years.[39]

From this, it is fair to conclude that support groups that do nothing more than let patients vent and share their feelings are unlikely to improve your odds of survival. But if they offer techniques that make you feel emotionally healthier, more in control, more socially connected, and less anxious, depressed, and isolated, and if they encourage healthy lifestyles they may well help you live longer.[40]

▶ **Restoring Control of Symptoms and Side Effects**
Mind-spirit techniques can help you cope with the side effects of treatment and the symptoms of the disease itself. As just one example, a number of studies have shown that progressive muscle relaxation, hypnosis, and guided imagery can reduce or eliminate nausea and vomiting in chemotherapy patients.[41] Other studies found that progressive muscle relaxation plus guided imagery was more effective than antiemetics alone in controlling severe nausea and vomiting during and in the four days after chemo.[42]

Mind-spirit techniques also reduce cancer-related pain.[43] Bone marrow transplant patients who practiced hypnosis or relaxation with imagery experienced relief from severe mucositis (mouth sores) induced by chemotherapy.[44] And focused relaxation, healing imagery, hypnosis, or a combination of these can dramatically improve and accelerate postsurgical repair.

Patients had such significantly reduced pain they had less need for pain meds; they experienced fewer complications, less blood loss, earlier return to normal digestion, and shorter hospitalization.[45]

▶ Revitalizing Your Life

"I sure didn't invite it, but cancer has given me a new opportunity!" If you've just been diagnosed with cancer, this will seem like a strange statement. If, on the other hand, you've spent as much time with cancer patients as we have at the Block Center, it may seem commonplace. Why is it that some cancer patients even refer to their malignancy as "an opportunity" or even "a surprising gift" and find that their disease opens up new vistas of understanding?

Let me be absolutely clear about one thing: just as cancer is not a punishment, neither is it, in reality, a gift. And patients whose disease is recently diagnosed, those whose disease has advanced quickly, or those who lack social support are not likely to see cancer as being a gift. But if you are lucky enough to have survived cancer for some time and have enough support to both meet daily challenges and reflect on them, you may one day find yourself saying something similar. Being faced with a threat to your life can make you reevaluate your goals, your priorities, and how you spend your time. We continually remind patients of the importance of doing what really matters—what is truly satisfying, what has value and meaning. And we emphasize that finding pleasure in life is vital to the energy and spirit of every cancer survivor. Although the goal of cancer treatment is survival, most patients hope to do more than merely survive. One patient told me in a letter how cancer had altered her perspective: "The difference between us and the non-cancer world is we no longer have illusions about life's predictability or our control of the future. I realize I have to live now and make the most of each day."

Some patients struggle to return to "the way things were," and find that how they were—what mattered to them, what gave them enjoyment—is how they decide to be again. But I find that the majority of patients use a diagnosis of cancer as an opportunity for positive change. This can mean repairing relationships, reconnecting with friends or family, rethinking the work you do, or discovering what truly engages and enthuses you.[46] Doing this is not easy or quick. It needs to unfold over time and over many stages of your recovery journey. But along with our center staff members, I have seen many, many patients do it—strengthening personal connections, trying out activities they always wanted to do but put off, and developing a commitment to internal harmony that sustains them.

CHAPTER 11

THE LIFE OVER CANCER CORE MIND AND SPIRIT CARE PLAN

How do you recover from the earthquake of cancer? What you need is a way to calm yourself, to curb and counteract the stress hormones coursing through your body, to give yourself a chance to take stock and evaluate your options. And there *are* definitely options. This chapter will give you the tools to do this. When you are just developing your mind-spirit practice, it can be helpful to keep a log, noting what you did and how it felt, and which techniques are more effective at different times or circumstances. Try out the variety of practices in this chapter and adopt those that work for you. On the LOC website, you can find a printable log for evaluating how well each technique works for you.

Recovering Calm, Creating Emotional Ease

I want to help you recover calm not just because serenity feels better than panic but because calm is a prerequisite for processing highly technical information, making good decisions, regaining your normal life, handling treatment side effects, and quelling the toxic stew of stress hormones that otherwise create the biochemical environment that cancer cells thrive in.[1]

The basis for recovering calm is to convince your body that the threat has passed, that it no longer must prepare for flight or fight, and that it can therefore dial down the release of stress hormones. Just think about it: something in your mind—hearing and thinking that you have cancer—has caused a dramatic response in your body, increasing your heart rate and blood pressure, making your breathing rapid and shallow, and magnifying your anxiety so that you can react with hair-trigger sensitivity to any sign of danger. Just as the mind can do all this, so it can ratchet down the secretion of the stress hormones and all that ensues. This is the basis of mind-body medicine and, in particular, of the relaxation strategies that can help you recover calm.

Relaxation techniques for reversing your body's stress response are not what many of us think of when we hear the word *relax*. They are not the same as sleeping or watching TV. True relaxation relieves chronic tension, allowing you to feel more alert, more focused, more clear-thinking. Regardless of the techniques you adopt, they should become part of your daily regimen and not some afterthought. The benefits of relaxation strategies, like most health-promoting activities, are cumulative—making regular, everyday practice a necessity. I recommend that you practice these and other methods in this chapter for ten to thirty minutes each day. If one technique doesn't work or doesn't appeal to you, try another. Don't give up even though the techniques can feel awkward and strange in the beginning. And don't worry if, while practicing relaxation techniques, your mind wanders or you fall asleep. Both reactions are common. So be persistent and don't get discouraged. Continue until the miraculous moment when you experience the relaxation response, a relaxed/alert state that brings a sense of pleasure, focus, refreshment, and general well-being, as well as reduced heart rate and respiratory rate and lowered blood pressure.

▶ **Relaxed Abdominal Breathing**

One of the three fundamental techniques of recovery, relaxed abdominal breathing is like a safe harbor you can find when you suffer shock or anxiety. In fact, you may hear your doctors or counselors encourage you to "breathe" when they detect signs of panic in a tense situation. Because breathing is the most direct link between mind and body, breath-work techniques may be one of the most valuable tools for inducing and maintaining relaxation. Research shows that relaxed breathing can promote strong immune function as well as blood pressure control.[2] By diminishing the intensity of nerve firing and raising the brain's oxygen uptake, deep, regular breathing can help you let go of fear, anxiety, anger, and resentment.[3]

1. To begin, sit or lie in any position that allows you to relax your body.
2. Close your eyes gently or focus your partially closed eyes on a small, non-moving object, without straining your neck.
3. Take a deep cleansing breath in through your nose or mouth and then sigh out through your nose or mouth. Feel as though you are completely emptying your lungs.
4. With the palm side of one hand resting easily against your chest and the other lightly on your upper abdomen, breathe deliberately, comfortably, and rhythmically, inhaling and exhaling through your mouth or, if more natural, exhaling through your nose.
5. As you inhale, your relaxed abdomen will expand, and as you exhale, your belly will contract or resume its normal shape.
6. The more relaxed you become, the slower your breathing rate will be.
7. You will begin to notice, as your breathing becomes relaxed and rhythmic, that the hand resting against your abdomen is moving in synchrony with your in-breath and out-breath, while the hand on your chest seems almost motionless.

8. If fear and apprehension arise, or if random thoughts about tasks and plans pop into your head, simply return your attention to the breathing, and allow it to slow and deepen once again. Concentrate on maintaining rhythmic, evenly paced inhalation and exhalation.

Some people find that counting helps them reach a comfortable breathing pace, but others find that counting makes them more tense. If you try counting, inhale while silently counting slowly to four, pause, then slowly exhale to the count of five. Repeat the slow inhale-pause-exhale-pause sequence for ten cycles. Some people find it helpful to adjust the number of counts in either direction, perhaps using five counts on inhaling and six or seven on exhaling. As you practice every day, you will gradually find your own rhythm and this technique will become easier. Although it seems simple, relaxed abdominal breathing takes practice to feel natural, not awkward, so you should definitely make it a part of your daily mind-spirit practice until it becomes second nature and you can call on it whenever you need. Once you become proficient, relaxed abdominal breathing can be used for as little or as long as you need, at any place or time.

▶ **Progressive Muscle Relaxation**
Progressive muscle relaxation takes longer and more sustained focus than relaxed abdominal breathing. Particularly effective if you're caught in a cycle of chronic or recurring stress and anxiety, progressive muscle relaxation is based on the physiological fact that you cannot be both relaxed and tense at the same time. By progressively tightening and releasing muscles throughout your body, you will find your body becoming more relaxed. Many people have found that progressive muscle relaxation is the most effective way to get into a state of deep relaxation when they're in the throes of chronic tension or insomnia.

1. Set aside ten to fifteen minutes for progressive muscle relaxation. You may find it easiest to do this lying down.

2. Take a deep cleansing breath through your nose, and "sigh" it out through your mouth. Let your whole body be at ease.
3. Inhale without effort through your nose and exhale through your mouth.
4. Begin at the toes. Contract them to a count of ten and then release the tension all at once.
5. Repeat this tensing and relaxing in your feet, ankles, calf, pressing the knees together, abdomen, lower back, hands, wrists, forearms, upper arms, shoulders, neck, jaw, mouth, eyelids, and forehead.
6. Do this at an unhurried pace, with deep refreshing inhalations and exhalations between each muscle group.

(i)   The LOC website offers a specific script for progressive muscle relaxation, which you could record for yourself or have someone read to you until you become familiar with the technique. As you become more skilled at progressive muscle relaxation, you will be able to tighten and relax whole muscle groups simultaneously—for example, all the muscles in the arms, or all the muscles in the legs. This is a time-saver, yet is still an effective way to achieve relaxation in the middle of a busy day.

Many patients like to pair progressive muscle relaxation with the "body scan," in which you mentally check every part of your body in the progressive muscle relaxation order to note where you harbor tension or discomfort. Note: if some spot hurts, do not contract that muscle group. Instead, picture yourself directing warm or cool air, whichever seems more soothing, to that spot, or use relaxed abdominal breathing to imagine that you are inspiring (literally) that spot with healing.

▶ **Comfort Space Imagery**
In comfort space imagery, you imagine a place that evokes for you a sense of tranquillity, ease, and safety—a beloved location in a park or wilderness, or fantasy setting, even an idyllic movie scene. One patient at our center imagined himself reclining in a canoe, gently bobbing on a slow stream with lush green trees arching overhead (and no mosquitoes).

1. Begin by imagining a sensation of relaxation spread from head to foot.
2. Once you are fully relaxed, envision entering your comfort space.
3. Use clear and vivid visual, auditory, olfactory, tactile, and kinesthetic details. How warm is it there? What time of day, the promise of dawn or the peace of evening? What do you see as you look around? What do you hear? Do you feel sun or cool breeze? Do you smell clean air or pleasing aromas? Are you alone, or is someone with you?
4. Remain in your comfort space for as long as you like or need to (some women find they can use this technique to get through hours and hours of labor and childbirth without anesthesia)—perhaps through a round of chemo or while undergoing a scan.
5. Before reopening your eyes, remind yourself that you can return to your comfort space any time you need to, and that you can carry certain, special sensations from your comfort space into the rest of your day or night.
6. Gradually, open your eyes.

See the LOC website for a list of tapes that provide instruction in guided imagery. (i)

▶ **Meditation**
There are many forms of meditation that reduce the stress response and bring relaxation, but let me mention one that my patients have had great success with, called mindfulness meditation.[4] In this meditative practice, you focus on everything happening inside and immediately around you in the present moment, noting every detail in a nonjudgmental manner. If you find your mind rummaging through past events and conversations or thinking ahead toward future concerns, you guide your attention back to where you are and what you are doing at that precise moment. In this way you witness whatever arises in your mind without reacting to or getting snared by memories or future worries. With practice—and I urge you to practice,

even if just for five minutes per day initially—mindfulness meditation can help you develop a more calm and nonreactive way of being and responding.

Many activities of your daily routine lend themselves to this style of meditative awareness. For example, while showering or taking a bath, note the smell of the soap, the temperature and feel of the water as it splashes against your skin, and how it feels when you towel off and are refreshed. Or while washing dishes, just calmly observe without internal commentary the temperature of the water, the way soap bubbles over the plate, the shine as you rinse away the detergent. Even walking in a comfortable rhythmic pattern and noting how your feet feel as you plant them consciously and deliberately in front of you and how your arms swing alongside your body can be a chance for mindfulness meditation. As you practice, you will be able to draw on mindfulness in many stressful situations. See the LOC website for a list of books on meditation techniques.

Reestablishing Equilibrium

Yes, there is a way to reestablish equilibrium. Beyond calming yourself in the face of disrupting news, establishing a new sense of "normal" now that you are a cancer patient boosts healing and well-being.

▶ **Expressive Writing**
In expressive writing you simply write about your disturbing thoughts and very private feelings.[5] No one need ever see what you write—even you don't have to read what flows from your pen. This process can let you vent feelings and reduce tension, face issues that seemed unmanageable, and admit to emotions that seemed inadmissible. Expressive writing is more about allowing disclosure than about the actual writing. It can also bring clarity to issues that felt overwhelming.

1. On a clean sheet of paper, write for twenty minutes each day for three consecutive days about your most distressing issue or upsetting experience.

2. Since this is not a writing exercise per se, do not worry about style. The aim is to write continuously without stopping and without worrying about grammar, wording, or logic. Just write, without hesitation, about your thoughts *and* feelings.

3. Explore your deepest thoughts and feelings without reserve. No one will read this, not even you if you choose not to.

4. Put what you have written safely away.

5. On the second day, using new paper, write again about your most distressing issue for twenty minutes. You can focus on the previous day's topic or you can select a different issue. But it is important that you explore your deepest thoughts and feelings. Again, after twenty minutes, put your writing away in a safe and private place.

6. On day three, the final day of your expressive writing experience, write *without any reservations* about your deepest feelings and thoughts on any distressing personal issue. Your topic could be the same issue as before, a related one, or a completely different one.

7. Again, when you have finished twenty minutes of freewriting, put your writing away. Keep or dispose of it in whatever way feels right to you. If stressful thoughts recur, we encourage patients to repeat the three-day process.

▶ **Cognitive Reframing**

This is a method for consciously and systematically altering your reactions to events, social interactions, physical symptoms, and your own self-defeating thoughts so that they do not automatically trigger distress. You can start it soon after your diagnosis and continue to use it to help you through every phase of your cancer journey.

Reframing is based on the well-established therapeutic approach called cognitive-behavioral therapy. Its core is teaching people to question the accuracy of immediate assumptions, consider different explanations, and rethink thoughts or interpretations that are self-defeating or irrational and replace them with adaptive thinking. This does not mean adopting false beliefs (see the discussion of the myth of thinking positive in the previous chapter). Instead, it means considering positive but *realistic* possibilities. For example, instead of assuming that a doctor's sideways glance signals unbearable news, you can realize that the doctor may be checking a pager that just beeped, or thinking through the most promising schedule for an effective treatment for you. Instead of seeing setbacks as evidence that you are doomed to suffer, you reframe them to be manageable situations that you can and will get through.

How we frame our thoughts and experiences determines our emotional response to them. In fact, it is the personal appraisal of the cancer—how each patient perceives his or her disease—more than the actual stage of disease that is most strongly correlated with the intensity of distress, as we have witnessed at the Block Center time and again.[6] One woman diagnosed with early stage breast cancer feels doomed, devastated, and helpless, for instance, but another woman with a more advanced disease, although concerned, views her disease as manageable and eagerly embraces a plan to eliminate it. The first woman remembers her mother's horrific and losing struggle with breast cancer; the second thinks of all the hopeful stories she has read about new therapies. With reframing, the first woman can unlearn her helpless/hopeless mind-set and replace it with one that allows her to move forward with energy, determination, and hope. At the center, we often find that one basic fact helps patients do this: if you are over thirty, your body has probably harbored cancer cells for years. Healthy body cells and renegade cancer cells can coexist in relative harmony for years. So envision your cancer as something you can again peacefully coexist with. As I tell patients, you do not have to cure your cancer or kill every cancer cell in order to live with it.

Another example: A sharp pain awakens you in the middle of the night. Before being diagnosed with cancer, you would have attributed this to a pulled muscle or strain. But now you interpret every ache, soreness, or burning sensation as a sign of cancer progression or recurrence. This is called catastrophizing. In this case, too, cognitive restructuring to examine other reasonable explanations can haul you back from the emotional precipice.

Ira: Talking with His Cancer

One of my patients showed me clearly how powerful reframing can be. Ira, who had been diagnosed with advanced prostate cancer that had spread to his bones, decided early on to strike a deal with his disease. In his diary as well as in his daily thoughts and meditations, he would carry on a conversation with the cancer: "It's okay if you survive, as long as you don't grow." Ira lived many years with his "little tumor," as he referred to it. Twelve years after being handed a death sentence, Ira told me he felt completely at ease with the idea that he could coexist with his disease. Instead of relating to the cancer as an unstoppable malignancy, he was content with the concept of keeping it in check while living a good, healthy life. Talking with those malignant cells made Ira feel less worried. His reframing was a crucial tool for easing the anxiety—and the resulting cascade of stress biochemistry—that would have otherwise plagued him.

Everyone needs to find his or her own peace with cancer. Establishing a dialogue with your own "little tumor" is only one possible way to move from fear to acceptance. Some others:

* Realize that your disease is not you. Instead of thinking, "I am a cancer patient," tell yourself, "I am [name], a person who has been diagnosed with a condition called cancer."
* Remind yourself that you *can* make it to the outer edges of the survival curve and be a survivor. Some patients defy the odds, and since you are embarking on the Life Over Cancer program, which contains many techniques and treatments that have been shown to shift the survival odds in your favor, there is no reason why you cannot be one of these "outliers." Tell yourself, "Once I make all these positive changes, grim statistics will not apply to me."
* When you find yourself in a "thought warp," as when a setback on your road to recovery pushes you into despondency, ask yourself whether you are *catastrophizing,* engaging in

emotional reasoning (assuming that emotional reactions reflect reality, so because you feel hopeless, the situation must be hopeless), or *overgeneralizing* (viewing a onetime negative event as likely to last forever, or assuming that an earlier problem will recur). If so, the first thing to do is recognize them as thought warps. Ask yourself, "What evidence contradicts this thinking? What are other explanations or interpretations?" Keep a record of thought warps so you understand what triggers them. (See the worksheet on the LOC website for an Automatic Thinking/Rethinking Record that will help you do this.) Then write down your experience as soon as it occurs, recording your thoughts without interpretations or amendments. Once you recognize the circumstances under which thought warps occur, you may head them off at the pass, so to speak. But if they keep coming, try these techniques:

Thought Stopping. In this technique, you deliberately allow yourself to wander into distressing ruminations, but *only for a limited time* that you set on a timer. For instance, you decide you will ruminate for ten minutes on being told that your cancer has spread. Explore how you'd feel, how you'd react, what you'd do—and then, when the timer goes off, *stop*. Change your position, shout "Stop," bolt out of your chair, flick your finger against the palm of your hand, or slap your hand loudly on a tabletop—anything to dramatically signal that rumination time is over. Replace these thoughts with any of the relaxation techniques. Breathe, practice muscle relaxation, or enter your personal comfort space. Then engage in a preplanned activity. The point is to prove to yourself, through practice, that you *can* call a halt to dark, destructive thoughts whenever *you* want. You are in control; unbidden thoughts do not control you. You will not be victimized by them.

Reimaging. Does the thought of chemo produce a thought warp because you see it as a poison being poured into your veins that will make you vomit? If so, reimaging can let you replace this negative perception with a positive one. One patient at our center felt traumatized by the incessant, thunderous noise of the MRI equipment in the scanning chamber, so she reimaged the pounding as the sound of a drum in a healing ritual. Another patient reimaged chemotherapy as a healing herbal solution pouring into her to cleanse her of cancer. With several chemotherapies being of botanical origin, this imagery is not far off from reality. Keep your new mental image in mind as you approach thought-warp situations.

► **Satisfaction Inventory**
By evaluating each day's activities, you can rediscover or enhance your sense of pleasure and mastery. Making a satisfaction inventory like the one on page 242 is a simple cognitive tool for identifying the positives in your life. All you have to do is, several times a day, examine your recent activities and record the level of pleasure and competence you experienced from each. Be generous with yourself. Realize that, depending where you are in your recovery, doing simple things can be a major accomplishment. List the focus of each hour and then rate each segment from one to ten for pleasure (P) and for mastery (M). Note moments of emotional brightness or personal meaning, and activities that score six or higher on mastery or pleasure. Take stock of what makes your life worth living.

This log can serve you well in two ways: it can give you evidence that despite very real limitations and challenges imposed by cancer, you are still able to experience a sense of accomplishment in specific projects or tasks and feel true pleasure, plus it will help you to identify what types of activities you should routinely include in each day to give you a renewed sense of vitality.

SATISFACTION INVENTORY, WEEK OF _____

Name and then rate each daily activity from P1 to P10, from least pleasurable to most, and from M1 to M10 for mastery.

Time	Monday	Tuesday	Wednesday	Thursday	Friday	Saturday	Sunday
6–7 A.M.							
7–8 A.M.							
8–9 A.M.							
9–10 A.M.							
10–11 A.M.							
11 A.M.–NOON							
NOON–1 P.M.							
1–2 P.M.							
2–3 P.M.							
3–4 P.M.							
4–5 P.M.							
5–6 P.M.							

Reconnecting: Support and Social Connectedness

If you have selected your A-Team, you have already been reconnecting your support and social network, which is crucial to your well-being and your ability to combat your illness. Here are some other ways to connect with people who "get it," so you are not alone in facing the challenges of cancer:

• Think of other important people in your life who are not on your A-Team. These may be people you have lost touch with or even became estranged from, or who are unsuitable for the A-Team but are nevertheless important to you. If you want to reestablish or enhance contact, you may find it easier to ask an A-Team member to initiate the first contact. ("Hi, this is Jill; I'm a friend of Lee's, who asked me to give you a call. . . .")

• Try making a new map of connections. Maybe you have an acquaintance who is a yoga fiend or a whole-foods aficionado. You never had much in common, but now you realize that these "fringe" interests can help in your recovery. They may never enter your intimate social circle, but it is definitely worth including them in your map of connections.

• I consider one aspect of your map particularly important. Most of us have lost contact with friends and family from the past. Many of my patients acknowledge what far too many of us experience: pain and injury from prior relationships. Whether we have injured others or been injured, a diagnosis of cancer provides a fresh opportunity and reminder of the importance for all of us to repair, to forgive, and to seek forgiveness. We have all made mistakes and errors in our lives. It is these vulnerabilities that make us human, and it is only through our efforts to go through change and to repair our errors that we grasp the possibility of fully healing. In many ways, healing is as profoundly important as recovering. It encompasses not merely our health but our humanity and compassion for each other as well.

• Consider a support group. Although these days it's considered almost abnormal if you're *not* part of a cancer support group, I would guard against peer pressure or any sense of compulsion to join. Depending on your personality and the quality of support provided by your inner circle and social network, you may not need a formal support group, or you may do better with one-on-one counseling. Some people simply don't feel comfortable with support groups, often because they don't feel comfortable sharing deep distress and difficult details with strangers. Others find such sharing reassuring and even vital. To get a sense of whether a support group is right for you, indicate whether you agree or disagree with the following statements:

Is a support group right for you?

Agree ___ Disagree ___ I rarely speak about my cancer and treatment, because I don't want to upset my family and friends.

Agree ___ Disagree ___ My family always wants to hear that I am doing well—they don't want to hear that I am dealing with dark emotions or experiencing distress.

Agree ___ Disagree ___ If I talk about my cancer difficulties, my spouse or partner, family, and close friends switch to another topic or try to minimize my concerns.

Agree ___ Disagree ___ My spouse or partner, family, or friends seem to be hiding their feelings from me—and even seem emotionally shut down or distant.

If you agree with two or more of the above, joining a well-led support group could allow you the comfort to deal safely and openly with difficult feelings and develop coping strategies shared by others who "get" the cancer experience.[7] (Otherwise you might benefit from one-on-one or family counseling to allow for more open private communication.) If possible, try out different groups to find one that feels right. You should feel comfortable with the group leader's style, professional assurance, and perspective, and find some connection to at least one person in the group. On the other hand, if you find that the other members' conversation and issues seem distant from yours, being in that group will possibly make you feel more isolated, not less. For instance, if the type or stage of cancer of the other patients is very different from yours, the group will not be a good match; if you have an early-stage cancer, listening to patients with very advanced disease and end-of-life issues will probably not be comforting. In this case, move on. You will be likely to get more out of a group whose members are in a situation similar to yours. Also, many people find same-sex groups more conducive to candid conversations about personal or intimate issues.

If you are not comfortable with a support group format, investigate one-on-one counseling. Or online support groups hosted by reputable organizations can give you access to many of the benefits of a sit-down weekly meeting. One of the advantages of going online, of course, is that you need not leave the comfort of your own home. Such support groups are run by several organizations, including the Wellness Community (www.thewellness community.org), the Association of Cancer Online Resources (www.acor.org), Oncochat (www.oncochat.org), and the Cancer Survivors Network (www.acscsn.org). See the LOC website for others.

Kate: A Support Group Transformed Her Life

Kate, who had been diagnosed with metastatic (stage IV) breast cancer, felt racked by anxiety between rounds of chemotherapy. With the help of our mind-spirit team, she realized that a big part of her distress stemmed from isolation—from feeling that no one in her circle understood what she was going through. She found a supportive outlet for her feelings in a group composed of people with advanced cancers. Five of the seven participants were women, and four of them had breast cancer. All were under our care or had received some components of Life Over Cancer treatment. For these reasons, Kate felt that the support group was a good fit for her. She felt an instant affinity and rapport with several of the participants. "Thanks to these women, I felt very comfortable and opened up to the group almost immediately," she told me. "They seemed to understand where I was coming from. They allowed me the space to feel vulnerable and talk about my fears and even laugh at some of my more bizarre experiences. After a few meetings, I no longer felt strange or alone."

Since all the members were using the Life Over Cancer system, the group helped Kate dissect specific problems, splitting them into more manageable parts, and find solutions. In well-run support groups with properly trained facilitators, there's a ripple effect: participants are fueled by the group dynamic to strive harder for their treatment goals.[8] They're more likely to eat, sleep, and exercise in ways conducive to health.

▶ **Restoring Control of Symptoms and Side Effects**

Drugs are not the only way to alleviate the pain, discomfort, or side effects of treatment. Mind-spirit techniques, especially in tandem with natural compounds, can treat or even prevent many symptoms of diseases and effects of treatment, and without the risks of grogginess, mood swings, and weakened immunity that pain medications and other drugs pose. (I cover natural therapies in Chapters 13 to 19.) Among the mind-spirit techniques our patients have found to be the most effective are progressive muscle relaxation, relaxed abdominal breathing, and comfort space imagery, as explained above. The mind-spirit staff at our center also recommend these:

- **Music therapy for pain relief.** For instance, patients who listened to music during colonoscopy required less sedation than control patients. A music therapist can help you devise a program that includes singing, humming, and chanting, as well as playing instruments (no special ability required).[9]
- **Hypnosis and self-hypnosis.** Under the guidance of a professionally trained practitioner, hypnosis allows you to enter a

deeply relaxed, focused state of attention—somewhat like the trance-like experience of guided imagery—allowing you to be more receptive to your own personal messages of healing and serenity. It has been found to reduce or eliminate anticipatory nausea and vomiting, which afflicts many patients before chemotherapy. Relaxation strategies and imagery, which are similar to hypnosis but can be done on your own, can also relieve nausea. They can also alleviate severe mucositis (drug-induced mouth sores).[10]

• **Systematic desensitization.** In this technique, you link relaxation with vivid mental images to decrease anxiety. To start, arrange a hierarchy of images associated with any procedure that you dread, starting with the least upsetting (finding a parking place at the clinic, perhaps).[11] Call up the first mental image, allowing the sensory specifics and fearful thoughts to develop in your mind until they seem as vivid and upsetting as the actual scene. Pair the image with a relaxation technique until you feel you can control the anxiety triggered by the image. Then move to the next image. For example, after the ride to the clinic and parking, you might move on to walking in the entrance, checking in with the receptionist, entering the chemo room, smelling the alcohol as the nurse opens the packet, and watching the nurse start the infusion. Don't move to the next image until you feel confident that you can maintain relaxation when "experiencing" the previous one. Repeat the entire sequence until the anxiety provoked by the images has faded. This strategy will equip you to maintain calm and ease when you experience the real thing, breaking the conditioned link between your intense apprehension and the queasy physical sensations that trigger anticipatory nausea and vomiting. It will also boost your sense of control and make the forthcoming treatment less formidable. The form on page 248 can help you organize your systematic desensitization stepladder.

To be clear, I am not opposed to medications. Suffering pain is not a good option. Pain meds and antinausea drugs—under the guidance and expertise of your medical team—can work in synchrony with mind-body approaches to bring you relief. I encourage you to consider nondrug methods as your first line against anticipatory nausea and vomiting, as well as pain and other side effects. But for more severe symptoms and side effects, mind-spirit techniques may not work well enough, so I do recommend pain medications or such antinausea medications as Aloxi, Ativan, Compazine, Emend, and Zofran or natural remedies such as the anti-inflammatory curcumin or the anti-emetic ginger.

SYSTEMATIC DESENSITIZATION

Description of Each Step	Tension Before Relaxation (1 = least, 10 = most)	Practice Used	Check When Confident	Tension After Relaxation (1 = least, 10 = most)
1.				
2.				
3.				
4.				
5.				
6.				

Revitalizing Your Life

Having a sense of meaning, purpose, and fulfillment in life doesn't require grand or public accomplishments. Even special attention to relationships can hold extraordinary significance. You may want to take this time to identify impasses and hurdles that stand in the way of achieving goals that you have yet to achieve, and to identify and affirm your internal resources and strengths.

▶ **Benefit Finding**
It may seem odd to think that cancer might have brought you any benefits, but don't dismiss this possibility out of hand. Instead, think about your cancer journey so far. Since your diagnosis, has there been any change, however slight, that you value? Perhaps a support group has helped you become more open in your relationships, or maybe the illness has brought you a deeper appreciation for the simple details of everyday life, from the brilliant colors of autumn leaves to savoring passages of a favorite novel. You can also try out new activities, such as those that you'd been "just too busy" to pursue. Many people discover that volunteer work—reaching out to make the lives of others better—can make their own circumstances easier to manage and even more meaningful. Helping out at an assisted living facility, coaching children, setting up a helpful blog, or working in a cancer service organization may be just the satisfaction you're looking for. Some patients have also enjoyed writing personal histories or working on an oral narrative. Taking time to renew activities that you gave up years ago can also energize body and mind: did you love doing sketches or wood carving when you were young, but let it drop in the busyness of career and family? Dusting off the parts of your life that have been misplaced can be a powerful tool for revitalizing your life.[12]

▶ **Changing Perspective**
Holding on to this bigger sense of your life's journey reminds you that you are much more than a "cancer patient." One strategy we use at our clinic is to encourage patients to draw two circles on a sheet of paper. One circle represents the cancer;

the other represents the whole self. In the beginning, the cancer circle can dwarf the self-circle, monopolizing the page as it does your life. The goal is to gradually adjust your perspective, so that the cancer circle becomes small relative to the self. Over time, as the reality of having cancer becomes less menacing and more manageable, the cancer circle will shrink, eventually occupying just a small spot on your page.

▶ **Making Meaning**

Cancer can spur you to reexamine what is important to you, what holds the greatest personal significance. We stress with every patient that finding true meaning can revitalize the spirit and transform the darkness of cancer. But how do you identify what brings joy and meaning? You might start by asking yourself, "When did I feel happiest and most enthusiastic in my life? What was I doing? What prevents me from doing that now? What did I hope to do but lacked the confidence for?" Finding meaning need not require revolutionary change. Sometimes it just requires pushing aside work to make space for family projects, or picking up an instrument you thought you would never have time to play. One patient mentioned her early dream of becoming an archaeologist; during her recovery from cancer, she took a course at a local natural history museum and toured an ancient dig just hours from her home. You can start your own search by going back to the satisfaction worksheet above, where you evaluated each day's activities for the sense of pleasure or mastery they provided, and build on those that pop up with a score of six or more. Or simply reflect on what you have been through and then write your life story or make a collage representing significant events.

After an experience that shakes the ground of our being, as cancer does, an instinct for transcendence comes naturally to many of us. Whether it finds itself in spirituality and mysticism or in the experience of losing a sense of ourselves in the flow of sports, dance, or absorption in work, this instinct can help you enlarge the meaning of your life. For some, this process manifests itself as a deeper or renewed connection with religious roots or a sense of having been guided by divine providence.

For others, a sense of spirituality that is not explicitly religious emerges, a communion with the energy of nature, other people, or commitment to repairing our world. There are ways to encourage internal harmony that are widely accepted by both religious and spiritual people. The many varieties of meditation, prayer, breath work, and acts of charity have been pathways to transcendent states for centuries. Exploring the paths that speak to your own religious or spiritual beliefs, and choosing people with whom you share this exploration, can enlarge your potential for inner personal growth.

▶ **Projecting Your Future**
A key step toward revitalization is to develop a positive future projection for yourself. Start by writing down your immediate and long-term goals. How would you like to see yourself one year, three years, and five years from now? Write a brief description of these images, using visual details and sounds, identifying the people around you, the focus of your time, and how you will evaluate whether you've reached your personal goals. (If you prefer a medium other than the written word, you can instead imagine this "as if" with photography, painting, or film. Since you will do this through creative mental imagery, you can use any visual art that works for you.) What will you be doing and where will you be? The vivid details will help you focus on your future goal. Seeing yourself as you want to be is a critical step to making it a reality.

Plan a 10-to-20-minute positive imaging session each day at a routine time, perhaps after a relaxation session. Each day, add another aspect to your imagined future life, health, and happiness. You will slowly create a more complete vision of what you hope to become. In so doing, you can reinforce your own mind-body-spirit connection to help potentiate this positive image and to engage in life-enhancing experiences.

CHAPTER 12

INDIVIDUALIZING YOUR MIND AND SPIRIT CARE PLAN

The cancer journey has more ups and downs than the stock market. Each new high and each new low brings different feelings and distinct psychological and emotional challenges. Practicing the mind-spirit program outlined in the preceding chapter can help you reduce stress and regain a sense of control; as I explained, everyone needs to find techniques that work best for him or her. But based on years of experience with patients, our center staff consistently finds that certain strategies are effective in particular situations along your path to recovery. What you need when you are overwhelmed by the crisis of a new diagnosis is not the same as what you need when you are in remission.

To get the most out of this chapter, first find where you are on this map of the cancer journey:

- **Critical stress points.** When you have just been diagnosed with cancer or learned that your cancer has recurred or is not responding to treatment.

- **Treatment preparation.** When you are anticipating surgery, radiation, chemotherapy, or molecular target therapies.

- **Side effect management.** When you are undergoing treatment and need ways (instead of or in addition to drugs) to manage its side effects.

- **Post-treatment.** When you are adjusting to the end of active treatment, usually after the final chemotherapy cycle. This situation can, perhaps surprisingly, prove quite stressful.

- **Remission maintenance.** Although definitely good news, remission introduces its own issues, most notably fear of recurrence. Remission is also when you will be most determined to take back your life from cancer.

I will introduce each of the five milestones on your cancer journey by listing the strategies we recommend, then explain each strategy in detail. Patients' mind-spirit needs are quite individual, and you don't need to use every single strategy. Choose which tools work best for you but do be willing to experiment.

CRITICAL STRESS POINTS : TOOLS AND STRATEGIES FOR COPING

Calling a time-out
Recruiting your A-Team
Assessing personal priorities
Assessing spiritual priorities
Determining your information ceiling
Listing questions for doctors
Tuning-in time
Conducting a body scan
Easing stress reactions
Reframing catastrophic thinking

▶ ## Calling a Time-Out
As you know only too well, being diagnosed with cancer or discovering a recurrence or other bad news can trigger a perfect

storm of emotions. This is definitely a case when you should listen to your heart: these emotions are a signal that you need to avoid making snap decisions, a signal that you need to get your bearings before proceeding. Otherwise, you will very likely find it tough to concentrate on technical details or evaluate medical options intelligently. Trying to absorb the rush of information, ramifications of your diagnosis, and treatment distinctions are issues that you should not rush into. Some patients do jump into discussions of complex treatments and medical strategies. I have seen this work for a few, but they are in the minority. If you feel as though you are bobbing on a tumultuous sea of emotions, you need to pause and find clarity before facing daunting decisions. Otherwise you may regret the choices you make. Don't let anyone tell you that postponing a decision for a short period to establish calm or get a second opinion can mean the difference between life and death: the vast majority of situations allow for at least a few days to reflect on your options. If you are told that an urgent decision is needed, don't hesitate to ask why and explore in detail what the advising physician feels are the consequences of a brief delay. True urgency is usually combined with advice for immediate hospitalization.

The misguided idea that you need to *act now* can mean that your decision is based on misunderstandings and poorly grasped information. A 2006 study found that men who were newly diagnosed with localized prostate cancer, for instance, were beset with confusion and misinformation.[1] That isn't surprising. Localized prostate cancer presents perplexing choices. There are several different treatments, none of which has a clear survival benefit over any others, and each has significant side effects, including sexual impairment. Many of the men, faced with confusing treatments and side effects, made decisions driven by fear, uncertainty, and a quest for rapid results even though early-stage prostate cancer is not an emergency (localized cancer grows very slowly). Most of the men did not seek second opinions, did not understand risk data, and were unable to consider their alternatives calmly and thoughtfully.

So if you have just been diagnosed with malignancy, progressive disease, or recurrence and are not in the midst of an acute crisis such as bleeding or shortness of breath, my advice is to slow down. Gather information, but hold off for days or a week, even two or three, until you can regain your equilibrium, before making critical decisions. Call a time-out. This simply means walking away from the clinical setting. Get away from the abstruse terminology of pathology reports, scans, and lab analyses, even from well-meaning friends and relatives who insist on evaluating details for instant action. Claim time and personal space for working with the calming techniques described in the previous chapter. This applies to your doctor, too: you should not feel shy about telling him or her that you need time to assimilate the bad news. Once the panic abates, you will be better able to engage in rational discussions, get a clearer understanding of the issues at stake without catastrophizing, and consider your options rationally and possibly get additional expert input.

Letters to Others. You may find that you will feel better if you ask your A-Team to do some research while you get grounded. This way, you'll have the comfort of knowing that people you trust are focusing time and effort on the particulars of your disease, and that once you are ready to assess your options and make decisions, you'll have the information you need to proceed wisely.

So that you don't have to explain to everyone why you aren't rushing full speed ahead into treatment decisions, you might try giving a "time-out letter"—asking people to allow you a short pause—to those who are actively or implicitly pressuring you to get a move on. See page 256 for a sample.

Facing the Critical Stress Your Own Way. Now that you have cleared personal space for processing all the emotions and new information, think about how you process disturbing information most comfortably.

- Alone?

- With someone close to you?

- In a supportive group setting?

> ## POSSIBLE TIME-OUT LETTER
>
> Dear ———,
>
> Please understand that I need to spend time processing, thinking, and dealing with my feelings about the shocking diagnosis I have just been given. I will need [a few hours, a few days, a week, or other] just to be by myself or to distance myself from the details of any treatment plans or cancer issues. If you feel it would be helpful to begin gathering information about treatment options or cancer generally, please do so. But I am not yet ready to read books or materials about cancer, or to make decisions about my medical care. Within [number of days], I will feel more able to engage in making decisions about which treatments make sense and what I need to do to help my recovery process.

- Sitting in a comfortable chair?

- Lying down?

- While engaged in vigorous physical activity?

- In private contemplative activity?

- Immediately and totally?

- In smaller components and intermittent moments?

There are no "right" answers. "Right" is only what feels right for you. The checklist above can be your personal guideline on how you will best process the news of a diagnosis or setback.

Just one note of caution: although delaying a decision for days or a week may have enormous personal and clinical value for making better choices, postponing a decision for too long—or indefinitely—can have equally worrisome consequences. Several new patients who came to our center over the years would have been better off making any choice as opposed to sitting paralyzed and unable to proceed in any direction.

Rejecting the "Medical Hex." I have explained in earlier chapters why statistics *do not apply to you.* Nevertheless, too many doctors act as if they do, telling patients they have only a brief time to live or that their cancer is "incurable." I do not believe in Pollyanna-ism. But the antithesis, a doctor's death sentence, can amount to what my friend and colleague Dr. Andrew Weil, in his book *Spontaneous Healing,* calls a "medical hex."[2] When medical experts state that your disease will kill you, their prognosis may inadvertently increase that chance, first by triggering a huge stress reaction that can cause an immune decline and physiological injury. This also disables your ability to sort through reasonable options for recovery. And without question, an expert's fatalism can decimate any hope that encourages you to move ahead with treatments and changes in your lifestyle that may, in fact, improve your outcome. So, please, do not believe everything you hear! I have seen any number of patients outlive such "medical hexes." Between dispiriting fatalism and Pollyanna-ism is genuine, constructive communication that offers hope. Tell your doctor that's what you want. One of my patients instructed her oncologist, "Don't tell me how soon I'm going to die! We're all going to die. I want to hear how to increase my odds of surviving."

▶ **Recruiting Your A-Team**
If you have already adopted the Life Over Cancer model, you probably have an A-Team lined up. If you do not, this is the time to do so. Follow the guidelines in Chapter 2. If you invite, but not pressure, those who are closest to you to choose a role they feel best equipped to perform, it's unlikely they'll feel burdened. Rather, they're more likely to want to help, and will feel frustrated if they can't. The A-Team arrangement will allow those who truly care about you to put that caring into action instead of sitting passively on the sidelines feeling useless. Plus, having your personal A-Team will bring you peace of mind.

▶ **Assessing Personal Priorities**
To place yourself squarely at the helm of your care—which can chase away any sense of helplessness—use the assessment below,

which is part of our Block Center patient questionnaire, to identify your personal priorities, and bring them up when your doctor presents you with treatment decisions. Rate how important each is to you and how satisfied you feel with each right now.

PRIORITIES

Rate the following from I (most important to you) to 8 (least important). Then indicate how satisfied you currently are with each, from 0 for very dissatisfied to 3 for very satisfied.

Order of Importance	Satisfaction Scale	Priority
		Vitality and performance
		Recognition/acknowledgment (for example, for your work)
		Associations/relationships (family, friends)
		Appearance
		Longevity
		Libido
		Freedom from pain
		Security/safety (physical and emotional)

Clark: The Importance of Identifying Priorities

Clark had been a young widower for a number of years before he met and married his wonderful new wife. Only months after their wedding, Clark was diagnosed with prostate cancer. One urologist insisted on immediate surgery. But Clark and his wife wanted to think beyond surgery. They realized that certain changes in how Clark ate, exercised, and lived could help ensure improved health, which is what brought them to our Evanston center. Filling out the priorities scale on our patient questionnaire, Clark marked a 1 under "order of importance" beside both libido and relationships. This told me that nerve-sparing surgery—which was not common in the late 1980s—would be essential to Clark's well-being. Otherwise, surgery would excise his spirit along with his tumor.

I firmly believe that doctors should not make medical decisions based solely on what procedures are the most common or easiest. Instead, they should match treatments to your priorities—but they usually will not know what your priorities are unless you tell them. Even with your list, you should allow your physician to explain his or her position and rationale regarding what he or she believes to be your best option. Hearing different positions in the face of knowing what you believe to be your personal priorities can allow you to better grasp your choices and the benefits and possible consequences of those decisions.

▶ **Assessing Spiritual Priorities**
Consider the following questions to determine if you would like your caregiver to understand and/or address the role of religion or spirituality during and beyond your cancer treatment:

- Would you like to discuss the spiritual or religious implications of your health care?

- If so, what aspects of religion/spirituality would you like your doctor to keep in mind?

- How do religious or spiritual beliefs influence your medical decisions?

- What is your source of strength during difficult medical episodes?

Use this inventory to guide your discussions with your doctor or other team members. If you uncover pressing spiritual issues, you may want to make an appointment with a hospital chaplain, appropriate clergy, or spiritual counselor.

▶ **Your Information Ceiling**

Do you like to be intimately involved in your treatment planning, to go on the Internet and research procedures, to go to cancer patient meetings, to bring your doctor reams of scientific papers? Or do the scientific and clinical details make you feel queasy, nervous, and besieged? If the latter, you might be more comfortable assigning major medical decisions to your doctor, or designating the appropriate member of your A-Team to act as go-between, synthesizing what the doctor says into a level of detail you are comfortable with and do not find overwhelming or confusing. If you feel bombarded with more technical information than suits your needs, you will be overwhelmed.[3] If, however, you don't get as much detail as you need to feel in control, you may become agitated and anxious. You can figure this out during your time-out, but remember, your needs are bound to fluctuate at different points along your path toward recovery.

▶ **List of Questions for Doctors**

At each consultation, figure out what you want to know from your medical team in order to make cogent decisions. Your A-Team can help with this. Here are some suggested questions that will elicit helpful answers.

- What is the medical explanation of your diagnosis?

- What is the rationale for each treatment recommendation?

- What is the medical reason for rejecting other options?

- What are the expected therapeutic benefits?

- Why are treatments and procedures sequenced this way?

- What are possible risks and how will the medical team address possible adverse consequences?

- What other options can you provide?

- Are there treatments you cannot provide?

- What would you consider if you had my disease?

- How supportive of an integrative regimen are you?

Is the doctor begrudging or encouraging in his or her answers? Remember, you have the right to choose a doctor who respects your views. If yours does not or does not provide satisfactory answers, ask your A-Team to search for one who will understand and support your values and priorities.

▶ **Tune-In Time**
Assessing your feelings and putting a label on them can be surprisingly helpful, allowing you to sort out which emotions really have you in their grip and which are not relevant at this time. Recognizing your emotions can help you communicate with your A-Team and your medical partners.

What are you feeling right now?

Afraid	Discouraged	Irritated
Apprehensive	Defeated	Edgy
Terrified	Hopeless	Confused
Anxious	Helpless	Uncertain
Panicky	Desperate	Dazed
Sad	Angry	Overwhelmed
Grieving	Infuriated	Embarrassed
Dejected	Distrustful	Alone or lonely
Depressed	Resentful	Isolated
Despondent	Bitter	Disconnected
Devastated		

You may also find it helpful to keep a journal. Becoming comfortable with how you feel, acknowledging it, and possibly sharing it with others, including your doctors, can be self-empowering and help you along the way to emotional healing.[4]

▶ **Body Scan**
The *body scan* is related to the emotional tune-in but relies on physical signs of emotional tension. Anxiety, anger, or despair may manifest itself as an uncomfortable muscle contraction someplace in your body, perhaps as a chronically clenched jaw or tight shoulders. Assess the level of tension in each muscle and use a technique such as the progressive muscle relaxation, imaging, or breathing described in the last chapter for relief. Identify the emotion behind the tension, bring it to the surface, confront it and revise any thought warps that lie behind it (with guidance from a therapist, if helpful).

▶ **Easing Stress Reactions**
The time-out during a critical stress point is the time to practice the three basic stress reduction techniques—relaxed abdominal breathing, progressive muscle relaxation, and comfort space imagery—described in the previous chapter. As I mentioned there, you can rely on these approaches for relief throughout your recovery. If you're looking for objective verification that what you're doing is really modifying your stress reaction, or if you're having difficulty achieving full relaxation, you might benefit from biofeedback. For this you will need a trained biofeedback therapist, who can teach you to use special computer equipment fitted with sensors that record skin temperature, muscle contractions, and even brain-wave patterns to control what are considered involuntary activities such as heart rate, blood pressure, and muscle tension. While some patients are put off by the electronic technology, biofeedback can be very effective for helping to better connect you to your automatic stress responses. It can also help with such chronic problems as pain, including phantom limb pain experienced by patients who have lost a limb to cancer.[5]

▶ **Reframing Catastrophic Thinking**

A crisis can easily throw you into the cognitive warp of cata-strophizing. If you have been diagnosed with a small early-stage breast cancer, for instance, your chances for survival after treatment are very high, but if you have close relatives who died of breast cancer or if you are naturally anxious, you may magnify the risks until you become as emotionally devas-tated as someone might if facing a stage III or IV cancer. In such a situation, you first need to get a reality check with your doctor or an authoritative website such as the National Cancer Institute's (www.cancer.gov). If your fears are out of line with the realities of your disease, look at the techniques in Chapter 11 for examining thought warps and using cognitive reframing. And even if your situation is very serious, remember that there are likely fresh treatment options to consider and that *statistics apply to groups, not individuals.* Refer to the discussion on page 216 if you need a refresher on this important point. By changing your lifestyle and your negative thoughts, and by ac-tively pursuing cutting-edge treatments and a comprehensive integrative plan, you can increase your odds of becoming a long-term survivor.

TREATMENT PREPARATION: TOOLS AND STRATEGIES FOR COPING

Orienting yourself to the treatment facility

Gathering information from your medical team

Listing questions for doctors

Twinning with an experienced patient

Reinforcing of self-calming techniques

Deciding on a support group

Scripting responses to queries

Learning sleep cues and techniques

Developing your personal imagery tape

Lining up practical support

As the day of your treatment approaches, if you are like most people, you will feel apprehensive about possible side effects such as pain, nausea, and fatigue. The Life Over Cancer detox-ification program, which I discuss in Chapter 29, can help counter the potential ill effects of therapies; just reading it will be likely to help you feel calmer and more confident. Your sense that you have some control over reducing long-term side effects can bring not only psychological benefits but also physical ones. Similarly, it is natural to worry prior to a major operation. These techniques can help:

▶ **Orienting Yourself to the Treatment Facility**
The familiar is less upsetting than the unfamiliar, and few things are more unfamiliar than chemo and radiation units. Visit the facilities where you will be treated so that when you do step in-side for your first infusion or radiation treatment, the setting and technology will not be startling. We frequently encourage patients beginning treatment in our chemotherapy center to visit, meet our full staff, speak with our other patients, and spend time getting comfortable with our spa-like environment. We find that taking a walk through our pharmacy, our treat-ment rooms, and the rest of the facility, as well as seeing the medications and technology used in treatments helps our pa-tients reduce tension and makes the first days much easier. This simple step alone can reduce your discomfort and stress.

▶ **Gathering Information from Your Medical Team**
A pre-treatment visit with your medical team can lower anxiety and reduce adverse reactions, so schedule an appointment to visit the clinic and talk with the doctors, the integrative staff if the clinic has any, and the nurses who will infuse your drugs. Clinics are used to this—or should be—so don't worry that you are asking for special treatment; your doctor can help you arrange it. Typically, the staff will show you around, and you'll have a chance to meet the clinical professionals responsible for your care, asking questions about the procedure. This will bol-ster your sense of control, countering feelings of vulnerability.

Your visit to the treatment clinic is a good opportunity to discuss using Life Over Cancer techniques to minimize side effects. Some of the mind-spirit, diet, exercise, and supplemental interventions that can help you do not require your medical team's involvement. You can, needless to say, practice comfort space imagery while receiving radiation without getting anyone's okay. But for others you will need your medical providers' support, collaboration, or at least knowledge. For instance, discuss with your doctor using headphones and a CD of music or positive suggestions during surgery. Explain that you would like to try lower dosing of antinausea medication for anticipatory nausea and vomiting, and instead try progressive muscle relaxation and focused imagery, so that increased medication will not automatically be written into your medical orders. Or you might desire more medication, taking every precaution to diminish risk of such side effects. The point is that communication is key. Don't hesitate to request to work with your nurses on managing mucositis with self-hypnosis or relaxed focused imagery (along with specific supplements), keeping your medication to a minimum. Ask how soon after surgery you can do exercises such as those described in the core fitness program in Chapter 8. This discussion will also help you determine how your medical team feels about integrative medicine.

▶ **List of Questions for Doctors**
To feel better equipped, you can formulate (and possibly even rehearse) a set of questions for the medical personnel administering your treatment, either before or during treatment. You will have different teams for surgery, radiation, and chemotherapy, so you will need to ask similar questions more than once.

- How many treatments are planned? Why? On what timetable?

- What are possible side effects?

- What measures are used to counteract side effects?

▶ **Twinning with an Experienced Patient**
In our clinic, when patients have agreed to participate, we "twin" a patient at an early stage of treatment with a "veteran" who can easily grasp the new patient's concerns and offer helpful insights and practical suggestions. Ask the personnel at your clinic whether they can suggest a patient with comparable issues who has coped effectively with treatment and who would be willing to speak with you (by phone, in person, or online).

▶ **Reinforcement of Self-Calming Techniques**
Many patients find it useful to keep a log of self-calming techniques to assess how well different ones work. You might want to copy the Personal Log of Mind-Spirit Strategies on the LOC website before you begin chemotherapy, radiotherapy, or doctor visits. If you fill this in daily for a few weeks, you will have a way to determine which situations in your therapy are most stressful and which techniques work best to allay the stress.

▶ **Support Groups**
We suggest joining support groups during your treatment and even after treatment, not right after diagnosis. After you receive upsetting news, you may still be reeling and feeling so overwhelmed by treatment decisions that you are unlikely to benefit from a support group.[6] But once you are in treatment, you will probably be more receptive to and benefit from a structured program that encourages (1) confidential expression of concerns, fears, and anger; (2) new or strengthened coping skills; (3) enhanced ways to communicate genuinely and effectively—affording a closer connection to those who matter most in your life and warding off isolation and disconnection; (4) relaxation, cognitive reframing, and self-hypnosis training; (5) meditation guidance; and (6) a chance to laugh with people who can readily appreciate the difficulty of finding special moments of joy. Your medical center may have support groups for patients with your cancer. In evaluating whether you should try one, refer back to the questions in Chapter 11.

▶ **Script Responses to Queries**

As a cancer patient, you will sometimes endure uncalled-for comments from friends and acquaintances who pressure you to take the latest herbal remedy they saw billed as a "cancer cure" on a website, offer stinging critiques of your chosen treatment, or tell you about a relative who supposedly had the same cancer as you and died an agonizing death within months of diagnosis (neglecting to mention that Aunt Phyllis was diagnosed with stage IV disease and refused all treatment, while you have stage I and are getting all reasonable interventions). Before you are subjected to any of these, think of polite but strong responses to affirm that (1) your team has investigated the best options and has chosen a treatment plan using a strong, combined approach; (2) you appreciate their concern, but if they have any questions or suggestions, please talk them over with the person on your A-Team who will field queries; and (3) you're sorry to hear about Aunt Phyllis, but fortunately your cancer diagnosis is very different. Or you can compose an e-mail or blog that heads off all of these comments, explaining what you have chosen to do and why and asking for full support without criticism. Plus, you can request that people not continue to call you about your condition, because you have been quite tired, so the relevant person on your A-Team will keep them posted on the status of your treatment and recovery.

▶ **Sleep Cues and Techniques**

In Chapter 8 I discussed the importance of sleep. Chemotherapy patients may find themselves with long-term sleep problems, especially those who have had sleep problems before. Good sleep hygiene is a must during treatment: go to bed at the same time every day, get daily exercise and exposure to natural daylight, remove distractions from the bedroom, limit naps to twenty minutes, and leave the bedroom after twenty or twenty-five minutes of restless tossing and go back to bed again after reading something that's boring or soothing. Keep the lights very dim, since bright lights will signal your brain to wake up. Take a hot bath one hour before going to bed, establish a regular bedtime, use relaxation techniques (such as progressive muscle relaxation, self-hypnosis, or comfort space imagery), or listen to quiet music just before bedtime, don't go on the Internet close to bedtime, and don't eat a large meal within two hours of bedtime. Consider sleep aids, including melatonin, which has strong anti-cancer properties. Your doctor may prescribe some of the newer sleep medications temporarily during this anxious time, but long-term use is less advisable than behavioral techniques.

▶ **Personal Imagery Tape**
Either hypnosis or guided imagery can reduce postsurgical complications, as I discussed in Chapter 10. A number of commercial CDs and tapes can help with this; see the LOC website. Or you can record your own tape or CD with personal messages and rapid recovery affirmations. These tapes offer more than simply relaxation messages or pleasant music; they communicate specific instructions to your body. At home prior to surgery, in the presurgical suite, or even during the surgery itself, you can listen to these recordings to "train" your body to direct blood away from the surgical site, heal the surgical wound more quickly, lessen nausea, and reduce pain. Though this may be surprising to you, hearing these suggestions when you are in a relaxed state appears to improve surgical outcomes.[7] You are well within your rights to ask if you can bring a CD that you find helpful into your surgical setting. Some hospitals provide headphones so that patients can listen to music of their choice during surgery. If yours doesn't, consider talking to your surgeon about bringing a CD player or iPod.

▶ **Lining Up Practical Support**
Chemotherapy, radiation, and surgery take time and drain you physically and emotionally, at least for a while. Arrange for transportation, child care, housework, meal preparation, and other regular responsibilities. You will probably need assistance not only when you are receiving chemo or radiation or in surgery but also during recovery. This is what your A-Team can organize. Be sure to ask them.

SIDE EFFECT MANAGEMENT:
TOOLS AND STRATEGIES FOR COPING

Minimizing physical effects
Controlling emotional reactions to treatment

Most of our patients are reassured by the knowledge that both nondrug therapies and specific medications are available for treating chemo-related side effects, including anxiety and emotional distress. There is no single right way to do relaxation and self-soothing exercises. The most important thing is to practice them every day, ideally for two 15-to-20-minute sessions. At the center, we recommend that patients make relaxed abdominal breathing—which occupies no more than five minutes—a morning essential and practice a body scan periodically throughout the day.

▶ **Minimizing Physical Effects**
Focused relaxation and progressive muscle relaxation can diminish chemo-induced nausea and vomiting. Practice for two weeks prior to chemo, an hour before treatment, then daily for five days after. Hypnosis, if you have access to a therapist who can do it or teach you self-hypnosis, can also help if you experience these side effects.[8] Focused imagery and hypnosis or self-hypnosis have been shown to significantly control mucositis, the severe mouth sores due to chemo. If you do experience other types of pain during treatment, hypnosis is an excellent option, as are focused imagery and any of the relaxation techniques. Breathing exercises, for instance, allow you to mentally float above pain signals. Even distraction, which can be as close as your DVD player, video games, or an absorbing book, can help because pleasant mental states block pain perception.[9] Pain is made worse by tension and anxiety, so daily practice of relaxation is a good preventive. If you experience persistent pain, talk to your doctor about more aggressive pain medication. Thankfully, current medical guidelines say that doctors must

give adequate treatment so that patients do not experience un-controlled pain.[10]

With anticipatory nausea, these techniques and systematic desensitization are good options. You can find a script and in-structions on the LOC website. You may be able to do this on your own, perhaps with the support of an A-Team member reading you the script. A psychologist at your medical center can also help. Or, since anticipatory nausea is a type of condi-tioned response, hypnosis can help disconnect this problematic association.[11]

▶ **Controlling Emotional Reactions to Treatment**

If you experience emotional distress during treatment, much of it will be transitory—short bouts of tension and anxiety. If you're relatively healthy and following your fitness plan, your body will bounce back fairly quickly from each fight-or-flight episode. If your disease is aggressive, or if the treatments you re-ceive are invasive or prolonged, the stress and tension can be-come chronic. If this occurs, you will need to be diligent about using the techniques in Chapter 11 (for example, meditation and breathing techniques) to help you feel less overwhelmed and to spare your body from the harmful effects of chronic stress, which can be debilitating and may even promote the growth and progression of cancer.

Emotions can also contribute to the perception of pain in sig-nificant ways. To the extent that you see pain as an indicator of threat or loss of control, your pain becomes magnified. Pain paired with anxiety becomes worse. If you suffer from persis-tent anxiety about your treatment and your future, you may find that a psychologist or a spiritual counselor can help you.

Some patients find that a common side effect of chemo or ra-diation that may seem to others inconsequential, such as hair loss, can tip them over the edge: it marks them even to strangers as "cancer patients." Plus, being hairless may leave you feeling exposed and vulnerable. You can avert some of this distress through advance planning, locating a natural-looking wig to match your hair, and even wearing it several weeks before you begin chemo. Other patients use scarves, interesting hats, or baseball caps. Check the LOC website for updates on hair- ⓘ saving treatments.

If you have been through treatment before and find yourself experiencing battle fatigue, please do not despair. As I will discuss later in this book, there are ways to detoxify, not merely from the chemicals of prior treatment exposure but from any psychological trauma that you may experience as well. While at times you may feel you are unable to take one more step toward recovery, do not underestimate the power of engaging in our mind-spirit program. It will help you dig deep to discover a place of healing and the psychological stamina required to continue.

POST-TREATMENT: TOOLS AND STRATEGIES FOR ADJUSTMENT

Support group
Satisfaction and mastery inventory
Future images and goal setting
Meditative practice
Finding a "new normal"
Discovering/revitalizing your personal vision

Lucy: Addressing Anxiety Over the End of Treatment

Lucy, who had an aggressive form of metastatic breast cancer, was just one day away from her last round of chemotherapy. All along she had anticipated the end of chemo—no more long car trips, no aftereffects of the drugs, no schedule disruptions—yet here she was feeling inexplicably tense. The anxiety she experienced prior to her *first* chemotherapy session had not surprised her, but the swelling panic as she approached her final chemo infusion was baffling. Knowing that her cancer had already spread to her liver once, she felt a nagging fear that the cancer might metastasize to some other vital organ. At least while receiving chemotherapy, she knew that something concrete was

being done to battle the disease and that she was closely monitored by the clinical staff. We reassured Lucy that although her
chemo was done, our care of her was not. To reinforce this, we
reviewed her integrative plan, moved her to our next phase of
care—growth control and containment—and scheduled regular
conversations for follow-up and support.

Lucy's distress is not uncommon.[12] During treatment, most patients focus on managing details of the chemotherapy, on immediate practical needs, and on coping with side effects. They
often feel assured that they are doing something to combat the
disease. With the end of chemotherapy and radiotherapy, you
may be torn: tempted to celebrate and to feel that you're okay
and able to resume your former life, but at the same time uncomfortable and vulnerable, since you are no longer under the
watchful eye of your medical team. Nor do you have chemo
drugs actively destroying cancer cells. For months after treatment, you may wonder whether it's possible or even desirable to
return to your former routine, whether you can ever recover the
sense of invulnerability you once took for granted, whether you
can resume a "normal" life. Many cancer patients finish their
conventional treatment and walk away from oncology centers
with a disquieting sense that now all they can do is wait passively and hope. Of course, the Life Over Cancer program of
ongoing nutritional, physical, and psychological self-care is designed to lower the risk of cancer recurrence; you should feel reassured that you are not a passive player in a waiting game, but
an active participant in defending against the return of cancer.

Fortunately, the mind-spirit techniques of the Life Over
Cancer program—thwarting thought warps and preventing
catastrophizing—can help at this stage in your recovery, too.
Once treatment ends, do not be surprised if you experience one
or more of the following:

- Anxiety over leaving the relative security of treatment, medical surveillance, and routine monitoring

- Pressure from family, friends, and coworkers to simply return to "normal," functioning, communicating, and relating to them as you did prior to diagnosis

- Self-imposed pressure to resume routine activities

- Fear of recurrence, especially when unexplained signs and symptoms arise

- Inability to reclaim a sense of control, competence, and mastery over daily life at home, in the community, and at work

- Anxiety before checkups, scans, or blood tests

- A sense of personal loss and of feeling flawed or defective, resulting in the need to discover a new self-image

- Altered sexuality, changes in self-image, and inhibition of sex drive

- Difficulty rebuilding a new sense of self and regaining self-esteem

How do you respond to these challenges? First, if people pressure you to get back to "normal" (as the husband of one of my patients did, telling her, "But you're done with cancer. Now we can get back to normal, right?"), gently but firmly explain that you are not back to your old normal, and quite possibly you may never be. That alone may be liberating. As for the sources of anxiety and fear listed above, rest assured that these feelings are not abnormal. Emotional distress does not evaporate with remission. So do not be surprised by the difficulty of readjusting to life when this phase of treatment ends. There are remission maintenance strategies (see Chapter 29) as well as monitoring that should continue well after treatment. Still, despite the normalcy of your reaction, this is the time to put into play other mind-spirit program tools.

▶ **Support Group**
The support group can be an ideal context for discussing strategies to improve life after cancer treatment. In fact, a formal

support mechanism may be even more critical after treatment than during it. Confronted with the continuing place of cancer in your life and wondering how to manage the presence of uncertainty, you might benefit from sharing your concerns with those who have parallel worries or who can tell you how they overcame them. These discussions can focus on problem solving—how to adapt to changes in your body, your family, your work, your priorities. Talk about physical and sexual changes, particularly ones due to procedures for breast, gynecologic, prostate, or colon cancer. As time goes on, your own experience can benefit others in the group, helping them regain a sense of competence and value, as well as social reconnection.

▶ **Satisfaction and Mastery Inventory**
Introduced in Chapter 11, this is a good way to identify special interests and pleasures possibly mislaid following diagnosis and during treatment. It can help you find activities that bring fulfillment and a sense of competence, allowing you to rediscover your life beyond cancer. On the other hand, if you find that your life is lacking in satisfaction and fulfillment, this can signal your need to seek counseling from a psychologist, life coach, or spiritual advisor.

▶ **Future Images and Goal Setting**
Begin to envision a positive future for yourself. You now know that the Life Over Cancer model can help you reduce your risk of recurrence. Using the technique outlined on page 251, you can replace the sense of loss with a sense of security and of controlling your destiny.

▶ **Meditative Practice**
Now that your treatment is over, you can begin healing your spirit with a practice that brings more than relaxation. Meditation can help you restore inner peace. There are many excellent meditation programs. You can find a course at a local health or activity center, contact one of the centers listed on the LOC website, or learn from a book (recommendations are on the LOC site as well).

▶ **Finding a "New Normal"**

The healing abilities of the human spirit are remarkable. As you move ahead, you will not be returning to your old "normal" but developing a new, healthier one. You will be eating more healthily, exercising smarter, and liberating yourself from thought warps. Don't feel distressed if you do not find a new normal immediately. If you work at it and are patient, it will come—perhaps when you realize that you have been so absorbed in planting your garden, fishing on a cloudless day, or laughing with your grandchildren that you did not think about cancer all day.

▶ **Discovering/Revitalizing Your Personal Vision**

The post-treatment adjustment period is when you can begin to reengage in your life with increased vitality and in every dimension of your being. Review the section on revitalizing in Chapter 11. Coping with the demands of treatment leaves most people without the energy needed to search for new or improved plans of living. But now that your treatment is over, you can refocus your attention. A good way to begin is to write down just one or two small benefits since your diagnosis—perhaps a stronger sense of special friendships. This may also be a good time to get involved in new activities. Revitalizing can be a long and fulfilling process, and now is the time to take the first steps.

REMISSION: TOOLS AND STRATEGIES FOR THRIVING

Cognitive reframing and thought stopping
Meditative practice
Satisfaction and mastery inventory
Exploring your dreams and visions
Finding inner spiritual meaning
Reenergizing hope

I believe that you can not only boost your odds of surviving cancer but thrive after your diagnosis and treatment. You are *not* in some morbid holding action. Now is the time to implement a plan for how you most want to be today and in the future. This means, as one of my patients put it, "Keep your eyes on the prize." You can do more than just make it through the daily hassle. You can, as another of my patients said, "find something good, something special, in each day." Here's how.

▶ **Cognitive Reframing and Thought Stopping**
If you've been in remission for five or more years, you are classified as cured. But this doesn't mean the impact of cancer is now absent from your life. Even six years out, patients still feel unease and uncertainty, shadowed by the fear of recurrence. When some innocuous pain or other feeling makes you think your cancer is back, practice cognitive reframing. As explained in the previous chapter, tell yourself, "I don't know what is causing my pain. I'll speak to the doctor in the morning. Besides, I did help my sister pack and move her books yesterday. In the meantime, I'll do some muscle relaxation and then go to my comfort space so I can get some sleep." Also, identify thought warps and write them in your Automatic Thinking/Rethinking record (see page ⓘ 240 and the LOC website), noting the accurate interpretation so you become adept at shifting from stress-arousing thoughts to calming or at least neutral ones. Practice thought stopping and reimaging to replace negative self-talk with more productive, rational thinking.

▶ **Meditative Practice**
If you have not yet found a form of meditation to practice regularly, remission is a good time to do so. Meditation can be an effective relaxation technique, and after regular practice it can also lead to continuing personal growth, inner peace, a deeper and more honest sense of self, insight, and a profound connection to a larger reality. As I mentioned in Chapter 11, meditation can help loosen the grip of exhausting ruminations over past events and future worries, allowing more vital living in the present. If meditation seems too exotic or poorly matched to your lifestyle,

remember that there are multiple ways to introduce a meditative practice into your life. Whatever routine activity you are engaged in can provide a meditative focus as long as your attention is fully absorbed in that activity or moment. At the Block Center, we explore different styles of meditation with patients, for example, prayerful or mindfulness, to find what fits best. I encourage you to look into the possibilities; the books listed on (i) the LOC website are a good place to start.

▶ **Satisfaction and Mastery Inventory**
During remission, it is important to work toward integrating changes in your goals and priorities, planning for the future, and taking stock of what makes life worth living. One patient told me, "I don't even recall how I started out in my work, or why I stayed with it." Discovering significant maladjustments in your life as a cancer survivor means it is time to make changes. Allowing sources of unbearable pressures to continue raising your level of stress hormones is not only a drain on your quality of life but also increases your risk of recurrence. Wherever and whenever possible, identify and establish new, personally meaningful life goals.

▶ **Exploring Your Dreams and Visions**
Now is also time for a simple inventory. Decide what really matters in your life and what you feel you can do without. Ask yourself, "Have I accomplished what I always wanted to do? How can I still move toward my goals despite the cancer-related changes in my life?" What enthuses you? Is there anything you hoped to do but somehow overlooked? Were there chances you missed? This is the time to take action on those missed chances and choices and, like many other cancer patients, move forward with a renewed investment in your future.

▶ **Finding Inner Spiritual Meaning**
Where do your spiritual or religious beliefs fit into your cancer journey?[13] Everywhere. Your spiritual or religious convictions may have provided the determination and strength to get you from your first, dizzying diagnosis to your recovery. Spirituality

and religion are not synonymous, although for many people they are interwoven. Spirituality is that element in our life that transcends the everyday business of existence and imbues life with a sense of meaning and purpose. Identifying your dream and revitalizing your vision therefore possess true spiritual significance. Listening to Beethoven's Fifth Symphony can be a spiritual experience, as can sitting atop a jagged peak at sunset or feeling connected to something larger than yourself. Religion rests on a particular system of beliefs and practices and is usually linked with an organized group, whereas spirituality often has no set of guidelines or precepts, and no specific congregation. A deep relationship with the divine and a connection to a practicing religious community can have a powerful impact on healing and wholeness. I encourage you to explore your religious roots. But I also know a number of patients who may not have strong religious ties but who do hold strong spiritual convictions.

If recovering from cancer has increased your desire to reconnect with spirituality or religion, you can find resources among health care professionals.[14] Hospital chaplains, community clergy, or pastoral counselors can provide a compassionate understanding of the spiritual aspects of health and illness. Art therapy, music therapy, and dance therapy can all help you explore profound aspects of being and living as a cancer survivor.

▶ **Reenergizing Hope**

Cancer recurrence can be even more devastating than the initial diagnosis. After doing all that was recommended, adhering to all medical regimens, undergoing multiple invasive procedures, and managing chemotherapy and its aftermath, you still did not beat back cancer for good. This is the time to find a doctor and health care team who believe in the potential of changing your internal environment so you can improve your odds of keeping cancer at bay. This is the time to work in earnest with a medical professional who thinks creatively and "beyond the box" (note: *beyond the box,* as opposed to *outside the box,* suggests that the box has its own importance and value and should be included), who is an expert in tailoring plans to meet your newest challenge.

Matt: Living Without Looking Back

A young man named Matt with a gastrointestinal stromal tumor was told by his initial oncologist that he probably would not make it to his next Christmas. Thankfully, his oncologist was mistaken. But Matt's medical path seemed more like crossing a minefield than a direct journey to recovery. Matt had been free of cancer for several years when he discovered that his cancer had returned. His spirits hit an all-time nadir. A cancer patient facing a recurrence must marshal inner stamina to undergo yet another bout of treatments, and Matt's will to continue was badly shaken. One of our Block Center mind-spirit specialists worked with him to help him marshal the determination to go the extra mile to curb his disease. He began a recently approved molecular target drug, Gleevec, with our oncology team, and the mind-spirit counselor worked with him day by day to stick with both his drug treatment and his full integrative program. Matt had a great response to Gleevec. With his body and spirit reinvigorated, he resolved to live without looking back. Matt even went on a skiing trip with his father for the first time in over a decade, an activity that brought him immense satisfaction and pleasure. Although he finally succumbed to his disease, Matt enjoyed another thirteen Christmases after that first dark year, navigating the challenges that cancer thrust into his path with reenergized hope and faith.

SPHERE 2

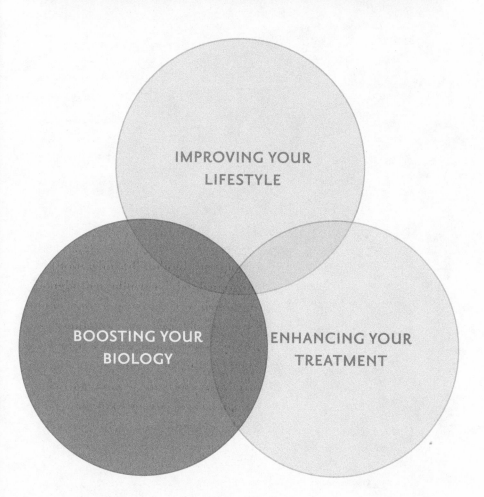

THE HEALING POWER
OF THE TERRAIN

When I was a medical student, I occasionally carried glass dishes full of human cancer cells from one lab to another. One day as I looked down at the little clumps of cells, I was struck by the disconnect between their fearsome reputation and their astonishing vulnerability. By vulnerability, I mean that despite cancer cells' immortality in the lab—scientists are able to propagate them indefinitely, under the right conditions—they are remarkably fragile. Unless they are nurtured as carefully as a hothouse orchid, just hours after being removed from a person they perish.

At that moment I understood instinctively that these cells can survive and cause such hellish destruction only when they are nourished, coddled, and protected by the biochemical terrain in which they reside. It would take years of my research and that of many, many others before I turned this realization into a coherent strategy for fighting cancer, but now it is a central focus of the Life Over Cancer program: your internal biochemistry can either nourish cancer cells or send them into molecular oblivion.

This is why targeting only the tumor is not enough to quash cancer. Conventional cancer therapies almost inevitably leave behind at least a small number of malignant cells. And remember that all cancers start with a genetic glitch *in a single cell*. It takes only one. That's why you have to do everything you can to keep that one—or those one thousand or one million—from proliferating and spreading.

The biochemical terrain—your body's internal chemical environment—plays an integral role in determining whether a tumor will regain its foothold after treatment, metastasizing to distant sites, or whether it will stay where it is without posing any threat. The internal biochemistry influences the microenvironment immediately surrounding the cancer cells. An inhospitable microenvironment impacts the disease. So, the biochemical environment matters. Which aspects matter? Inflammation, for one. In a 2005 study of 2,438 people who were followed for more than five years, those who had the highest levels of C-reactive protein, a marker of chronic inflammation, developed cancers of the breast, lung, and colon at higher rates than people without chronic inflammation.[1] Insulin and blood sugar also matter. Among 237 breast cancer patients, those who had high levels of blood sugar and insulin, characteristic of type 2 diabetes, had larger tumors that were more advanced and that had a worse prognosis than nondiabetic patients, a 2006 study found.[2]

Let's look at it another way, from the standpoint of people whose biochemical terrain is hostile to malignant cells. A number of studies have shown that many people who die of causes other than cancer had an undiagnosed malignancy, but one that, despite being present for years if not decades, had no effect on their health or survival. In one autopsy study, 86 percent of elderly African American men had undetected very early prostate cancers.[3] Yet something about their biochemical terrain kept the tumor in check. Whether your biochemical terrain coddles or combats cancer cells has a huge effect on whether you beat cancer for good or let it return.

If your body harbors malignant cells—and many of ours do—then the strategy is clear: make your biochemical environment hostile to their growth and spread.

In previous chapters I explained how diet, exercise, and mind-spirit interventions can affect this biochemical terrain by, for instance, reducing the inflammation that cancer cells thrive on. I hope you are adopting the suggestions in those chapters. What I want to do now is introduce even more powerful ways to make your terrain inhospitable to cancer. For although the Life Over Cancer diet program is designed to take full advantage of cancer-fighting foods and food concentrates, such as the green vegetable, fruit, and berry drink containing the Healthy Dozen food families that we give our patients at the Block Center, you need stronger weapons in your dietary arsenal if you are to make your terrain as hostile as possible to cancer cells. If you have cancer, it is a sign that your terrain has probably been imbalanced for years, which means you need help to restore your biochemistry to a cancer-fighting state. In addition, cancer and its treatment deplete your nutrient stores and amplify your nutritional needs beyond what is reasonable to expect from a diet. Nutritional supplementation, in tandem with the Life Over Cancer diet, offers another logical option.

Making your biochemical terrain hostile to cancer will have the additional benefit of improving your quality of life. Oxidation, for instance, nourishes cancer cells and makes them resistant to chemotherapy, but it also causes fatigue.[4] Inflammation promotes the growth of cancer cells, but it also causes pain and edema.[5] A disrupted immune system robs you of your body's natural cancer-fighting machinery, but it also makes you susceptible to infection.[6] By creating a biochemical terrain that is hostile to cancer, you will also be creating one that prevents unpleasant and even life-threatening complications.

Failure to target the biochemical terrain, including the impact of conditions such as obesity, is one reason we have been losing the "war on cancer" that President Nixon declared in 1971.[7] Billions of dollars later, research has yielded powerful anti-tumor drugs. But although the drugs shrink or even (apparently) eliminate the tumor, they often do not improve patients' survival.[8] How can this be? Surely if your tumor is gone, or a lot smaller, you have a better chance of survival. Unfortunately, it turns out that as long as the original cancer-coddling biochemical environment remains unchanged, cancer can—and often does—come back in full force. Not only can tiny numbers of residual cancer cells grow back into a tumor, but both chemotherapy and radiation produce enormous numbers of inflammatory molecules and free radicals that promote the growth of malignant cells and blunt the effectiveness of these same conventional treatments.[9] Since cancer uses the body's own resources to grow and multiply, we must use every aspect of your internal biochemistry to rein it in. Only by transforming the conditions that allow cancer cells to thrive can we hope to overcome the disease, especially over the long term.

Let me give an example of why and how we target one aspect of your internal biochemistry, through something I mentioned in the chapters on diet. Free radicals—reactive biochemicals that are by-products of oxidation—increase the rate at which cancer cells accumulate mutations. Each mutation has the potential for making the cell more resistant to chemotherapy or radiation.[10] Diets high in animal fats increase levels of free radicals, which help explain their cancer-promoting effects. But a low-fat diet, natural foods rich in antioxidants, "nutraceuticals," and botanical medicines limit free radicals and hence may reduce the genetic instability that increases the aggressiveness of cancer cells.[11] Putting together these and other interventions to make your terrain hostile to cancer is the basis of the Life Over Cancer terrain plan.

Five Cancer Challenges

Drawing on my clinical experience, I've identified five major cancer challenges that must be addressed. Your biochemical terrain will determine whether your body can successfully meet them.

1. **Reducing tumor growth and spread.** The state of your terrain affects your risk of developing cancer and, if you do develop it, how aggressive it is, whether it metastasizes, and whether it recurs after going into remission.

2. **Reducing tumor bulk and improving treatment response.** The state of your terrain can either interfere with or enhance the effectiveness of conventional treatment. For example, in-

flammation can turn on genes that can make radiation less effective at shrinking a tumor.[12]

3. Tolerating conventional treatment. The terrain can either aggravate or minimize side effects, which determine whether you can complete your treatment. For example, nerve pain can be minimized by reducing free radicals;[13] insomnia can be alleviated by reducing stress hormones.

4. Optimizing daily functioning. Your terrain can have a tremendous impact on your clinical condition and quality of life. Although fighting the disease is the first priority, seemingly minor quality-of-life issues are just as vital to your well-being. Energy swings, fatigue, and emotional lability, for instance, can often be corrected by regulating blood sugar.[14]

5. Reducing the risk of life-threatening complications. Most patients do not die from their cancers; they die from the *consequences* of cancer and its treatment. For example, many patients die from wasting syndromes with marked muscle loss and nutritional decline, which is fueled by inflammation. Others die from a blood clot that can break loose from where it forms and travel through the blood to hit major organs such as the brain or a lung, causing a stroke or embolism. Still other patients die of pneumonia or sepsis, the result of a suppressed immune system. Pain itself can send patients into a decline, setting off a series of clinical problems. With proper attention to your internal biochemistry, many of these complications can be prevented, and prevention is a far better strategy than trying to treat them after they arise.

To meet these challenges, it is necessary to optimize six defining features of your biochemical terrain. Cancer thrives on each of these, and the chapters that follow will tell you how to address each in turn:

1. Oxidation
2. Inflammation
3. Immunity

4. Blood coagulation
5. Glycemia
6. Stress chemistry and biorhythms

As you will see, many of the healing solutions overlap, so one intervention helps reduce inflammation as well as oxidation, for instance. In my experience, when patients correct disruptions and simultaneously repair and renew all six of these, they can tip the balance of power from malignancy to health.

Flora: Biochemical Health Makes Remission a Reality

Flora, fifty, had metastatic cancer. Her doctors could not find or even identify the original tumor, but it had spread to other parts of the body. These types of cancer are referred to as CUPs, or cancers of unknown primary. Before coming to our center, Flora had lost twenty pounds. When we saw her, she had no appetite, and her blood level of albumin (a measure of bodily proteins) was 2.1 g/dL, alarmingly low, and synonymous with a poor prognosis.

When we treat patients with such marked weight loss and low albumin, we track protein levels in the blood as well as body weight and lean muscle composition. When protein stores become depleted, patients can start a downward spiral to severe malnutrition that is difficult to reverse and makes continuing treatment impossible. Flora's previous oncologist prescribed a commercial protein-calorie drink and Megace (megestrol acetate), an appetite-stimulating drug. But this produced no improvement in her weight, protein stores, or albumin, leaving Flora vulnerable to a progressing cachexia and its attendant inflammation. Even low levels of chronic inflammation promote tumor growth, invasion, and metastasis. Indeed, the level of inflammation can be a reliable indicator of a cancer patient's prognosis, a 2000 study found.[15] Inflammation is also often the root cause of malnutrition, causing lack of appetite and cachexia.[16] This is probably why the previous oncologist's strategy failed: most high-calorie formulas that target cancer malnutrition were developed years before the medical world recognized that inflammation is the underlying mechanism of cachexia, so they contain inflammation-fueling refined sugars and omega-6 fats.

For these reasons one of the first things we did was test Flora's inflammatory markers. Sure enough, they were elevated. We immediately started her on a customized program initially built around selected supplements. We replaced the commercial formula with a whey-based shake that provides calories and protein in combination with other micronutrients but contains very low amounts of omega-6 fats. This much will be familiar from the chapters on diet. But that would not be enough. I also gave Flora a highly potent formulation of curcumin, a compound in the Indian spice turmeric, other plant extracts, and fish oil designed to increase her ratio of healthful omega-3s to omega-6s and support her body's natural inflammation responses.

After a short period, Flora recovered from her cachectic condition. Her appetite returned and, with it, her strength and vitality. Retesting her inflammatory markers, we found they were near normal. Her albumin level rose back into a near normal range, 3.5 g/dL, and she returned to her pre-cancer weight. Because Flora was so much stronger now, we were able to pursue other integrative treatments, including conventional anticancer therapies, which she was unable to tolerate before and which her inflammatory state would have made her cancer resistant to. Her metastatic disease went into complete remission. Today, as of this writing, Flora remains free of any detectable cancer.

Supplements: Positive and Negative Interactions

Some patients arrive at my office with a bag full of supplements, hoping that one (or all) will function as a magic anti-cancer bullet. Others disdain supplements, believing that a healthy diet is all they need. The first approach makes no sense, because without a sound scientific basis for choosing which supplement to use when, you can put yourself at risk of interactions or serious harm, or at best limit your benefits. The second approach ignores the many scientific studies supporting the value of supplements in modifying the internal terrain, fighting cancer, and enhancing treatments. For example, when researchers in Australia studied the interaction between a low-fat diet and fish oil supplements, they found impressive synergies: a low-fat diet *without* fish oil supplements produced no improvement in blood stickiness (a measure that is relevant to cancer growth, as I will discuss in Chapter 17), a low-fat diet *with* fish oil supplements reduced blood stickiness in most volunteers, and a high-fat diet *with* fish oil supplements nullified the beneficial effects of supplementation.[17] This is why you need a healthy diet *plus* smart supplementation, or you can inadvertently erase the beneficial effects of one through negative interactions from the other. (Interestingly, there is also evidence that fish oil can make cancer cells more vulnerable to chemotherapy agents, increasing their cancer-killing effect, a major reason we often suggest that patients take fish oil with chemotherapy.[18])

CAUTION: WHAT IS IN THAT SUPPLEMENT?

Just what goes into the supplements you take can be of major importance to your health. The research that has most impressed me indicates that the closer supplements are to whole, natural foods and botanicals, the more likely they are to be safe and healthful. Many supplements are made synthetically or by extracting a single phytochemical from an herb or food and packing it into capsules for sale. In whole plants and herbs, however, phytochemicals come in complex mixtures. If you take just one phytochemical out of a plant, you risk missing out on important synergies and beneficial effects, and may even cause harm. There are, for instance, eight different chemical forms of natural vitamin E in foods and all eight make critical contributions to health. Most commercial vitamin E supplements, however, include just one form, alpha-tocopherol. Taking only alpha-tocopherol crowds out other beneficial forms, such as gamma-tocopherol, and may actually be harmful. Mixed tocopherols, which include all eight forms, are much closer to natural vitamin E. The same applies to beta-carotene and the wide variety of carotenoid phytochemicals in vegetables and fruits. One reason I believe most research on supplements has not yet demonstrated impressive results is that the majority of studies focus on a single nutrient or phytochemical. This model neither represents the natural state of phytochemicals, nor results in a supplement that might address the multiple molecular defects and biochemical disruptions and pathways in cancer. When we start researching supplements that are closer to whole-plant natural foods and traditional formulations, I expect the data to look more impressive.

Another concern: some supplements may not contain what is stated on the package. Many tests have shown that some have less of the key component or components than the label claims. Some contain substances that are not on the label at all—such as sawdust. It's therefore of major importance to select a high-quality supplement from a reputable source. You can find a comprehensive discussion of supplement quality on the Life Over Cancer website.

It is important to note that some supplements can have negative interactions with your medical treatments. St. John's wort, for instance, stimulates the activity of liver enzymes that break down drugs in the body. The heightened enzymatic activity leads to low blood levels of some drugs—including chemotherapy drugs.[19] Other supplements have the same kind of physiological effect as prescription drugs and so can magnify their

effects. Several supplements magnify the effect of anticoagulants (blood thinners), for instance fish oil, feverfew, garlic, ginseng, vitamin E, vitamin C, ginger, and ginkgo.[20] Still others
may magnify the effect of sedatives or tranquilizers, including
the herb valerian. If you are taking supplements and prescription or over-the-counter drugs at the same time, you need to
have your pharmacist or doctor check them for negative interactions. Because of the possibility of drug interactions, you need
to have your supplements checked each time you start a new
drug. My research staff and I developed a professional consultation model in which we can assess potential drug-supplement
interactions. Besides evaluating patients for adverse interactions, we also search for favorable combinations and synergisms to improve results. You can learn more about scheduling
a consultation on the website.

Some foods also interact with medical treatment. Grapefruit,
for instance, inhibits the activity of the same enzymes that St.
John's wort stimulates, as well as enzymes that transport drugs
through the intestinal lining. Drinking grapefruit juice with
some oral medications can therefore affect blood levels of the
drugs, leading to either diminished or increased activity.[21] In
the latter case, you may also experience an increase in the
drugs' side effects. Turmeric, garlic, licorice, chile peppers, and
leafy green vegetables can negatively interact with anticoagulant drugs; your doctor or pharmacist should be watching for
these effects. However, don't assume that you must eliminate
these healthful foods. You just need an experienced practitioner to help you establish a safe and healthy balance of your
food, supplements, and medications. Needless to say, the following chapters do not recommend any supplements with
proven toxicity, although herb toxicities can be difficult to pin
down—the relaxing herb kava has recently been associated
with liver toxicity, for instance. So has black cohosh, an herb
that reduces hot flashes. In both cases, there are still significant
doubts that the associations have any validity.[22] I do tend to err
on the side of caution in cases of possible toxicity. I will have
more to say about supplement-drug interactions in Sphere 3,

where I discuss supplements that might be used during chemotherapy.

A final point about supplements: if you are scheduled for surgery, you will need to stop your supplements ahead of time.[23] If the surgery is done on an emergency basis, have a list of the supplements you are taking so the surgical team can take into account the anticoagulant effect of any supplements, since that could affect bleeding; and the sedative effect, since that could affect anesthesia.

Life Over Cancer Supplementation Strategies

The program I describe in the next six chapters takes into account all of these interactions in order to safely combine therapies and improve your prognosis. It does not simply pile nutrition advice on top of surgery, chemotherapy, and radiotherapy. Different dietary components are combined in a carefully orchestrated fashion, all with the goal of making your body hostile to cancer. The foundation is a healthy diet such as the Life Over Cancer diet described in Chapters 4, 5, and 6, since there's little sense gulping fish oil if your diet consists of burgers, pastries, and shakes: the inflammation-promoting diet will swamp the anti-inflammatory omega-3s in the fish oil. The second layer is the Healthy Dozen food families, food concentrates that can be taken separately or in such combinations as green vegetable, fruit, and berry drinks; concentrated fish oil; and vitamin-mineral formulas like those we give patients at the Block Center.

The third layer is the Terrain Support Program, the subject of the next six chapters. This focuses on supplements aimed specifically at the six most important aspects of your biochemical environment, listed on pages 287 and 288. The foundation of Terrain Support is a broad-spectrum supplement that contains a selection of agents that address all six aspects of your biochemical terrain:

BROAD-SPECTRUM SUPPLEMENTATION FOR TERRAIN SUPPORT

Dosage Range	Nutraceutical	Terrain Factor
25–75 mg	Grape seed extract, standardized to 90% oligomeric proanthocyanidins	Oxidation
250–500 mg	Alpha-lipoic acid	Oxidation and inflammation
500–800 mg	*Curcuma longa* (turmeric) extract standardized for curcuminoids	Inflammation
500–700 mg	*Agaricus blazei* (royal sun agaricus)	Immunity
500–1,000 mg	*Scutellaria baicalensis*, standardized for flavones (baicalin)	Inflammation
10–20 mg	Oregano essential oil (*Origanum vulgare*), 85% carvacrol, 0.5–4.0% thymol	Immunity
1,000–2,000 mg	Gingerroot extract, standardized for gingerols and shogaols	Blood coagulation and inflammation
100–200 mg	Cinnamon (a water-soluble, standardized cinnamon extract that has been through clinical testing should be used, as taking ordinary cinnamon long-term can be problematic)	Glycemia
100–200 mg	Siberian ginseng (eleuthero or eleutherococcus), standardized for 0.8% eleutherosides	Stress chemistry

I recommend taking a single broad-spectrum formula that includes as many as possible of these agents every day as the first step toward making your internal biochemistry as hostile as possible to cancer cells. But be careful to scrutinize where you are getting your formulations from, since quality can make the difference between a beneficial impact and none. (See www.lifeovercancer.com to learn how to determine supplement quality.) Work with your integrative medical practitioner to select appropriate supplement dosages and formulas. Use combination formulas that include the needed agents, so you can minimize pill-taking. ⓘ

Then, depending on your situation, I recommend building on this foundation with specific terrain boosters and modifiers, which target one or more particular aspects of the terrain. How do you know which aspects of your terrain you most need to target? Laboratory testing, which is how we make that determination at our clinic, is best, but there are also ways to make this identification on your own.

Determining Your Terrain Disruption

The most accurate way to determine which aspect of your internal biochemistry you most need to target is through lab testing. For this, you will need a medical partner, a health practitioner (integrative physician, oncologist, nutritionist, naturopath) who can order lab tests for you, who has the expertise and experience to help you to interpret the results, and who can make optimal decisions about selecting nutraceuticals and adjusting dosages. Here are a few of the tests I use to assess each of the six crucial aspects of a patient's terrain (the "Medical Partnership" section of the following chapters addresses each in detail):

Terrain Testing

Oxidative assessments: lipid peroxide levels and/or oxidized LDLs

Inflammatory assessments: C-reactive protein and/or fibrinogen

Glycemic assessments: fasting blood sugar, baseline insulin, and/or IGF-I levels

Blood coagulation assessments: VEGF, D-dimer, and prothrombin factor I.2 levels

Immune assessments: natural killer cell activity

Stress chemistry/biorhythms assessments: cortisol and melatonin rhythms

---

If you don't have immediate access to lab testing, you can still get a general idea of what features of your terrain may be out of balance by using the two lists below. The first shows, for different cancers, which aspects of the terrain are most often imbalanced. Some cancers, such as lung cancer, are more likely to cause problems with, say, blood coagulation, and make patients prone to blood clots, whereas others, like breast cancer, are worsened by high insulin levels, indicating disruption in glycemia. The second table shows which terrain imbalances are probably present based on cancer symptoms and treatment side effects. For instance, insomnia and depression often reflect disrupted circadian rhythms and stress chemistry, while cachexia and disabling fatigue are associated with inflammation.

To determine which aspect of your terrain you need to prioritize, look first at the diagnosis table and write down the terrain features associated with your cancer. Then look at the symptoms and side effects table. Look for overlaps: that's where you should focus first, starting by turning to the relevant chapter or chapters. To keep your supplementation reasonable, I encourage you to focus on one or two chapters. For the combination support supplements shown in these chapters, use a single formula that combines a few or even all of the listed supplements. For the terrain modifiers, you will use one or two single-agent supplements. If you have more than two disrupted aspects of your terrain, either ask a health professional with expertise which to tackle first or consider the following: if a symptom is potentially life-threatening, such as cachexia, or is making your life very difficult, such as pain, address the terrain features associated with that symptom first.

Once you get that symptom under control, you can move to your next priority, and go back and read the other terrain chapters that relate to your diagnosis. I do encourage you to read each of the terrain chapters, since the overall state of your terrain determines your clinical condition and the success of your treatments.

Diagnosis and Terrain Factors

Lung cancer: inflammation, blood coagulation, oxidation, stress chemistry

Breast cancer: glycemia, stress chemistry/biorhythms, inflammation

Prostate cancer: inflammation, glycemia

Colorectal cancer: inflammation, glycemia

Pancreatic cancer: glycemia, blood coagulation, inflammation

Melanoma: immunity

Bladder cancer: immunity, oxidation

Kidney cancer: immunity, glycemia

Ovarian cancer: inflammation, blood coagulation

Gliomas or brain tumors: inflammation, blood coagulation

Esophageal cancer: inflammation, blood coagulation

Endometrial cancer: glycemia, blood coagulation

Myeloproliferative cancers (such as chronic myelogenous leukemia): blood coagulation

Lymphoma: inflammation

Symptoms or Side Effects and Terrain Factors

Cachexia or accelerated weight loss: inflammation, glycemia, immunity

Slow surgical healing, pain, or swelling: inflammation, glycemia

Neuropathy: oxidation, inflammation

Heart damage from chemo: oxidation, blood coagulation

Nephropathy (kidney damage): oxidation

Insomnia or depression: stress chemistry/biorhythms, inflammation

Mood swings or emotional lability: glycemia, stress chemistry

Recurrent colds/flu, pneumonia, or other infections: immunity, inflammation

Fatigue: inflammation, oxidation, glycemia

Blood clot or embolism: blood coagulation, inflammation

Moderate to marked anxiety: stress chemistry/biorhythms

Using the Terrain Chapters

Each terrain chapter has three sections. First is an explanation of how the specific terrain factor affects your ability to respond to cancer's challenges. Next is "Your Self-Care Program," a section on diet, lifestyle, and supplements that you can implement on your own. Whether or not you have a medical partner, you should read and follow these lifestyle instructions. This section typically comprises four steps:

1. Eliminating terrain disrupters such as smoking and eating unhealthful foods
2. Adjustments to your fitness regimen that are important to the particular terrain feature
3. Ways to improve your dietary intake to optimize the terrain aspect
4. Recommendations for which supplements to take to address problems with that terrain factor

Each of the supplement ingredients has a recommended dosage or dosage range. These dosages are based on our analysis of clinical trials, my clinical experience, and other scientific literature. They tend toward the lower end of acceptable doses. This is done as a precaution, since they may be combined with other botanicals or phytochemicals that have synergistic activity. Patients at the Block Center may receive larger or at times smaller doses based on clinical care, laboratory results, disease symptoms or treatment side effects, drug interactions, and our ability to observe the patient's response to the supplement. As a reader of this book, you are strongly advised to work with your integrative practitioner in making decisions about supplement formulations and dosages for every aspect of Sphere 2. Your integrative practitioner can also help you choose which terrain factors you should concentrate on. Remember that you should be taking a broad-spectrum terrain support formula and following the lifestyle and supplement recommendations for only one or two terrain factors.

Finally, the "Medical Partnership" section explains the lab tests that are used to identify trouble within each terrain factor, how to interpret the results, and what supplements and foods to take if that terrain factor is disrupted. This section also describes special supplements and prescription drugs that may help restore that terrain factor to health. I recommend being retested every three months or so. That way you'll know whether you need to adjust your regimen or whether you've licked the problem.

CHAPTER 14

OXIDATION: FIGHTING CANCER-PROMOTING FREE RADICALS

E very cancer patient knows the feeling. As the day of your next scan or other test approaches, your anxiety mounts as you worry that the tumor has barely shrunk or that the cancer has returned. What would you say if I told you that you may be able to improve your odds of getting good news? By simply taming a common but vicious biological process, you may be able to counter both what drives the growth of cancer and what makes cancer resistant to drug therapies. This biological process is oxidation. And you can turn it way, way down by making changes in how you live and, especially, in what you eat. What I am proposing is that you undertake a serious lifestyle change, spurred by the real possibility that doing this will buy you additional ammunition in your battle with cancer.

Oxidation occurs during metabolism and many other biological processes. The problem is that oxidation generates free radicals, highly reactive molecules that damage DNA. As you recall, cancer starts with DNA damage, and each additional mutation increases the likelihood that the cancer will develop resistance to radiation or chemotherapy. A body with high levels of free radicals is said to be under oxidative stress, one of the key aspects of a terrain that nourishes cancer. But it is possible to mop up the free radicals in your body through antioxidants, in both foods and supplements. This not only improves your chances of going into and staying in remission but also can increase your survival. This chapter explains how you can reduce oxidative stress. I will use the term synonymously with "an unhealthy abundance of free radicals."

Oxidative Stress

Iron rusts, a sliced apple turns brown, and skin wrinkles: all are processes of oxidation. Oxidation in the body isn't exactly the same as rusting, and doesn't necessarily involve oxygen, but it can be as damaging to biological molecules as rusting is to iron. Oxidation means the loss of an electron from an atom or molecule. Because atoms and molecules like to have their full complement of electrons, the loss of one (or more) makes them seek replacements. In less anthropomorphic terms, the atom or molecule becomes a highly reactive free radical, driven to combine with other molecules in order to grab their electrons. Free radicals are like addicts who have had their drugs confiscated. Desperate and on the prowl, they'll do anything to get their drugs—electrons—back. For a free radical, any molecule is a potential target, including DNA. If a free radical reacts with DNA, the result can be a mutation that initiates cancer, promotes growth and progression, alters the cell in a way that makes it resistant to radiation or chemotherapy, or makes it metastasize.

Where do free radicals come from? Many are formed when we breathe oxygen and digest food, things you definitely do not want to stop doing. Ironically, given that free radicals are especially pernicious for cancer patients, cancer itself can increase their production. Cancer cells produce free radicals at a much higher rate than normal cells, and the chaotic blood flow in tumors causes periods of low oxygen to alternate with reoxygenation, a process that generates free radicals. These radicals in turn fuel further growth, promoting a vicious cycle of more radicals and more growth. Also, tumors are often infiltrated by immune cells called macrophages, which may deliver free radicals as part of an attempt to kill the cancer cells.[1] That's great if it works, but often it doesn't, with the result that the barrage of free radicals has merely damaged the cancer cell, making it more aggressive and resistant to treatment.

Oxidation and the Challenges of Cancer

As a cancer patient, you face major challenges. Oxidative stress throws obstacles in the way of overcoming these challenges.

Challenge	Consequences of Oxidative Stress
Reducing tumor growth and spread	Increases mutagenesis and DNA mutation rate. Upregulates angiogenesis, leading to faster tumor growth. Increases the risk of spread; more likelihood of metastases.
Reducing tumor bulk and improving treatment response	Accelerates tumor sculpting. Increases resistance to radiation and to many chemotherapies.
Tolerating conventional treatment	Tissue damage to heart, nerves, liver, ear, and gut. Increases risk of neuropathy, cardiotoxicity, liver toxicity, kidney damage, hearing loss, and gut damage.
Optimizing daily functioning	Disrupts mitochondrial functioning. Causes fatigue.
Reducing the risk of life-threatening complications	Causes progressive weakness, leading to inactivity that promotes muscle wasting, which raises the risk of pneumonia and death.

Let's examine each one of these challenges and how oxidative stress impairs your ability to overcome them.

▶ **Reducing Tumor Growth and Spread**

Only in the last few years have scientists come to recognize how powerfully oxidative stress can raise a tumor's malignant potential. Free radicals can disable genes that suppress cancer growth (tumor-suppressor genes) or activate genes that promote tumor growth (oncogenes).[2] How can free radicals exert such opposite effects, disabling one gene but turning on another? The explanation is that free radicals are like unguided missiles. They break strands of DNA, alter the molecules that constitute DNA, and mix up chromosomes during cell division—all at random. So while there is a mathematical possibility that a free radical will disable an oncogene and activate a tumor suppressor gene, the sheer number of them makes it far more likely that one will eventually do something damaging and not beneficial. (Sure, the monkey has a statistical chance of typing *Hamlet,* but it has a greater chance of typing *tktkzqu euety eyth. . . .*)

Free radicals do not stop with DNA. They can also damage the endothelial cells that line blood vessels, making it easier for tumor cells to enter and exit the bloodstream—their highway to metastasis.[3] Free radicals help tumors release metastatic cells, promote angiogenesis (growth of blood vessels that feed tumors), and damage the cancer cell's internal communication network by increasing the level of signaling molecules responsible for out-of-control proliferation.[4]

These processes have real-world consequences. In a 2002 study of 363 breast cancer patients, those with the highest blood levels of oxidatively damaged fat molecules were twice as likely to develop a recurrence as women with the lowest levels.[5] And women with metastatic breast cancer had twice as much free radical damage to the DNA in their breast tissue as women with localized cancer: a 1996 study found a clear correlation between the growth of metastatic tumors and the extent of free-radical-induced DNA damage.[6]

Given the power of free radicals to promote the growth and spread of cancer, they need to be in your crosshairs. Unfortunately, mainstream oncology has yet to fully recognize how important it is to support patients' antioxidant defenses. My clinical experience, however, suggests that optimal use of antioxidants

can spell the difference between thriving and merely surviving—
or not surviving at all.

► Reducing Tumor Bulk and Improving Treatment Response

Radiation and many chemotherapy drugs kill malignant cells
by generating lethal oxidative stress. That is, they generate such
an avalanche of free radicals that the cells are destroyed. The
problem is that there are always some survivors. Cancer cells
that are exposed long-term to free radical levels that are high,
but not high enough to kill them, adapt. In a perverse case of
Darwinian "survival of the fittest," some cancer cells may mu-
tate in a way that makes them more and more resistant to treatment.[7] It is very much like mosquitoes developing resistance to
DDT: survivors of the initial spraying become invulnerable to
the poison, and their offspring inherit the same resistance until
the entire population shrugs off DDT. So it is with cancer cells.
If even a few develop resistance to treatment, all of their de-
scendants have it, too.

This is why it is so important to alter your oxidative environment. Otherwise, the terrain is right for the cancer to come
roaring back after treatment, even to evolve into a more aggressive form. Indeed, cancer's ability to continually adapt is one
reason why chemotherapy and radiation are not more effective
against cancer: the treatments also produce free radicals that
support the disease process, allowing any cells that survive the
barrage of radiation or chemo to thrive. That does not mean rejecting conventional treatments. On the contrary, I believe that
conventional therapies may be made safer and sometimes even
more effective by combining them with specific antioxidant
strategies. This is a somewhat controversial view. Some oncologists believe that antioxidants will counteract the effectiveness
of chemotherapies that work by creating free radicals. But after
combing the scientific literature for studies in which antioxidants were given along with chemotherapy in randomized
trials, in a study published in August 2007 in *Cancer Treatment
Reviews,* my staff and I found no case where survival or tumor
shrinkage was significantly worse in the antioxidant group. In
fact, the antioxidant group did better—in nearly half of the

studies, significantly better.[8] There is simply no evidence that antioxidants make chemo less effective, and there are strong hints that they may make it easier for patients to receive their full doses of drugs without having to stop due to adverse side effects. This appears to impact response to treatment and survival.

▶ **Tolerating Conventional Treatment**
While the processes that drive malignant growth are invisible, other effects of oxidative stress can cause tangible misery in the day-to-day life of a cancer patient undergoing treatment. As noted above, both chemo and radiation generate free radicals to destroy malignant cells. Unfortunately, there are more than enough free radicals left over to attack healthy tissue, too. This causes some distressing chemo side effects.

The most common is neuropathy, which arises from damage to nerve cells and is experienced as tingling, numbness, and pain, often in the extremities. It can arise when free radicals generated by several chemotherapy drugs attack nerve cells.[9] Oxidative stress can also cause chronic radiation proctitis, inflammation of the rectum that results in diarrhea, rectal pain, rectal bleeding, and/or fecal incontinence.[10] Oxidative stress can also damage your heart muscle. The chemo drug Adriamycin (doxorubicin) generates powerful free radicals by interacting with iron in your body, which is why I routinely give heart-protecting antioxidants to patients who receive Adriamycin.[11]

Ideally, treatment would minimize the free radical damage to normal tissues without diminishing the lethal effects of free radicals on malignant cells. In most cases, though, some damage to normal tissue may occur. That's why following conventional therapy, I advise my patients to use every technique in the Life Over Cancer tool kit to reduce oxidative damage to normal tissues.

▶ **Optimizing Daily Functioning**
In addition to causing the side effects described above, oxidative stress can impair many cellular functions essential to your health and vitality. For instance, free radicals break down cells' outer membranes, making them more permeable to noxious

invaders. Among the invaders are—you guessed it—free radicals. Penetrating deep into the cell, they attack energy-generating structures called mitochondria. The cell becomes less able to utilize glucose and oxygen to generate energy.[12] This may be one of the causes of "chemo brain," resulting in memory and cognitive impairment, and of muscle weakness and fatigue.[13] Cancer-related fatigue can rob you of the fighting spirit you need to overcome disease.

▶ **Reducing the Risk of Life-Threatening Complications**
Fatigue caused by oxidative stress can trigger a vicious cycle. It can make you become physically inactive, which leads to muscle wasting. As you lose muscle, you are bound to be even more sedentary. Muscle loss also weakens your respiratory function, leaving you vulnerable to respiratory infections such as life-threatening pneumonia, and depletes your stores of glutamine, an amino acid essential to mounting a strong immune response.[14]

The Life Over Cancer program can, by reducing oxidative stress, help you rise to these challenges.

YOUR SELF-CARE PROGRAM

When you are healthy, the body's natural antioxidant mechanisms can usually keep up with free radicals, limiting oxidative stress and even mopping up the damage it causes to DNA and cells. To keep this system robust, all you usually need to do is eliminate harmful habits such as smoking, reduce stress, and adhere to a low-fat diet high in antioxidant phytochemicals. But when you have cancer, you need to do more to control and reduce oxidative stress. This is because oxidative levels tend to be higher in people with cancer, partly because of the radiation and chemo treatments that work by generating free radicals and partly because tumors themselves generate free radicals. By "doing more," I mean boosting the body's natural antioxidants with those available in foods and supplements, and engaging in lifestyle and stress-reduction practices so you do not add to your body's free-radical burden.

Studies show the benefits of reducing oxidative stress. In a 1994 study of sixty-five patients with bladder cancer, the five-year survival rate of those who received the higher doses of antioxidant vitamins in conjunction with conventional treatment was double that of patients who received vitamin supplements at Recommended Daily Allowance levels.[15] Similarly, a 1992 study of eighteen patients with small-cell lung cancer who received antioxidant supplements in addition to standard treatment found that the two-year survival rate was 33 percent, double the usual 15 percent.[16]

So how do you go about managing oxidative stress? You have basically two options: decrease the production of free radicals from processes that you can control, and increase the production of antioxidants that mop up free radicals.

▶ **Eliminate Oxidative Offenders**
Minimize your exposure to oxidants and maximize exposure to antioxidants. As you can see in the list below, the first part of this is totally under your control.

Oxidative Offenders

Tobacco and alcohol consumption (a single puff of cigarette smoke contains more than one hundred billion free radicals)[17]

Sedentary lifestyle and excessive body fat

Overly strenuous aerobic exercise

Psychological stress

Ionizing and nonionizing radiation, such as from excessive sun exposure or tanning booths

High storage levels of iron as ferritin, usually due to chronic inflammation or overconsumption of dietary iron

---

Don't Smoke, and Stay Away from Secondhand Smoke. Cigarette smoke is loaded with free radicals and can also change antioxidants into pro-oxidants.[18] (This may explain why, in two large studies of smokers and former smokers, taking beta-carotene supplements was linked with an increased risk of dying from lung cancer: the very nutrient that helps non-smokers by acting as an anti-cancer antioxidant hurt smokers by acting as a cancer-promoting pro-oxidant.[19]) Interestingly, in a 2008 report in the *International Journal of Cancer,* a randomized study showed that beta-carotene increased cancer recurrence and mortality in a group of patients with head and neck malignancies—but only among those who smoked during treatment. Nonsmokers, or those who stopped for the duration of treatment, had no ill effects from the beta-carotene supplements (a fact generally overlooked in press coverage of this study).[20] There are no two ways about it: if you have cancer and continue to smoke, you are far more likely to experience accelerated tumor growth, but if you quit, your chances of survival will increase.

Zero Out Alcohol Consumption. Liquor has an adverse effect on the liver's antioxidant systems, increases oxidative stress, and can interact with key nutrients in a detrimental way. Alcohol does a Jekyll-and-Hyde number on the important antioxidant beta-carotene, turning it into a pro-oxidant that promotes the generation of free radicals.[21] A possible exception is red wine, which packs a strong antioxidant punch. Drink red wine only with a meal, since drinking it on an empty stomach can make your blood sugar surge, and drink in moderation[22] or less.

Avoid Iron-Rich Foods. Red meat and other iron-rich foods can also fuel oxidative stress when the iron reacts with hydrogen peroxide in the body to generate hydroxyl ions, which are free radicals that damage DNA.[23]

Reduce Psychological Stress. Psychological stress has been associated with oxidative damage. For instance, workers who reported high levels of job-related stress also had higher levels of oxidative damage to DNA than their colleagues. Stress management, as described in Chapter 10, can help here.[24]

Avoid Radiation Exposure. Common sources of radiation include sunlight and tanning booths, as well as work-related radiation exposures, which you should, of course, minimize. Oxidative damage by radiation is one of the steps in the induction of skin cancer by excessive sun exposure.

▶ **Fitness Adjustments**
Follow the fitness regimen appropriate to your needs, as described in Chapter 9. Although short-term, intensive exercise raises oxidative stress, developing a routine with regular moderate workouts will reduce it over the long term.[25] Even four hours a week of exercise can significantly increase your body's resistance to free radicals.[26] Doing only an occasional, very strenuous exercise (e.g., episodic marathon training), however, is linked to low antioxidant protection. That's why I advise my patients to avoid the "weekend warrior" syndrome. Exercising at least a few times a week, if not daily, is much more beneficial than cramming four hours of exercise into a Saturday and Sunday, a pattern that promotes oxidative stress and, if the exercise is particularly intense (as it tends to be when people feel they have to make up for lost time), increases your need for antioxidants. On the other hand, a sedentary lifestyle contributes to excess body fat, which is linked to chronic inflammation, another source of antioxidants. Moderate, regular exercise is, again, the key to normalizing your antioxidant capacity.

▶ **Improve Dietary Intake**
Reduce the Total Fat Content of Your Diet. Fats are the main dietary oxidizers. As the fat content of your diet goes up, so does the oxidative damage to your tissues, cells, cell membranes, and DNA. One recent study, for instance, found that women who consumed higher levels of fat had significantly more damaged DNA in their tumors than women on a low-fat regimen. Another study of breast cancer patients found a 16 percent increase in the risk of mutated DNA for every

additional gram of fat in these patients' daily diet; for every extra gram of saturated fat, there was a 30 percent increase in the
risk of mutated DNA.[27]

Avoid High Doses of Single Antioxidant Supplements. Don't be
fooled by the word *antioxidant* on a bottle of pills. Not all antioxidants are created equal. Some are stable, and others are
what I will often call *labile*. Labile antioxidants—which include
vitamins A, C, and E, selenium, and beta-carotene—can change
into pro-oxidants, as I mentioned in the no-smoking advice
above.[28] Thus they can increase the oxidative stress of your terrain and, if used without proper supervision, enhance the
growth and spread of cancer cells. Used in the right dosages and
combinations, however, they can help control malignancy. See
"Take an Antioxidant Support Supplement" below.

Refine Your Dietary Intake. Following the LOC nutrition program as outlined in Chapter 5 will boost your antioxidant intake automatically. A few reminders:

• **Eat plant foods in a rainbow of colors.** Antioxidants
function as a "mutual support" network in the body. Eating a
wide variety of foods, especially colorful fruits and vegetables,
will help you maintain the network.[29]
• **Consume organic foods whenever possible.** Although you
certainly want to reduce exposure to carcinogenic pesticides,
there is another reason for a cancer patient to go organic: studies have found that some organic fruits and vegetables contain
considerably more phenolics and other antioxidant compounds
than does conventionally grown produce.[30] Many supermarkets
carry organic produce, as do farmers' markets.
• **Choose grains for their antioxidant capacity.** Barley, millet, and oats have higher antioxidant levels than some other
whole grains.[31]
• **Choose proteins for their antioxidant capacity.** Aim for
two to three servings a week of salmon, which contains the carotenoid antioxidant astaxanthin, and one daily serving of soy-

beans (e.g., tofu, soy milk, tempeh). Among vegetable sources of protein, pinto beans, black beans, broad beans, kidney beans, and small red beans have the highest antioxidant capacity; get one or more servings a day.[32]

• **Choose oils and nuts that are high in antioxidants** and not easily oxidized, such as almonds, walnuts, pecans, extra-virgin olive oil, walnut oil, high-oleic safflower oil, and almond oil.[33]

• **Choose drinks for their antioxidant capacity,** such as green tea, white tea, and rooibos tea.

• **Spice up your meals** with high-ORAC spices and seasonings. Oregano has more than forty times the antioxidant capacity of apples, more than ten times that of oranges, and four times that of blueberries. This means one tablespoon of fresh oregano has antioxidants equivalent to one medium apple or two oranges. Other high-ORAC seasonings include dill, fresh garlic, fresh gingerroot, rosemary, cloves, sage, cumin, and paprika. The whole-leaf or unground versions have the highest antioxidant power.[34]

• **Use powerfood concentrates.** Supplement the antioxidants you get from food by having one to two servings a day of a green-vegetable-and-fruit drink with ingredients such as those I described in Chapter 5. Food concentrates of this type are high in lycopene, lutein, and other antioxidants, which are especially effective at quenching free radicals.

▶ Take an Antioxidant Support Formula

Since many times oxidative stress cannot be completely corrected by the preceding modifications, at the Block Center we use an antioxidant support formula composed of micronutrients and plant extracts, in addition to whole-food concentrates. A good antioxidant support formula should contain a diverse group of antioxidants from natural sources: The diverse antioxidants in a good support formula come in moderate doses, to reduce the chance that any labile antioxidant will become a pro-oxidant and make it more likely that the antioxidants will act synergistically. Lung cancer patients in particular, especially former or current smokers, should avoid megadoses of particular antioxidants such as vitamin E and beta-carotene, as well as vitamin A. Some studies have indicated risks to these patients and to smokers from pro-oxidants formed in the hazardous internal environment that smoking causes.[35]

The support formula recommendations below take advantage of the networking properties of antioxidants in the body.[36] Vitamin E (alpha and gamma tocopherol), for instance, works best paired with vitamin C and alpha-lipoic acid. In addition, the antioxidants below target many types of free radicals of concern in cancer—hydroxyl radicals, superoxide radicals, singlet oxygen, and nitrogen free radicals—while improving your overall antioxidant capacity. You should take an antioxidant support supplement in addition to a foundation of the Healthy Dozen powerfoods and a broad-spectrum formula that addresses each aspect of your terrain. I recommend using a combination formula containing multiple agents that support normal oxidative stress status by adjusting several different mechanisms.

RECOMMENDATIONS FOR A COMBINATION ANTIOXIDANT SUPPORT FORMULA

Nutraceutical and Dose	Oxidative Targets
Grape seed extract: 50–150 mg (standardized to 90% oligomeric proanthocyanidins)	Total antioxidant capacity of the bloodstream[37]
Vitamin C: 500–1,000 mg with citrus bioflavonoids	One of the body's main antioxidants; reduces lipid peroxidation, especially in people with high oxidative stress levels[38]
Lycopene: 7–10 mg	Scavenges oxygen free radicals[39]

Pycnogenol: 50–100 mg	Scavenges the dangerous hydroxyl radical that causes DNA mutation[40]
Rutin extract/citrus bioflavonoids: 300–600 mg	Scavenges the superoxide radical[41]
Aged garlic extract: 500–1,800 mg	Scavenges free radicals including the superoxide radical[42]
Alpha-tocopherol: 200–400 IU	Squelches free radicals[43] Best obtained from mixed tocopherol formula
Gamma-tocopherol: 200–400 mg	Squelches nitrogen-based radicals[44] Best obtained from mixed tocopherol formula
Beta-carotene (natural): 5,000–10,000 IU	Scavenges the singlet oxygen molecule[45] Best obtained from mixed carotenoid formula
Alpha-lipoic acid: 300–800 mg	Has been described as the major "recycling" antioxidant, extending the metabolic life span of the other antioxidants[46]

Search for a supplement containing a combination of as many as possible of these herbs and phytochemicals for antioxidant support, or at least take one or two. Be sure to work with your integrative practitioner in selecting agents and dosages and in minimizing the pills you take. Note also that ongoing research may modify these suggestions.

Especially if you are undergoing chemotherapy, your doctor, pharmacist, or other health practitioner should check any formula for interactions with your drugs. Because of the anticoagulant effects of garlic and vitamin E, you may need to omit supplements that contain these if you develop a low platelet count—particularly less than 60,000 cells per microliter—while taking chemotherapy; consult with your oncologist about this. (i) More information about antioxidants is available at www. lifeovercancer.com.

MEDICAL PARTNERSHIP

Once you've laid the foundation for reducing oxidative stress with the self-care program, the next step is to acquire information about your disease and your nutrient and biochemical status to fine-tune your antioxidant supplements. Since this information comes from lab tests, you will need to find a physician or nutritionist who can help you determine which ones to order. (If lab testing is not possible, return to Chapter 13 and review the section "Determining Your Terrain Disruption.") At the Block Center, we run not only assays that test your total antioxidant capacity but also specific tests to identify which antioxidant nutrients are low. This enables us to adjust our supplement recommendations: if you have rock-bottom levels of ascorbate in your system, for instance, we recommend doses high enough to bring you into the normal range and then monitor you to make adjustments up or down.

▶ **Measuring Antioxidant Status**
At the Block Center, we run a panel of oxidative stress markers to help us determine which ones are elevated in our patients. With continual monitoring and reevaluation, this enables us to provide the right supplements and adjust doses. Following are the tests for oxidative stress you should ask your medical partner about.

1. **Total antioxidant capacity** is a snapshot of the overall antioxidant protection circulating in your blood. Any weakness in this test indicates a need to reduce oxidative stress. A normal level for the test currently used in the Block Center is over 1 mmol/L.

2. Oxidized LDLs and lipid peroxides measure long-term oxidative stress, including how much cellular damage has occurred in the last few months. Normal levels of oxidized LDL are 200 to 800 mg/dL; anything over 1,000 is cause for concern. The normal level of the lipid peroxide test currently used at the center is less than 0.45 mmol/L.

3. Vitamin C, vitamin E (alpha- and gamma-tocopherol), vitamin A, coQ_{10}, and carotenoids such as alpha-carotene, beta-carotene, lycopene, and lutein can be measured in blood. I like to see beta-carotene levels (in nonsmokers and nondrinkers) well above the reference range of 1 mmol/L, not only because it is an important antioxidant but because I use it as a marker for vegetable consumption: if this marker soars, I know the patient is eating lots of veggies.

4. Serum zinc and selenium are crucial for proper functioning of the body's antioxidant enzyme systems. Deficiencies are common in advanced cancer patients, particularly those undergoing chemotherapy.[47] However, blood levels of selenium above about 1,000 mcg/L can be toxic, and levels of zinc above about 30 mmol/L may suppress your immune system. So it is necessary to monitor blood levels to ensure optimal dosing.

5. Serum ferritin, a measure of iron stores, monitors iron in the body. Excessive iron can generate dangerous hydroxyl radicals that damage tissue, worsen treatment-related side effects, increase DNA mutation, and further promote malignant growth. Serum ferritin should be below 150 mg/dL; levels above 200 mg/dL warrant medical intervention.

An important point about interpreting your tests: Many times the "normal" laboratory range is derived from a sample of healthy people. Because cancer patients may require a more therapeutic level, at the center we devise individual dosing regimens intended to produce levels of critical antioxidants such as lycopene *above* the normal range and levels of deleterious oxidative markers such as lipid peroxides *below* the normal range.

The results of this and your other terrain tests will help you evaluate whether the terrain factors that you picked out from the tables in Chapter 13 are actually disrupted. If your results for these tests are consistently normal, you can proceed to the chapter on the next aspect of terrain you need to target. If one or more antioxidant tests are abnormal, however, you should go to the next section, on terrain modifiers.

► **Terrain Modifiers**

Once you know from these tests which (if any) measures of antioxidant status are impaired, you can address the problem more precisely than you could with a combination antioxidant support formula. After your integrative oncologist, your nutritionist, or another medical partner has gone over the results of your tests, the next step is to fine-tune your program with a terrain modifier by finding the supplements or food sources that can best address any readings that fall outside the therapeutic range. Below is an abbreviated version of food and supplement recommendations suitable for terrain modification. Your medical partner should be using appropriate caution to screen these for negative drug interactions among patients taking medications. Because many of the body's important antioxidants come from what you eat, you can use food as well as supplements as terrain modifiers.

ANTIOXIDANT TERRAIN MODIFIERS

Lab Test Results	Consider
Low total antioxidant capacity	*Supplements:* anthocyanidin extract, green tea polyphenols (EGCG), mixed mineral ascorbates. *Foods:* increase the foods from the dietary refinements list on page 310.

High levels of oxidized LDLs or lipid peroxides	*Supplements:* grape seed extract, beta-carotene, alpha-tocopherol succinate (a form of vitamin E), carnosine.
Low levels of vitamin C	*Supplements:* ascorbic acid or mineral ascorbates. Note: if you are on anticoagulation therapy or you have low platelet counts, keep vitamin C intake to under 1,800 mg/day.
Low levels of vitamin E (alpha-tocopherol and gamma-tocopherol)	*Supplements:* mixed tocopherols. Note: if you are on anticoagulation therapy or you have low platelet counts, keep vitamin E intake to under 200 IU/day.
Low levels of vitamin A	*Supplements:* pre-formed vitamin A sources such as cod liver oil or retinol. Avoid excessive dosing of pre-formed vitamin A (above 25,000 IU daily). *Foods:* To increase vitamin A, eat soy products, cod liver oil, whole eggs, most animal foods, sweet potatoes, carrots, spinach, squash, cantaloupe, apricots, and any other foods high in vitamin A. If you have abnormal liver enzymes or functions or your vitamin A levels are too high, reduce consumption of these foods.
Low levels of coenzyme Q_{10}	*Supplements:* coenzyme Q_{10}. Note: coQ_{10} might reduce the effectiveness of Coumadin therapy.[48]
Low levels of alpha-carotene	*Supplements:* alpha-carotene. *Foods:* carrot juice, cooked carrots, Swiss chard, pumpkin, winter squash, tomatoes, green beans, cilantro.

Lab Test Results	Consider
Low levels of beta-carotene	*Supplements:* natural beta-carotene. *Foods:* many of these are the same as for alpha-carotene, such as spinach, carrots, carrot juice, sweet potatoes, kale, turnip greens, winter squash, and collard greens. Overconsumption of beta-carotene can make your skin yellowish, usually on the soles of the feet and the palms of your hands. Carotenodermia is harmless and will reverse itself when you lower your beta-carotene intake. If levels are too high, reduce the consumption of these foods.[49]
Low levels of lycopene	*Supplements:* tomato extract or lycopene. *Foods:* tomatoes, watermelon, apricots, papaya, guava, pink grapefruit. If levels are too high, reduce consumption of these foods.
Low levels of lutein	*Supplements:* lutein. *Foods:* eggs, spinach, collard greens, broccoli, zucchini, corn, brussels sprouts.
Low levels of zinc	*Supplements:* zinc. If levels are too high, reduce or stop supplementation. *Foods:* pumpkin seeds, sesame seeds, green peas.
Low levels of selenium	*Supplements:* selenium. If levels are too high, reduce or temporarily stop supplementation. Note: do not take more than 400 mcg a day. *Foods:* barley, rye, oats, salmon, spinach, yellowfin tuna.

High levels of serum ferritin (iron)	*Reduce intake* of animal foods, spinach, chard, romaine, blackstrap molasses, tofu, greens, mustard, mushrooms, turnip greens, green/snap/string beans, leeks, and some spices and herbs high in iron such as thyme, basil, cinnamon, oregano, turmeric, black pepper, dill weed, cumin, parsley, rosemary, and coriander seeds.

After you have been taking the relevant terrain modifiers for about three months, have blood tests done again. If test results have normalized, you can continue your basic support, including a cancer-specific multivitamin, fish oil, a green-vegetable-and-fruit drink containing the Healthy Dozen food families, and the broad-spectrum and antioxidant support supplements that support the entire terrain, but drop the specific terrain modifiers. Get retested approximately every three months to see if your oxidative markers remain normal.

▶ **Pharmaceutical Therapy**

If dietary supplements do not right your antioxidant imbalance, you should discuss with your physician whether you might increase your dosage of the support supplement or whether prescription medications might help. These would include off-label use of approved drugs—that is, using the drug to treat a condition for which the manufacturer has not requested approval from the Food and Drug Administration, but for which there is reasonable clinical evidence of safety and efficacy. This can be especially crucial when you are undergoing chemotherapy or radiation, since both can markedly raise oxidative stress and cause side effects so toxic you have to quit treatment.[50]

Here are some examples of situations in which off-label use of pharmaceutical-grade antioxidants is warranted:

• Platinum drugs such as cisplatin, which are widely used chemotherapy agents, can induce brain toxicity through oxidative stress, especially in people who are bedridden. Animal studies show that free radical scavengers including the drug allopurinol can inhibit cisplatin-induced damage to the cerebral cortex, although this subject needs more research.[51]

• Cisplatin can also cause kidney damage. In a clinical trial, intravenous glutathione reduced the incidence of kidney damage among cancer patients receiving cisplatin, without interfering with the chemo's anti-tumor effects.[52]

• Radiation and chemo kill cancer cells with toxic free radicals. As I noted above, free radicals also attack healthy tissue. In some studies the drug Ethyol (amifostine), injected alongside chemotherapy or radiation treatment, protects against side effects and blocks this damage by scavenging free radicals. In fact, patients with metastatic lung cancer who received amifostine along with conventional treatment had better response rates and prolonged survival.[53] There is a small (3 percent) possibility that Ethyol might impair anti-cancer efficiency of radiation. Whether you want to explore trying these drugs is something you should discuss with your physician, who will have to work with you in choosing and obtaining the medications.

Freddy: Managing Oxidative Stress

Freddy traveled to the Block Center all the way from his home in Argentina for treatment of metastatic (stage IV) renal cell carcinoma. The original tumor, in his left kidney, had been discovered early in 2000 during a routine exam. Freddy had the kidney removed, but the tumor had grown into surrounding fat, requiring removal of his pancreas and spleen, too. After being discharged from the hospital, Freddy was given no additional treatment beyond a brief course of an experimental hormone therapy designed to reduce the risk of recurrence. Freddy didn't ask many questions. He used denial as a coping strategy to stave off depression and intentionally avoided learning too many details of his illness. Six months later, Freddy got shocking news: a CT scan revealed kidney cancer near the site of the surgery. This time, Freddy was put on a regimen of interleukin-2, an immune cell product (cytokine) that stimulates a cascade of immune reactions, including production of T helper cells, drivers of the immune assault on kidney cancer. A standard and often effective treatment for advanced kidney cancer, interleukin-2 can also be highly toxic.[54] After Freddy began his five-days-a-week injections, he experienced fevers, chills, severe fatigue, and weight loss.

Freddy did enough reading and investigation to make some appropriate dietary changes, in hopes of improving his flagging health during his treatments. He had some success, experiencing few of those debilitating side effects during his second cycle of interleukin-2. After three six-week courses of treatment, he finally received some good news: although the kidney tumor was still there, it had stabilized. But a few months later, after more drug treatments, Freddy's energy and general health began to deteriorate again. It was at this point, in 2002, that Freddy came to the Block Center. He wanted a more comprehensive way to fight his cancer, he told me, and a way to recover his lost vitality.

I mapped out the Life Over Cancer program, explaining how it integrates conventional treatments, which we continued with the help of his oncologist in Argentina, and an individualized program of complementary therapies that help reduce the side effects of and improve response to treatment. I explained how my staff would work with him to achieve an optimal internal biochemistry, one inhospitable to cancer, through nutrition, supplements, fitness, and other changes in lifestyle. Freddy listened, nodding, as I told him that he had a serious malignancy and that regaining his health would require his full participation. I also told him that there were probably emotional, social, and stress-related contributors to his condition, and he would have to make a sincere effort to address these.

Freddy told me, "I am on my third marriage, and have been divorced twice. I am the father of six children, ages twenty-four, twenty-two, twenty-one, fifteen, and twins who are seven. My past marriages and divorces were very stressful. I felt bad for a long time, and I blamed myself for their failure." Brightening, he continued, "But my current marriage is great! I feel comfortable; she is wonderful. But I still have the stress of my job. I am an engineer, and the standards are rigorous and deadlines are always tight."

Having heard what the Life Over Cancer program entails, Freddy had no doubts about undertaking the changes that would be necessary to fight his cancer. "This is why I decided to visit your center," he said. "I expect to be one of your successful patients. I am sure I can follow a dietary therapy and a healthier style of living. I want to be a vigorous person again, one who has decided to live." I was taken by Freddy's powerful will to live and his ability to express it. On that agreeable note, Freddy and I began our journey.

As part of his Sphere 1 interventions, our staff helped Freddy implement the diet, support supplements, exercise program, and mind-spirit treatments described previously. To initiate Sphere 2, I ordered comprehensive lab tests of Freddy's nutritional status, including levels of oxidative stress and blood levels of various antioxidants. Fatigue is often associated with abnormal levels of oxidation, and indeed, the lab tests showed that Freddy's oxidative stress was sky-high and that he had worrisomely low levels of anti-cancer nutrients and antioxidants. Add to this his weight loss and diminished energy, and it certainly looked as if his elevated levels of free radicals had taken a toll.

Because his oxidative stress was so high, our dietitians also recommended supplements that target this aspect of the biochemical terrain:

- A combination antioxidant formulation to quench free radicals

- A time-release version of vitamin C designed to keep blood levels elevated throughout the day

- High-dose green tea extract, a powerful antioxidant

Since kidney cancer is one of the most immunogenic cancers, meaning kidney cancer cells can be detected and eliminated by cells and biochemicals of the immune system, we also recommended immune-supporting vitamins, minerals, other nutrients, and plant-based medicines, including mushroom extracts known to support immunity. For a short period, he added an experimental vaccine to his treatment plan.

After six months on his Life Over Cancer program, Freddy's markers of oxidative stress were significantly lower, within normal range. His levels of the antioxidants retinol (from vitamin A) and carotenoids including lycopene (from tomatoes) were *above* normal—not a bad thing when you have cancer—reflecting his increased intake of vegetables, fruits, and "healing foods" such as the green drink supplement. Fourteen months later, two of the three main measures of antioxidant capacity had improved even further. As I reviewed Freddy's nutrition diary, I saw that he had stuck to our nutrition and supplement program, which left me confident that his biology was changing for the better. Freddy returned to Argentina, and we continued to coordinate his treatments and care through his local physician. In August 2002, seven months after he had begun his integrative program at the Block Center, we received a letter from his oncologist, saying Freddy had no symptoms, was in good general health, had high levels of energy—and had *no evidence of cancer.* As of this writing, in 2008 Freddy remains cancer-free, despite having had a cancer with a median survival of about a year at the time it recurred.

As I have said repeatedly about statistics, they do not apply to individuals. Freddy's case shows this with crystal clarity. By making his biochemical terrain hostile to cancer, I am convinced, we allowed him to derive the maximum benefit from conventional treatments, altered the biological environment through lifestyle interventions and nutrition to defend against growth, and beat the odds.

CHAPTER 15

INFLAMMATION: OVERCOMING CANCER'S FIERY SIDE

This book is, of course, about what to do when you have cancer rather than how to reduce your risk of developing cancer. But some of the mechanisms that initiate the cascade of molecular events that lead to cancer also promote the growth and increase the aggressiveness of existing tumors. One of these is inflammation.

When I was a medical resident, one of my patients insisted that a melanoma on her toe was the result of chronic injury and inflammation there. I was dubious. But as the years passed I came across more and more case reports and studies supporting her claim: inflammation is indeed associated with malignancy. If a cellular mutation is the spark that lights the malignant fire, then inflammation is the fuel that keeps the fire growing and spreading.

Evidence of the ability of inflammation to both initiate and fuel cancer has been accumulating since at least the 1980s. Several studies show that rheumatoid arthritis increases the risk of lymphoma and lung cancer; the longer you've had arthritis, in fact, the greater your likelihood of dying from cancer.[1] Patients with chronic infections of the bone (called osteomyelitis) or even bedsores are prone to aggressive carcinomas and sar-comas.[2] Diseases that end in -*itis*—arthritis, bronchitis, fasciitis, colitis—as well as eczema and asthma all stem from chronic in-flammation; left to their own devices, many -*itis* disorders can increase the risk of cancer. Approximately one in every ten pa-tients with ulcerative colitis, for instance, will eventually de-velop colorectal cancer, according to a 2000 study. By another estimate, chronic inflammation may precede at least one-third of all cancers.[3]

And once you have cancer? Inflammation is still the bad ac-tor. Your inflammatory state can be measured by blood levels of C-reactive protein, or CRP for short, in addition to other fac-tors such as fibrinogen. Excess levels of CRP are associated with more aggressive or advanced tumors. In general, the higher your CRP levels, the more unfavorable your prognosis. Indeed, in advanced cancers, CRP levels are often the most reli-able indicator of prognosis, particularly with colorectal, lung, pancreatic, and prostate cancers. Among women with breast cancer, high CRP levels not only correlate with a more ad-vanced stage of disease but also may predict the onset of bone metastases.[4]

The converse is also true: controlling inflammation can re-duce the risk of and decrease the aggressiveness of cancer. Three studies, for instance, have shown that women who take non-steroidal anti-inflammatory drugs (NSAIDs) such as aspirin or ibuprofen have a significantly lower incidence of breast cancer than women who do not.[5] In a study that followed eighty thou-sand women for a decade, taking aspirin at least three times a week was associated with a 23 percent reduction in the risk of getting breast cancer, and women who regularly took ibuprofen (found in such products as Advil and Motrin) twice a week or more had half the rate of breast cancer of women who did not. A 1999 study found that women who had breast cancer and were long-term users of NSAIDs were significantly less likely to have large tumors and positive lymph nodes—two critical indi-cators of prognosis. Finally, a 2007 study observed that breast cancer patients who took NSAIDs were 36 percent less likely to die of cancer than those who took none.[6] This chapter will tell you how to control inflammation and thereby improve your prognosis.

Inflammation and the Challenges of Cancer

Inflammation has a very specific connection to each of the key cancer challenges.

Challenge	Consequences of Inflammation
Reducing tumor growth and spread	Increased cancer development, angiogenesis (growth of blood vessels which feed tumors), and metastasis[7]
Reducing tumor bulk and improving treatment response	Increased resistance to treatment due to COX-2 functioning and stimulation of other molecules that promote inflammation; interference with programmed cancer cell death (apoptosis)[8]
Tolerating conventional treatment	Increased risk of blood clots and radiation-induced fibrosis (lung scarring); delayed surgical healing due to cytokines (cellular messaging molecules) that promote further inflammation[9]
Optimizing daily functioning	Increased pain caused by inflammation-mediating molecules; inflammation-induced fatigue and malaise; edema (excessive fluid retention), anemia, fever, and anorexia (lack of appetite)[10]
Reducing the risk of life-threatening complications	Inflammation-induced cachexia, associated with severe weight loss, malnutrition, and protein wasting, in turn leading to low albumin levels[11]

▶ **Reducing Tumor Growth and Spread**
Although inflammation is your immune system's healthy, natural—and critical—response to an injury or illness, when the

inflammatory response persists, the white blood cells and macrophages that swarmed all over the invading pathogens can inflict long-term damage on tissues and encourage the growth and spread of cancer through a number of mechanisms:

• **Activation of tumor-promoting macrophages.** These immune-system cells produce biochemicals that promote tumor growth, including TNF-alpha, PGE2 (prostaglandin E2), and LTB4 (leukotriene B4), all critical biochemicals in the inflammatory response. In pro-inflammatory environments, macrophages can also trigger insulin resistance, a condition in which excessive insulin circulates in the blood. Insulin is a well-known stimulant of cancer growth.[12]

• **Activation of inflammatory molecules called cytokines,** which trigger production of a biochemical called NF-kappaB, a powerful promoter of tumor growth and metastasis.[13]

• **Weakening of immune competence.** In general, the greater the inflammation, the greater the immune suppression, which means your natural defenses against rogue cancer cells are diminished.[14]

• **Increased blood supply for new tumor growth.** A number of inflammatory mediators, such as vascular endothelial growth factor (VEGF), promote angiogenesis, the growth of new blood vessels that let tumors grow and spread.[15]

• **Increased blood vessel permeability.** This enables a protein called fibrinogen to pass from the blood into a wound area, where it is converted to fibrin, which appears to play an important role in angiogenesis.[16]

• **Breakdown of the fibrous material that surrounds cancer cells** by proteolytic enzymes. This allows the malignant cells to pass into the blood and metastasize.[17]

▶ **Reducing Tumor Bulk and Improving Treatment Response**

Molecules that promote inflammation appear to interfere with programmed cancer cell death (apoptosis). One reason involves an enzyme called COX-2: the target of the so-called COX-2 inhibitor drugs such as Celebrex (celecoxib), Bextra (valdecoxib), and Vioxx (rofecoxib); the latter two were withdrawn from the market in 2005 because they unduly raised the risk of cardiovascular events such as stroke and heart attack. Several herbs, such as turmeric and ginger, also inhibit COX-2, but there is no sign that they raise cardiac risks.[18] COX-2 triggers production of prostaglandins, which are responsible for the pain and swelling of arthritis inflammation. Blocking COX-2 therefore reduces that inflammatory response. But COX-2 is also involved in resistance to radiation and chemotherapy, apparently by increasing synthesis of another major inflammatory molecule, NF-kappaB, which both amplifies the inflammatory cascade and increases tumor resistance to radiation and chemo.[19] This may be why the response of lung cancer patients to conventional therapy is correlated with their level of inflammation: in one study, thirty-two out of sixty-one lung cancer patients with a significant drop in their levels of C-reactive protein benefited from radiation therapy, whereas patients with high levels of CRP did not.[20]

▶ **Tolerating Conventional Treatment**
Radiation can cause a host of inflammation-related side effects, including fibrosis (abnormal fibrous tissue in the lungs), mucositis (mouth sores), cystitis (bladder inflammation), enteritis (GI tract inflammation), esophagitis (inflammation of the esophagus), pneumonitis (lung damage), and proctitis (inflammation of the rectum).[21] What seems to happen is that when the radiation damages a cancer, there is collateral damage to normal tissues. The normal tissue responds as it does to any injury, igniting the inflammatory response. Which inflammatory condition results depends on what kind of tissue the radiation hits.

Chemotherapy produces its own set of inflammatory side effects, such as lethargy, sleepiness, loss of appetite, and increased risk of deep vein thrombosis, hemorrhaging, clotting, and hand-foot syndrome.[22] The last is a painful inflammatory disorder that causes swelling and peeling of the skin on the extremities. These side effects are caused by several different mechanisms that include increased production of inflammatory molecules called cytokines, produced when chemotherapy switches on certain inflammation-producing genes. A

2008 study showed that chemotherapy resulted in high levels of inflammatory molecules such as VEGF or interleukin-6 in some patients.[23] Even surgical complications, notably slow wound healing and swelling, are exacerbated by localized inflammation.

▶ **Optimizing Daily Functioning**
Dolor, rubor, calor: these Latin words for "pain, redness, heat" are how, for centuries, medical students have learned to identify inflammation. For our purposes, the significant word is *dolor,* "pain." Inflammation hurts. That is why aspirin and other non-steroidal anti-inflammatory drugs (note the *anti-inflammatory* in the name) alleviate pain: they reduce inflammation and its attendant swelling by going after inflammatory chemicals. Less inflammation, less pain.

▶ **Reducing the Risk of Life-Threatening Complications**
Inflammation can bring on cachexia, the severe wasting syndrome common among patients with solid tumors and, especially, metastases. Cachexia, which is particularly common in cancers of the pancreas, colon, and lung, can lead to the rapid breakdown of muscle, including the heart muscle. Before the 1990s, most oncologists believed that cachexia occurred because cancer siphons away the body's energy stores, beginning with glucose and fat and then moving on to the proteins in muscle. We now recognize that cachexia stems mainly from out-of-control inflammation. What happens is that inflammatory cytokines cause reduced appetite in addition to abnormal metabolism of proteins, fats, and carbohydrates, leading to loss of muscle and weight.[24]

YOUR SELF-CARE PROGRAM

I hope that the above persuades you of the importance of reducing inflammation as part of your battle with cancer. Just as reducing oxidative stress makes your biochemical terrain inhospitable to malignant cells, so does reducing inflammation. The rest of this chapter is about how you can reduce this fiery side of your biochemical terrain. Some sources of inflammation come with the cancer territory: cancer cells produce high quantities of inflammatory biochemicals; tumors are infiltrated by macrophages that release more inflammatory biochemicals; and surgery, radiation, and chemotherapy can all worsen inflammation, as can their side effects. There is not much you can do about these sources of inflammation. But others are well within your control.

To begin the self-care program for quelling inflammation, make sure that you are following the LOC recommendations for Sphere 1 as well as possible, including taking a green-vegetable-and-fruit drink containing the Healthy Dozen power-foods, or systematically including them in your diet.

▶ **Eliminate Inflammatory Offenders**
Using the list below, identify the main sources of inflammatory offenders in your life.

Inflammatory Offenders

Smoking

Alcohol consumption

Indoor and outdoor pollution

Sleep deficit

Extreme exercise

Unhealthy dietary fats: overconsumption of omega-6s and saturated and trans fats

Unhealthy carbohydrates: overconsumption of high-glycemic-index foods

Unhealthy cooking methods: high-flame or high-heat methods, such as charcoal grilling and deep frying

Being overweight, especially with excess abdominal fat

Avoid Tobacco Smoke. If you don't smoke, you are already ahead of the game. If you do, I don't know how to say this any more clearly: *you have to stop smoking.*[25] Inflammation is aggravated by exposure to cigarette smoke. Smoke from regular cigarette and pipe tobacco, as well as from marijuana, exacerbates the activity of your body's inflammatory cells. Tobacco smoke also accelerates the formation of highly toxic and mutagenic substances, not only fueling inflammation but accelerating the growth of existing tumors.[26] Continuing to smoke can undermine your battle against cancer and shorten survival.[27] There are many quitting strategies now available, such as nicotine gum and herbal gums designed to reduce cravings. Hypnotherapy can be effective, and possibly acupuncture.[28] Ask your doctor to recommend smoking-cessation programs, a hypnotist, or an acupuncturist. Secondhand smoke also causes your body's inflammatory cells to swing into action.[29] Stay away from areas where other people are smoking, something that is considerably easier now that many localities have banned smoking in restaurants, workplaces, and other public places.

Avoid Excessive Alcohol Consumption. An occasional glass of red wine is fine; compounds in red wine have anti-inflammatory effects. But excessive drinking, especially of hard liquor, raises your body's inflammatory level by increasing oxidative stress and altering enzymes that modulate the inflammatory response.[30,31,32] Result: a drop in your body's production of anti-inflammatory chemicals. If an evening cocktail (or two) is an ingrained part of your daily routine, try bubbling springwater on the rocks with a twist of lime. Your body will thank you.

Maintain Normal Weight. Body fat, or adipose tissue, is a major source of interleukin-6 (IL-6), a cytokine that promotes chronic inflammation, as well as arachidonic acid. As you might expect, overweight people have a higher level of inflammatory compounds in their blood, regardless of lifestyle or medical history.[33] Low-grade, chronic inflammation is par for the course if you are overweight or obese. I don't need to tell you how difficult it is to lose weight and keep it off, and this is not a weight-loss book. But to reduce your body's fat stores, I recommend the basics—a low-calorie, high-fiber diet plus moderate aerobic exercise. Over the years we have had excellent long-term success getting patients to their ideal body weight with persistent adherence to the LOC core diet and exercise plan.

Get Enough Sleep. Sleep deficit, which for most people is less than six hours a night, can increase pro-inflammatory chemicals such as IL-6 and TNF-alpha. Sleeping less than four hours a night for ten nights straight can make levels of C-reactive protein soar.[34] If you have trouble getting enough sleep, please refer back to the tips in Chapter 19. Don't use your bedroom as an office or for watching television, and avoid erratic bedtime hours.

Minimize Exposure to Pollutants. Chemical pollutants can induce inflammation through a variety of mechanisms, including oxidative stress, disrupting liver detoxification, triggering allergic reactions, and production of pro-inflammatory molecules such as TNF-alpha. Chronic inflammatory reactions can also result from regular exposure to diesel exhaust, ozone, mercury from coal-fired power plants, and other air pollutants. Since we in the West live in a sea of chemicals—in the air, water, and consumer products—avoiding them altogether is not feasible. But you can take steps to minimize your exposure.[35] For example, keep your home and work environment free of toxic materials by using nontoxic cleaning agents (avoid oven cleaners in particular) and having plenty of air-filtering houseplants. For a selection of comprehensive guides, see the LOC website.

▶ **Fitness Adjustments**
The "weekend warrior" syndrome, in which an intense bout of jogging, bicycling, or other exercise is packed into two days to make up for a sedentary five days, is an excellent way to trigger the inflammatory response. That's why you hurt: the assault on muscles unaccustomed to such demands releases inflammatory cytokines.[36] Aches and pains are *not* a natural, let alone healthy,

part of getting in shape. So stick to a regular, moderate fitness regimen, exercising at least every other day, and ideally daily, as described in the core fitness program. If you've had to reduce your workouts due to cancer or the side effects of treatment, when you get back up to speed (as discussed in the fitness chapters) do so gradually. Give your tissues time to recover before exercising again. You can figure out the right exercise-and-recovery schedule by trial and error: if you are sore after working out, especially the next morning, you've overdone it. Transition gradually into any new activity or into one you're just resuming after an interruption of more than a week. As you continue to exercise, you will find that you can do more and more without getting sore.

▶ **Improve Dietary Intake**
Adjust Your Intake of Fat. This is by far the most important way to control inflammation through diet. In one study of people who ate a typical fast-food breakfast of sausage, egg sandwich, and hash browns, blood levels of pro-inflammatory chemicals soared and stayed high for up to four hours after eating. (Levels of free radicals, a marker of oxidative stress, as described in the previous chapter, doubled and remained high for the same period.[37]) Inflammatory mediators are triggered by the imbalance of omega-6 fatty acids in our cells—that is, too many omega-6s and too few omega-3s. That ratio is determined almost exclusively by what we eat. A diet and supplement plan that produces an optimal level of omega-3s compared with omega-6s is critical for undoing persistent inflammation and making your terrain hostile to cancer.[38] A Japanese study published in 2008 showed that a diet high in vegetables, fruit, soy products, and fish was associated with lower levels of CRP.[39]

Unfortunately, we in the West have been going in the wrong direction on this one. We have dramatically increased consumption of omega-6s such as arachidonic-acid-rich animal fats and linoleic-acid-laden vegetable oils while decreasing consumption of omega-3-rich fish and green leafy vegetables. To reduce arachidonic acid, avoid beef, milk, cheese, pork, egg yolks, and poultry, all of which are hefty sources. To reduce linoleic acid,

zero out corn oil, safflower oil, sunflower oil, and other vegetable oils in favor of the following:

- Canola oil
- Flaxseed oil
- Olive oil (extra-virgin)
- Walnut oil

As I explained in the diet chapters, you *want* omega-3s. So
while a low-fat diet is desirable, you need not go overboard: a
very-low-fat diet, defined as one in which fat calories amount
to 10 percent or less of total calories, rarely provides enough
omega-3 fat and so can lead to an unhealthy ratio of omega-3s
to omega-6s. Fish oil supplements are a must at this fat percentage. I've seen many patients who thought they were doing
themselves a favor by cutting nearly all fat out of their diet.
Instead, their inflammatory problems escalated. I therefore recommend two to three servings a week of salmon, mackerel, herring, or sardines, all excellent sources of omega-3s. Also cut
back your egg consumption to one to two weekly, and these
should be omega-3-enriched eggs or, better, egg whites.

Eliminate trans fats, which appear on food labels as partially
hydrogenated fats or oils.[40] Abundant in processed foods, they
lower your body's production of anti-inflammatory chemicals.
Avoid margarine, vegetable shortening, hydrogenated oils,
commercial peanut butter, baked goods, fast food, cookies,
crackers, snack foods, french fries, prepared mixes, candy, and
commercial waffles.

Steer Clear of Refined Carbohydrates. Refined carbohydrates
(found in many of the trans-fat-containing foods listed immediately above) aggravate inflammation by causing insulin
production to spike.[41] Because refined carbs and other high-
glycemic-index foods are directly related to blood levels of
C-reactive protein, that marker of inflammation, emphasize
whole grains, high-fiber foods, legumes, vegetables, and fruit,
as described in the chapters on the Life Over Cancer diet. High-

fiber foods and whole-grain products prevent the inflammatory effects of surges in blood sugar and insulin.

Choose Foods That Actively Fight Inflammation. Some foods are especially high in anti-inflammatory compounds, so if your inflammatory markers are particularly elevated, I recommend getting even more of the following foods than in the core Life Over Cancer diet.

• **Salicylate-rich foods.** A natural anti-inflammatory compound, salicylate is one of the key active ingredients in aspirin. It is produced by a wide variety of plants when they are attacked by pathogens, in a kind of immune response. But unlike aspirin, natural salicylates do not prevent clotting and thus pose no risk of gastrointestinal bleeding. Among the best sources of natural salicylate are wintergreen, turmeric, and tomatoes. As with other disease-fighting phytocompounds, salicylates tend to be present at higher levels in organic foods than in those treated with pesticides, so buy organic whenever you can.[42]

• **Flavonoid-rich vegetables and fruits.** Flavonoids are not only potent antioxidants, as described in the previous chapter.[43] They are also anti-inflammatory, inhibiting the same COX-2 molecules that Celebrex, corticosteroids, and ibuprofen do and suppressing key cytokines that are essential cogs in the inflammatory network and are off the charts in many cancer patients.[44] It's easy to pack your diet with flavonoids—go for color. Cherries and raspberries have the highest COX-2 inhibitory effect, with fresh blueberries, blackberries, and strawberries close behind. The flavonoid quercetin, which reduces levels of inflammatory TNF-alpha and interleukin-8, is present at high levels in onions and apples. Aim for at least two to four servings (one to two cups cooked) a day of these anti-inflammatory-rich vegetables:

Artichokes	Spinach
Broccoli	Sweet potatoes
Cucumbers	Tomatoes
Onions	Zucchini
Parsley	

Aim for one to two cups a day of these fruits:

Apples	Cranberries
Apricots	Prunes
Blackberries	Raspberries
Blueberries	Red grapes
Cantaloupe	Strawberries
Cherries	Tart cherries

Even spices can boost your anti-inflammatory intake. The best sources of anti-inflammatory compounds are in the whole-leaf or unground form of:

Basil	Nutmeg
Bay leaves	Oregano
Cayenne pepper	Rosemary
Gingerroot (fresh)	Sage
Mint	Thyme
Mustard	Turmeric (curry)

Prepare Foods Healthfully. Food preparation is just as important as food selection. Long cooking time and high-temperature methods such as deep frying and charcoal grilling increase a chemical process called glycation. This is basically a gumming up of proteins by carbohydrates; the result is an abundance of "glycotoxins," highly inflammatory compounds. You can **reduce glycotoxins** by avoiding deep-fried, scorched, burned, caramelized, or charred foods.[45] Instead, use low-temperature, moist-cooking techniques such as stir-frying, poaching or steaming with seasoned water or vegetable broth, stewing, boiling or using a slow-cooking Crock-Pot.

▶ **Take Supplements**
I also advise multivitamin, mineral, and cofactor formulations designed for cancer patients to restore essential micronutrients. For instance, vitamin E has anti-inflammatory properties of its own, but it also protects the anti-inflammatory benefits of fish oil. These two supplements should therefore be taken together.

Look for a multivitamin with vitamins C and quercetin or green tea polyphenols, which can block the activation of NF-kappaB, the inflammatory molecule.[46] An easy way to provide yourself with a solid anti-inflammatory foundation is to take a green-vegetable-and-fruit drink that contains the Healthy Dozen powerfoods (or focus on these foods in your diet), as discussed in Chapter 5.

If you have abnormal, chronic inflammation, as measured on a test of C-reactive protein, and 30 percent or more body fat, an aggressive fish-oil supplementation program will be necessary to displace the arachidonic acid stored in your adipose tissue.[47] I recommend 8 grams daily for two or three months, at which point another test of C-reactive protein will show whether your inflammation has been normalized to a healthy level.

I encourage the use of a combined support supplement in addition to all the above.

RECOMMENDATIONS FOR A COMBINATION SUPPORT SUPPLEMENT

Nutraceutical	Inflammatory Targets
Mixed tocopherols: 400 IU with standardized amounts of alpha-, beta-, gamma-, and delta-tocopherols[48]	CRP, IL-6, NF-kappaB
Tart cherry concentrate: 1–2 tablespoons standardized to contain at least 5% flavonoids[49]	CRP and PGE2
Gingerroot extract composed of both lipid and aqueous components with standardized levels of gingerols[50]	PGE2 and LTB4

Nutraceutical	Inflammatory Targets
Turmeric (*Curcuma longa*) extract: 500–1,200 mg with both hydroethanolic and supercritical components of turmeric rhizome containing a standardized amount of curcumin and aromatic fractions[51]	PGE2, TNF-alpha, and NF-kappaB
Boswellia extract: 150–300 mg standardized to 65% boswellic acids[52]	LTB4
Stinging nettle leaf concentrate: 1,000–1,500 mg 4:1 hydroalcoholic extract[53]	TNF-alpha
Alpha-lipoic acid: 300–800 mg pharmaceutical grade, tested for purity[54]	NF-kappaB

Search for a supplement containing a combination of as many as possible of these herbs and phytochemicals for support of a healthy inflammatory response or at least take one or two. Be sure to work with your integrative practitioner in selecting agents and dosages and in minimizing the pills you take.

MEDICAL PARTNERSHIP

▶ **Measuring Inflammatory Status**
Once you have settled into the inflammation-fighting self-care regimen, the next step is to customize your anti-inflammatory

battle. Lab tests can reveal which specific inflammatory molecules are present in high levels. Many cancer patients have high levels of PGE2, for instance, as a result of overactivation of the COX-2 enzyme.[55] With such knowledge, you can target PGE2, or any other inflammatory molecule, with specific supplements. At the Block Center, we designed a panel of inflammatory markers to help us determine which markers are elevated in our patients. With continual monitoring and reevaluation, this enables us to provide the right supplements and adjust doses. (If lab testing is not possible, return to Chapter 13 and review the section "Determining Your Terrain Disruption.") Among the tests for inflammation you should ask your medical partner about are:

1. **C-reactive protein.** CRP rises in response to inflammation more than other molecules do, and so is a particularly sensitive test of this condition.[56] I like to see results under 1.0 mg/L. A physician or nurse should interpret the test results.

2. **Erythrocyte sedimentation rate (ESR)**, or settling rate of blood cells. An older measure of inflammatory state, normal levels are 0 to 30 mm/hr, depending on your age and gender. I like to see levels below 15 mm/hr.

3. **Fibrinogen.** High levels can also be a marker for elevated risk of cardiovascular disease and abnormal blood clotting. I like to see levels under 300 mg/dL.

4. **PGE2 (marker of overall COX-2 activity) and LTB4 (marker of overall 5-LOX activity).** In addition to measuring your blood levels of these inflammatory enzymes, you can have tumor tissue tested for overexpression of markers for these enzymes. Overexpression means that the tumor is producing even more of these inflammatory mediators than most tumors, making it all the more crucial that you tame the inflammatory terrain. These tests are research-oriented and can be difficult to find.

For PGE2 I like to see levels under 400 pg/ml, and for LTB4 under 100 pg/ml.

5. **Interleukin-6.** Aim for under 10.0 pg/mL.

6. **TNF-alpha.** Aim for under 8.0 pg/mL.

The results of these tests will help you evaluate whether inflammation is indeed a terrain factor you need to focus on. If not, then proceed to the next factor you identified in Chapter 13. If one or more of your inflammation tests are abnormal, however, you should proceed with taking a relevant terrain modifier.

▶ **Terrain Modifiers**
Once you know from these tests which (if any) measures of inflammation are abnormal, you can address the problem more precisely with the right terrain modifier. Below is an abbreviated version of supplement recommendations suitable for terrain modification. Your medical partner should be using appropriate caution to screen these for negative drug interactions among patients taking medications. Here is how we match supplements to specific lab results:

ANTI-INFLAMMATORY TERRAIN MODIFIERS	
Lab Test Result	**Consider**
High CRP or ESR	Higher intake of omega-3 fish oil with some gamma-linolenic acid (dosed according to lab test monitoring), alpha-tocopherol (total of 800–1,200 IU a day), cherry extract
High fibrinogen	Bromelain, vitamin C, garlic extract

TNF-alpha	Higher intake of omega-3 fish oil with some gamma-linolenic acid (dosed according to lab test monitoring), stinging nettle leaf extract, resveratrol, luteolin, quercetin (water soluble is best), curcumin
PGE2 (marker of COX-2 activity)	*Phellodendron amurense* bark, bromelain, ginger extract, curcumin, grape seed extract, quercetin (water-soluble is best)
LTB4 (marker of 5-LOX activity)	Higher intake of omega-3 fish oil with some gamma-linolenic acid (dosed according to lab test monitoring), boswellia extract (standardized), flower pollen extract, ginger extract, quercetin (water-soluble is best)
IL-6	Higher intake of omega-3 fish oil with some gamma-linolenic acid (dosed according to lab test monitoring), vitamin K1 or K2
NF-kappaB	Alpha-lipoic acid, curcumin, mixed tocopherols

After you have been taking the terrain modifiers for about three months, have blood tests done again. If test results have normalized, then you can continue with your basic support, including a cancer-specific multivitamin, fish oil, a green-vegetable-and-fruit drink containing the Healthy Dozen power-foods, and a broad-spectrum supplement that supports the entire terrain, but drop the specific terrain modifiers. Get retested approximately every three months to see if your inflammatory markers remain normal.

▶ **Pharmaceutical Therapy**
If dietary supplements do not right your inflammatory imbalance, you should discuss with your physician whether you might

increase the dosage of your anti-inflammatory support supplement and terrain modifier, or whether prescription or off-label drugs might help. *Off-label* refers to the use of approved drugs to treat a condition for which the manufacturer has not requested approval for from the Food and Drug Administration, but for which there is reasonable clinical evidence of safety and efficacy. Physicians are permitted to use a drug for a condition not indicated on the label as long as the patient is adequately informed of possible benefits and risks, understands and consents. In addition to nonsteroidal anti-inflammatory drugs such as ibuprofen, among the most potent pharmaceutical anti-inflammatories are statin drugs, such as lovastatin and fluvastatin, which reduce cholesterol. A recent test of a statin found that it lowered CRP, TNF-alpha, and NF-kappaB.[57] Since COX-2 enzymes are inflammatory, you might imagine that COX-2 inhibitors would be potent anti-inflammatories, and indeed Celebrex (celecoxib) is; the increase in heart attack risk with Celebrex does not appear to be so severe as with other COX-2 inhibitors, such as Vioxx (rofecoxib), which has been removed from the market. Statin drugs also have potentially serious side effects.

You may ask, "Why not just take COX-2 inhibitors and statins rather than adjust my diet to damp down inflammation?" I have had patients who were taking COX-2 inhibitors yet still had inflammatory levels off the charts. Although these drugs can be a useful part of your inflammation-fighting arsenal, they treat the smoke rather than the fire. It is much more beneficial to get at the root causes of inflammation: disease, treatment, lifestyle, and the habitual consumption of meats, dairy products, trans fats, and omega-6s.

Shannon: Overcoming Chronic Inflammation

Shannon was a fifty-year-old mother of four when she received the results of her CT scan just before Thanksgiving 2000. She had non-small-cell lung cancer, which has recently overtaken breast cancer as the number one cause of cancer mortality among women. For Shannon, who had smoked for ten years before quitting in 1974, the very idea of Thanksgiving seemed a grim irony. It was increased by the fact that Shannon had been a founder of and therapist with the Wellness Community in Santa Monica, California, which counsels cancer patients to take an active role in their struggle to recover from cancer.

After surgery to remove the nine-centimeter tumor from her lung, Shannon began chemotherapy. Two months later, extreme shortness of breath sent her back to the hospital for a CT scan, which showed an inflammatory buildup of fluid in her chest. Even worse, the cancer had spread to her liver, which meant— according to her oncologist—that chemo could, at best, extend her life twelve to fifteen months. He explained that she could choose to do nothing, since chemotherapy would probably cause many painful and debilitating side effects, or she could try an alternative clinic. Shannon chose us rather than an alternative clinic.

By the time Shannon came to the Block Center, four months after her surgery, she was suffering from severe cachexia marked by fatigue, chronic pain, debilitating loss of muscle, complete loss of appetite, and profound weakness. "I feel so awful, I want to die," she told me. She went on to tell me that she'd grown up eating a typical American diet, had parents who smoked heavily, and was married to a smoker.

In addition to assessing Shannon's nutritional status, fitness level, and quality of life, I began terrain testing, suspecting from her history of cachexia that she suffered from a high level of inflammation. Her lab tests indeed showed that her levels of the inflammatory markers fibrinogen and C-reactive protein were high, in spite of the prescription COX-2 inhibitor she was taking.

Supporting the function of biochemical pathways that affect CRP is a challenge with food alone, so I recommended fish oil at a starting dose of 8 grams daily with ongoing adjustments based on her lab test results. Shannon took a fish oil we have been researching at the Block Center which has shown exciting inhibition of lung cancer cells in testing at M. D. Anderson Cancer Center laboratories, and which provides twice the concentration of omega-3s of most fish oils on the market.[58] Because Shannon had high levels of C-reactive protein, I also advised her to take extracts of turmeric (curcumin), boswellia, and ginger. While we need to learn more about these herbs, research suggests they may support normal inflammatory functioning. Shannon also took a vegetable-fruit drink containing abundant green and cruciferous vegetables and therefore carotenoids, lycopene, lutein, flavonoids, and other phytocompounds. After one week on this regimen, Shannon noticed a dramatic change. "I had an appetite for the first time since the surgery," she said. Her pain, malaise, and fatigue lifted. Later lab tests showed that her fibrinogen level dropped more than 150 points in three months; her other inflammatory markers also dropped remarkably.

As I have said before, many cancer patients die not of the disease itself but of its complications and treatment-related side effects, of which cachexia is one of the chief killers. None of the anti-cancer therapy I could offer Shannon would make any difference if we could not keep her from dying of cachexia. Once she was strong enough for treatment, I recommended an innovative type of radiation therapy called radiofrequency ablation that in under an hour—today less than ten minutes—eliminated Shannon's liver tumor (itself a major cause of inflammation) with few side effects, and I started her on the comprehensive Life Over Cancer program. Our staff helped Shannon to implement diet and supplement changes, exercise, and a mind-spirit program.

Although Shannon was strongly considering skipping chemotherapy altogether, I asked her to keep an open mind. I suggested we work first on rebuilding her lost muscle and weight and on getting her strength back. Once diet, fitness, mind-spirit interventions, and a vegetable-fruit drink had pulled Shannon out of her inflammatory tailspin and restored her strength, she was able to receive a planned seven cycles of chemotherapy at the Block Center. She responded well. Then, over a year later, a routine CT scan of her brain showed three small tumors. An innovative radiation treatment eliminated them. Shannon survived more than three years longer than she was expected to with her initial diagnosis, turning back the disease again and again before finally losing her battle.

Shannon's story demonstrates that it is possible to produce a shift in your inner biochemical environment from one that nourishes and supports cancer growth to one that deprives and resists malignancy. Snuffing out the fires of inflammation is a major step in this process.

There is still much to learn about how natural interventions may affect this terrain factor. We are closely following the advancing science in this area and also further pursuing our own research projects.

CHAPTER 16

IMMUNE SURVEILLANCE: MOUNTING THE IMMUNE BARRICADES

It happens all the time. I am sitting with a new patient in my consulting room, and he or she says, "Dr. Block, I'm concerned about the side effects of chemotherapy and radiation. I want to do everything possible to get well, but I would much prefer to treat my cancer naturally, by boosting my immune system. Can you help me?"

I am certainly sympathetic to the desire for "natural" or "alternative" cures for cancer, but I have to tell patients the truth: there are a few intriguing experimental research approaches, but an all-natural immune-based cure for cancer is for now still more dream than reality.

The notion that boosting your immune system through diet, supplements, or another approach can eradicate cancer is a common and troublesome myth promulgated in some sectors of the alternative medicine community, but it is fatally flawed. For one thing, the immune system is not the only or even the primary factor influencing cancer. It is just one of a multitude. For another, contrary to popular wisdom, the immune system does not automatically recognize cancer as a potential threat.

Instead, cancer cells are so similar to normal cells that the immune system often does not register them as dangerous. Also, cancer constantly adapts to the immune system, finding ways to thwart it by, for instance, adopting molecular disguises that make malignant cells indistinguishable from normal cells.[1] In fact, the longer a tumor has been growing, the better able it is to escape immune surveillance, the constant monitoring of your body for signs of cancer, viruses, and bacteria. Since most cancers have been growing for years by the time they are diagnosed, most alternative and even experimental immune-based treatments are ineffective at best, and could delay effective treatment. In particular, so-called non-immunogenic cancers— such as breast, lung, prostate, and colorectal—are able to escape routine immune surveillance.

Even when the immune system does recognize cancer cells as dangerous invaders, cancer cells are not necessarily doomed. For instance, immunogenic cancers—kidney and bladder cancer as well as melanoma—can be readily recognized as foreign entities by the immune system. As a result, they are often responsive to immunotherapy, which increases cancer-targeting cells of the immune system and directs them against the cancer. Still, self-care techniques alone cannot rev up routine surveillance enough to overcome immunogenic cancers. To do that requires more potent medical therapies. Interleukin-2 and interferon-alpha, for instance, activate the immune system and are common treatments for advanced melanoma and kidney cancer. A preparation of killed bacteria called bacillus Calmette-Guérin jump-starts immune cells and can be successful against bladder cancer.[2] Bottom line: your immune system can help you fight cancer, but to do so it will need outside help.

If you were diagnosed with an immunogenic cancer, such as kidney cancer or melanoma, your primary treatment after surgery was probably an immune-based therapy. Adding an integrative regimen to bolster your natural defenses might seem superfluous. But because the immune system has so many components, a single strategy rarely calls all of them into action. An integrative program of nutrition, exercise, and mind-spirit

techniques can. For instance, the immunogenic cancers secrete cytokines and prostaglandins, hormone-like substances
that can shut down the activity of natural killer cells that approach them.[3] An integrative program can curb these substances, leaving the cancer more vulnerable to immune system
attacks.

What this all adds up to is that for most cancers, current
immune-based therapies alone—whether pharmaceutical or
"natural"—are not sufficient to cure you. Having seen a number
of patients over the years who came to me in trouble after having relied on alternative immune strategies while disregarding
conventional ones, I am convinced that many placed themselves
at unnecessary risk. Some had early-stage breast cancers that
could have been easily treated with surgery, but because they refused this procedure their cancer spread and they found themselves facing a life-threatening malignancy. I am convinced that
you may place yourself at serious risk if you avoid appropriate
conventional therapies in the misguided hope that immune
manipulation will eradicate your cancer. In most cases, if your
cancer is accessible you are best off having the tumor treated
conventionally, and *only then* exploiting the immune system's
resources. As I will discuss in Chapter 26, the more active immune strategies do have an important role, but to date they are
more for containing growth or sustaining a remission than
shrinking or eliminating tumors. Immune-enhancing alternative
therapies alone are most often just not potent enough to eliminate established tumors, let alone advanced or metastatic disease.

Your Immune System and the Challenges of Cancer

This is not to say that you cannot enlist your immune system in
your battle against cancer. This chapter explains what you can
realistically expect from your immune system during and after
conventional treatment. Specifically, here is what you can do to
help yourself meet the challenges of cancer:

Challenge	Impact of Improving Immune Function
Reducing tumor growth and spread	Improve your immune system's ability to prevent cancer metastases or recurrences once you are in remission by picking up escaped cancer cells in the bloodstream and lymph system. Raising NK activity may help eliminate micrometastases and mop up cancer cells that remain after surgery, chemo, and radiation. Shifting macrophages so they are more cancer-killing as opposed to cancer-supporting and raising the immune system's ability to identify cancer cells may inhibit tumor progression.
Reducing tumor bulk and improving treatment response	Healthy NK cells, macrophages, and/or T cells may decrease vulnerability to metastases immediately following surgery.
Tolerating conventional treatments	Healthy white blood cells and, specifically, neutrophil counts decrease opportunistic infections, reducing your risk of flu, colds, and infections of the respiratory, urinary, and GI tracts.
Optimizing daily functioning	T cells may cause post-treatment fatigue syndrome. Cytokine therapy such as IL-2 or interferon can cause depression. Use LOC mind-spirit strategies for support.
Reducing the risk of life-threatening complications	A strong immune system reduces the risk of fatal complications such as pneumonia or sepsis.

▶ Reducing Tumor Growth and Spread

Four kinds of cells of your immune system play a role in reversing the growth and stopping the spread of cancer:

- **Natural killer cells** are adept at killing cancer cells. When they encounter cells that bear proteins (called antigens) that they do not recognize as being a normal component of the body, they recognize them as foreign and destroy them. NK cells have a special ability to clear the bloodstream of metastatic cancer cells and therefore play a crucial role in preventing the recurrence and spread of cancer.[4] In fact, long-range survival can be predicted on the basis of NK activity, especially for patients with lung, breast, bladder, and colon cancers. Unfortunately, NK activity may be suppressed in as many as half of all patients with metastatic cancers, hurting their chances of making a full recovery.[5] There are a number of reasons for low NK activity. It can be inhibited by chemotherapy and surgery, the repeated infections that plague many cancer patients, poor diet (especially inadequate protein, excessive fat, and deficiencies of key vitamins and minerals), emotional distress, and cachexia. Exposure to toxic compounds, chronic fatigue syndrome, and lack of physical activity can also impair NK activity.

- **Macrophages** act as phagocytes, literally "cell eaters," killing cancer cells when they detect foreign antigens. Some macrophages roam through the bloodstream and can help with immune surveillance of cancers. Some settle in tumors, where they secrete substances that can help "turn on" immune functioning and destroy tumors, especially early in tumor development; this is one way that small tumors are eradicated before they become a problem.[6] But macrophages within tumors can also become turncoats, churning out inflammatory molecules that stimulate angiogenesis, tumor growth, and metastasis. The balance of help and harm may be dictated by which part of the tumor macrophages settle in (the turncoats are more common in areas that lack blood vessels), and possibly by diet.[7]

- **Two types of T lymphocytes** coordinate the responses of other immune cells by relaying instructions about which antigens are foreign to the body. One variety, T helper cells, alert T killers, macrophages, and natural killer cells to kill cancer cells. T killer cells can destroy cancer cells by triggering programmed cell death (apoptosis), though some tumors secrete substances that thwart this cell-killing capacity.[8]

The immune system has two distinct modes.[9] In the Th1 or anti-cancer mode, the T cells instruct macrophages, T killers, and natural killer cells to attack cancer cells, and relay information about what antigens to search for.[10] In the Th2 mode, T cells communicate more with a different set of cells, the B cells, which produce antibodies. This process is useful in repelling bacterial infections and in mounting allergic reactions. However, the ability of the immune system to kill cancer cells in the Th2 mode is limited. Tumor cells have their own self-preservation capacity and can switch the immune system over to produce fewer Th1 cancer-killing cells and more Th2 cells, suppressing anti-cancer defenses. This Th1/Th2 imbalance can increase as a cancer progresses. Our job is to shift the balance back to encouraging Th1 cells in order to combat malignant cells. The Th2 mode is also triggered when immune cells are exposed to high amounts of the inflammatory prostaglandin PGE2.

Because immune surveillance does a better job detecting and destroying individual cancer cells than large tumors, your immune system will help you most after surgery, radiation, or chemotherapy has removed the bulk of your tumor.[11] Your immune cells may be able to destroy micrometastases, nests of cancer cells that could grow back to haunt you, in addition to eliminating cells floating in the bloodstream looking for someplace to settle and grow into metastases. The LOC program may aid surveillance, although we need more advanced research in this area.

▶ **Reducing Tumor Bulk and Improving Treatment Response**
Surgery, and specifically anesthesia, can suppress the activity of the immune system.[12] Experimental studies and preliminary clinical trials show that administering an immune system stimulant, interferon-alpha, during surgery restores the activity of NK cells and T cells, enabling them to potentially clean up some of the micrometastases that remain after surgery and to kill cancer cells that are released into the blood during surgery.[13] This technique is still quite experimental, though, and it is not likely that your surgeon will use it. However, by doing all you can to prepare for surgery by making sure your immune system is healthy, using the suggestions in this chapter, you may be able

to bounce back more quickly after surgery and reduce the likelihood that cancer cells will escape after surgery.

▶ **Tolerating Conventional Treatment**

Neutrophils are immune-system cells that search for invading bacteria, engulfing and destroying them. When their numbers are low (in a condition called neutropenia, usually due to chemotherapy), it can allow life-threatening bacterial infections to proliferate. Symptoms include fever, chills, shaking, sore throat or mouth, white patches in mouth, cough, shortness of breath, earache, diarrhea, nasal congestion, increased vaginal discharge or itching, burning during urination, frequent urination, cloudy urine, and inflammation at the site of an injury or cut. If you develop any of these, especially when your white cell count is low, contact your doctor right away. On the other hand, if you take steps to maintain a healthy neutrophil count, you reduce your risk of infections, which, if serious enough, can require hospitalization. Poor nutrition, inflammation, and low serum albumin predispose cancer patients to developing severe neutropenia during chemotherapy, so you may be able to reduce your risk of neutropenia by following the LOC program.[14] In particular, if you develop low levels of albumin during chemotherapy (this will show up in your lab results), follow the instructions for nutritional interventions to raise albumin in Chapter 6. The suggestions in the section of this chapter called "Your Self-Care Program" should also help maintain your nutritional status and avoid excessive inflammation, which can burden your immune function.

Avoiding Infection If You Develop Neutropenia
Avoid
• Undercooked fish and other animal products
• Unpasteurized juice
• Raw honey

- Buying foods in bulk bins

- Contact with people who have colds or infections

- Situations likely to result in cuts, scrapes, or bruises

- Children who have recently been immunized with live-virus vaccines and so may be shedding viruses for three weeks afterward

- Sampling open foods in grocery stores

- Raw fruits and vegetables, especially salad bars

- Cleaning out cat litter boxes

- Construction areas, which may stir up fungus-laden dust

- Live plants or fresh flowers left in standing water in your room

- Squeezing pimples

- Scratching yourself with your fingernails

Do

- Eat only well-washed cooked fruits and vegetables

- Refrigerate perishable foods immediately upon arriving at home

- Check "use by" dates on packages carefully and do not buy out-of-date food

- Wash your hands frequently, scrubbing under your fingernails

- Take good care of your mouth and teeth daily, using a soft toothbrush

- Use only prescription mouthwashes if you have mucositis (inflammation of the mouth), not commercial ones

- Ask your doctor whether you should wear a face mask in certain situations, such as walking through hospitals or flying in airplanes

- Keep the rectal area and the perineum scrupulously clean; women should wipe from front to back after urination

- If you are constipated, add fiber to your diet and use a stool softener to avoid straining, which can tear the rectum

---

• Use a water-soluble lubricant during sex

• Breathe deeply and cough hard periodically to clear your lungs

• Ask a family member or someone from your A-Team to clean cat litter and clean up after your dog

• Get plenty of rest

▶ **Optimizing Daily Functioning**

Many cancer patients face fatigue not only during treatment but for long periods afterward. While there are many reasons, the immune system plays a role. For example, patients in remission who continued to report fatigue had higher levels of blood T cells than non-fatigued patients.[15] In addition, interferon or interleukin-2 therapy may not only produce severe fatigue but also cause depression.[16] Should you feel a change in your emotional state during such treatments, talk to your doctor. You should also reread the sections of Chapter 11 that discuss depression, particularly cognitive reframing and thought-stopping.

▶ **Reducing the Risk of Life-Threatening Complications**

Aging, malnutrition, multiple treatments, and repeated episodes of neutropenia can make you more vulnerable to a serious infection such as pneumonia or sepsis. A significant drop in your white blood cell count accompanied by fever of 101 degrees or higher should be treated as a life-threatening situation. If you do develop sepsis, you will be hospitalized and immediately placed on intravenous antibiotics, which can save your life. This is no time to tough it out: call your doctor at the first sign of fever if you have such predisposing factors, or go to the nearest emergency room. This is not something that can be treated with self-care. When you are recovering from one of these episodes, you should follow the Treatment Support diet or the High Intensity Nutritional Support diet according to your needs, until you have returned to your pre-crisis state.

Shortly after chemo, when your immune cells may still be below par, it makes sense to take infection-fighting herbs and supplements, especially if you are exposed to someone with an infection. But a few cautions. The use of immune-stimulating products if you have leukemia or lymphoma is controversial. There is some concern that they may stimulate the source of the cancer, so I advise against them for now; you can check the LOC website for updates. Do not take echinacea to fight colds (something the jury is still out on) for more than a few weeks; it may impair production of immune cells, although lab data do not consistently support this concern.[17] A better choice is the herb kan jang, *Andrographis paniculata,* which according to an analysis of seven randomized trials helps with the symptoms of upper respiratory infections and, possibly, in prevention. One of its active compounds increases the proliferation of white blood cells and the production of interleukin-2.[18] Another herb, *Pelargonium sidoides,* decreased the severity and duration of bronchitis and strep throat in clinical studies.[19] These are encouraging, if somewhat preliminary, results.

To meet the cancer challenges described above, I recommend an immune support program, which I describe in the rest of this chapter. Please remember, however, that your immune system is not an island. Excess free radicals, chronic inflammation, disrupted circadian rhythms, and chronic stress can all depress immune function.

YOUR SELF-CARE PROGRAM

To begin the self-care program for immune surveillance, you should make sure that you are following the LOC recommendations for Sphere 1, including the Healthy Dozen powerfoods in your diet or in a green-vegetable-and-fruit drink. Then make the following refinements to diet and lifestyle.

▶ **Eliminate Immune Surveillance Offenders**
Let's first look at common sources and causes of immune suppression—the immune surveillance offenders.

Immune Surveillance Offenders

Smoking

Alcohol consumption

Emotional distress

Unhealthy weight loss

Sedentary lifestyle

Poor nutrition

Unhealthy dietary fats

Dairy

Iron-rich foods

Referring to the list above, identify the main sources of immune offenders in your own life.

Avoid Tobacco Smoke. If you don't smoke, you are already ahead of the game. If you do, *you must stop smoking.* Smoking tobacco or marijuana hinders macrophage activity.[20]

Avoid Excessive Alcohol Consumption. Alcohol makes natural killer cells sluggish, reducing their arsenal of perforin, the chemical bullet they use to kill cancer cells. Although an occasional glass of red wine can increase NK activity, I advise you not to consume alcohol regularly. Habitual consumption of alcohol impairs macrophage activity and reduces T cell counts, including T helper cells, pushing the immune pathway to produce more Th2 cells than cancer-fighting Th1 cells.[21]

Minimize Emotional Distress. Stress can impede the activity of natural killer cells. A number of situations—poor social support, anxiety over the huge disruption that cancer causes, depression, apathy, lethargy, and even job loss—are linked to depressed immune function.[22] Stress can also cause you to eat and exercise poorly, lose sleep, and abuse tobacco, drugs, and alcohol, all of which can further impair immune function. Be especially diligent, therefore, about following mind-spirit strategies such as relaxation techniques. Even something as simple as humor therapy can enhance your natural killer cells: in a study of healthy adults, researchers found that those who viewed a funny video had higher NK activity than those who saw a tourism video. The more the participants had laughed, the more robust their NK activity was.[23]

▶ **Fitness Adjustments**
Avoid Unhealthy Weight Loss. Dropping pounds, intentionally or not, tends to decrease numbers and activity of natural killer cells. Both can be restored if you exercise as part of any necessary weight-loss program.[24] Yo-yo dieting can also lower NK cell activity.

Get Active. Failing to engage in physical activity is associated with lower NK cell activity and impaired T cell function. In one 2001 study, for instance, elderly men who exercised did not experience the age-related decline in T helper cells seen in sedentary men, and had higher numbers of NK cells. Walking, running, and other exercises enhance NK activity.[25] However, I have mentioned several reasons not to overdo exercise, and here's another: excessive exercise or an abrupt change in exercise patterns can depress your immune system.[26] Follow the guidelines in Chapter 8 to build up gradually to a healthy fitness level, maintain consistency, and include yoga or qi gong.

▶ **Improving Dietary Intake**
Reduce Dietary Fat. Follow the low-fat LOC diet: a high-fat diet can decrease the cancer-cell-killing power of NK cells. Minimize your intake of saturated fats: T cells show poorer functioning when exposed to high levels of saturated fats, and high levels of "bad" cholesterol, or LDLs, are the result of a diet high in fats and low in fruits and vegetables.[27] It is these LDLs that, in concert with stress hormones, can create "turncoat" macrophages that support tumors. Choose the right fats for a

healthy ratio of omega-3s to omega-6s by using walnut, flaxseed, or canola oil while reducing consumption of omega-6s (most other vegetable oils): high consumption of omega-6s is associated with increased production of inflammatory prostaglandins, which armor tumors against attack by NK cells and switch on the Th2 immune response, disabling your immune system's attack on cancer.[28] See Chapter 5 for a daily plan of healthy fat intake.

Reduce or Eliminate Dairy. Casein, a cow's milk protein, can shift the balance of the T helper cells toward the Th2 response at the expense of the cancer-killing Th1 response.[29] As I have said before, patients with advanced-stage cancers should therefore reduce or even eliminate consumption of dairy products; see Chapter 6 for recommendations based on your stage of care. Get your protein instead from plants and fish, which contribute to immune health. In contrast to casein, whey protein from cow's milk can increase NK activity, and may also help cancer patients bounce back from the immune-suppressive effects of chemo and radiation.[30] But because other components of cow's milk are detrimental to other aspects of your terrain, you should get whey in supplement form rather than from dairy products.[31]

Reduce Iron. Too much of this mineral can have an adverse impact on your immune system. High blood levels of iron enhance the number and activity of suppressor T cells, which can call off the cancer-killing immune response and reduce the number and activity of cancer-killing Th1 cells. Iron also raises levels of oxidative stress, which can suppress your immune system.[32] I therefore recommend that you avoid red meat; a vegetable-rich diet such as the Life Over Cancer core diet will keep iron levels in check.

Build Your Diet Around High-Fiber, Low-Fat Foods. Studies of breast cancer patients show that following a diet high in whole grains, legumes, vegetables, fruits, and some fish led to a higher ratio of T helper cells to T suppressor cells, which is desirable for eliminating cancer cells that remain after surgery and chemo or radiation, and increases the activity of NK cells.[33] Aim for a dozen servings a day of phytochemical-rich vegetables and fruits. Carotenoid-rich vegetables appear to be an especially good way to maintain healthy T cell function.

Use Immune-Boosting Spices and Seasonings. Garlic shifts the immune pathway toward greater production of anti-cancer T cells.[34] I recommend that patients trying to boost their immune defenses take garlic extract equivalent to one to three cloves daily.

▶ **Take Supplements**
I also advise multivitamin, mineral, and cofactor formulations designed for cancer patients to restore essential micronutrients.[35] Look for a multivitamin with vitamins E, C, and B_6; zinc, magnesium, and selenium; also use fish oil, carotenoids, and medicinal mushroom extracts. Many cancer patients are deficient in these nutrients; deficiencies can shift the balance of T helper cells toward the Th2 pathway at the expense of the cancer-fighting Th1 pathway. CoQ_{10}, an enzyme that stimulates the immune system generally, increases blood levels of T lymphocytes.

Because so many Americans are deficient in omega-3s, and have an unhealthy omega-6/omega-3 ratio, taking fish oil can be beneficial. Studies show it can increase the ratio of T helper cells to T suppressor cells in patients with advanced cancers.[36] Since deficits of omega-3s can worsen after surgery, I advise taking 6 g of fish oil in supplement form in the weeks before and after surgery, stopping only for one week immediately prior to and one week after surgery so as not to increase the risk of bleeding.[37] One caveat with fish oil: several studies find that high-dose fish oil depresses NK activity in healthy people. Taking vitamin E with fish oil may counteract this problem, which is why we include vitamin E when giving fish oil supplements. Studies of people with advanced cancer, however, found beneficial effects on immune function.[38]

An easy way to provide yourself with a solid immune foundation is to either use a green-vegetable-and-fruit drink containing members of the Healthy Dozen powerfoods, discussed in Chapter 5, or be sure to use these in your daily diet.

Many times immune function cannot be completely corrected through the above diet and lifestyle steps. For this reason I encourage the use of a combined immune support formula. An immune-boosting formulation should contain micronutrients and plant extracts, with low to moderate doses of agents to boost the main immune cells. Here are suggested components for combined immune support formulas.

RECOMMENDATIONS FOR A COMBINATION IMMUNE SUPPORT SUPPLEMENT

Nutraceutical	Improves These Immune Functions
Vitamin C: 1,000–2,000 mg	Cytotoxic activity of NK cells;[39] macrophage activation and T cell functioning[40]
Zinc: 10–25 mg	NK activity, macrophage and neutrophil phagocytosis, lymphocyte development, T cell functioning[41]
Selenium: 50–200 mcg	NK activity[42]
Astragalus membranaceus extract (Chinese name huang qi): 1,000–2,000 mg of a solid extract at a 5:1 concentration ratio	NK activity, T cell functioning, T cell activation[43]
Ligustrum lucidum extract (glossy privet): 500–1,500 mg of a solid extract at a 5:1 concentration ratio	Macrophage functioning[44]

Agaricus blazei (royal sun agaricus): 500–1,000 mg	NK cells, macrophages[45]
Lentinula edodes mycelia extract (shiitake mushroom): 200–500 mg	Macrophages, T cells[46]
Ganoderma lucidum with standardized amounts of triterpenes and polysaccharides (reishi mushroom): 1,000–3,000 mg	NK cells, T cells, neutrophils, macrophages[47]
PSP, a concentrated, standardized extract of *Coriolus versicolor* (turkey tail mushroom): 400–1,200 mg	T cells, neutrophils, macrophages[48]
CS-4, a concentrated, standardized extract of *Cordyceps sinensis* (caterpillar mushroom): 500–1,000 mg	T cell functioning[49]

Search for a supplement containing a combination of as many as possible of these herbs for immune support, or at least take one or two. Be sure to work with your integrative practitioner in selecting agents and doses and in minimizing the pills you take.

What do we know about whether specific supplements can help redress immune imbalances? In one study, thirty advanced-stage cancer patients who took reishi extract (1,800 mg three times daily) for twelve weeks showed a significant increase in natural killer cell activity.[50] This is remarkable, since NK cell activity typically shows a dramatic decline in advanced-stage cancers. This is one example of why I routinely include selected mushroom and immune formulas in my patients' regimens.

MEDICAL PARTNERSHIP

Because many cancer patients experience immune suppression during chemotherapy or other treatments, it is advisable to work closely with your doctor and/or integrative practitioner to overcome immune deficits. If they are marked, in most cases you will need medications.

▶ **Measuring Immune Function**
Once you have settled into the immune support self-care regimen, the next step is to customize your efforts. At the Block Center, we run a panel of immune markers to help us determine which ones are abnormal in our patients. With continual monitoring and reevaluation, this enables us to provide the right supplements and adjust doses. (If lab testing is not possible, return to Chapter 13 and review the section "Determining Your Terrain Disruption.") Among the tests for immune function you should ask your medical partner about are:

1. **Complete blood count (CBC).** If you are receiving chemotherapy, or if your doctor is concerned about your ability to fight infections, he or she will order a CBC to measure your red and white blood cells. White blood cell (WBC) counts below 3,000 are common after intensive chemotherapy; lower levels increase risk and if below 1,800, particularly with fevers, medical attention is essential and urgent. Anything above 9,000 can indicate an acute infection. Note: If you are taking Neupogen or Neulasta, you can expect your WBCs to be elevated well over 10,000. Don't confuse this with an infection.

2. **Flow cytometry for immunophenotyping.** This test measures the different types of T cells. A typical normal range for T helper cells is 400–3,040 cells/mm^3, with values below 400 common in immune-suppressed patients. A typical normal

range for T suppressor cells is 220–865 cells/mm^3; anything above that range is an indication of potential immune suppression. A typical normal range for total T cells is 930–3,250 cells/mm^3; if you are below that range, your overall immune response is potentially impaired. Make sure that any repeat tests are run at the same lab and that the blood is drawn at the same time of day, since T cell counts can vary over the course of a day.

3. Natural killer cell cytotoxicity. This assay measures how well NK cells can kill cancer cells. Results are presented as a percentage of cancer cells that the NK cell is able to destroy. In healthy people without cancer, NK activity ranges from 43 percent to 100 percent, while a cancer patient's NK activity may be only 2 percent to 8 percent. A typical normal range for natural killer cells is 75–300 cells/mm^3; below that, your tumor-cell-fighting battalion is insufficiently active and too depleted to help you.

If the results of these tests are normal, or have normalized after taking a combination support supplement, then you can move on to other aspects of your biochemical terrain that you selected in Chapter 13. If one or more of your test results are abnormal, however, you should proceed with taking a relevant terrain modifier.

▶ **Terrain Modifiers**
Once you know from these tests which (if any) measures of immune status are abnormal, you can address the problem more precisely and include the right terrain modifier. Below is an abbreviated version of food and supplement recommendations suitable for terrain modification. Your medical partner should be using appropriate caution to screen these for negative drug interactions among patients taking medications.

IMMUNE SURVEILLANCE TERRAIN MODIFIERS	
Lab Test Result	Consider
Low white blood cell count/low PMNs (a measure of neutrophil levels)	Alkylglycerols[51]
Low NK cell activity	Inositol hexaphosphate,[52] melatonin,[53] extracts of medicinal mushrooms (see page 458), echinacea,[54] ginseng,[55] aged garlic[56]
Low T cell count	Vitamin E,[57] zinc,[58] arginine (except in breast cancer, where there is a suggestion that it might stimulate malignant cells)[59]

After you have been taking your combination immune sur-veillance support supplement for about three months and adding the relevant terrain modifiers, you should have blood tests done again. If the abnormal test results have normalized, then you can continue with a broad-spectrum all-terrain for-mula and your basic support formulations, which include the Healthy Dozen powerfoods (or green-vegetable-and-fruit drink), concentrated fish oil, and a cancer-support multiple. This will help with all aspects of the terrain while allowing you to drop the specific terrain modifiers. Get retested approxi-mately every three months to see if your immune markers are still where you need them to be.

▶ **Pharmaceutical Therapy**
If dietary supplements do not right your immune imbalance, you should discuss with your physician whether you might in-

crease the dosage of your immune surveillance support supplement and terrain modifier or whether prescription medications might help. My staff and I have identified two prescription drugs for which there is evidence of an immune-enhancing effect. In general, these agents are best used immediately after surgery, radiation, or chemotherapy, when there is a strong likelihood of immune suppression. Again, ask your physician if either of these might be right for you.

Tagamet (cimetidine), an antiulcer drug, has been shown to promote the cancer-cell-killing Th1 pathway. In clinical trials of patients with advanced colorectal and other gastrointestinal cancers, it restored NK activity after surgery. Tagamet also may bolster the ability of lymphocytes to infiltrate colorectal tumors, perhaps by overcoming the immune-suppressive effect of chemicals produced by the tumor. Other studies have shown improved three-year survival among patients with gastric cancer who received Tagamet, and improved ten-year survival among colorectal cancer patients who received the drug in conjunction with 5-FU chemotherapy, one of the standard drug treatments for this cancer.[60]

COX-2 inhibitors, such as Celebrex (celecoxib), are prescribed for arthritis. As mentioned above, immunogenic cancers such as kidney, bladder, and melanoma cancers secrete prostaglandins, hormone-like substances that can shut down the activity of natural killer cells. But all is not lost: because prostaglandins are manufactured by the COX-2 system, COX-2 inhibitors can halt production of prostaglandins, allowing the immune system to return to action. This is why natural and pharmaceutical COX-2 inhibitors, notably Celebrex, are being studied for treating melanomas and kidney and bladder cancers.[61] I believe the evidence is strong enough that COX-2 inhibitors can protect and enhance the anti-cancer immune activity of interferon or interleukin, which activate natural killer cells, that you should discuss with your medical partner adding these drugs to your anti-cancer arsenal. Extended use of Celebrex may not be wise due to potential cardiovascular effects, particularly if you are at risk, which your doctor will discuss with you.

Greg: Integrative Immune Therapy

Like his father and grandfather before him, Greg Rogers raised cattle in Colorado, often working sixteen to eighteen hours a day seven days a week. He ate red meat twice a day and lots of milk, cheese, and sweets, and had smoked since he was a teenager. He also had a family history of bladder cancer. In the summer of 1990, Greg noticed a hard mass in his abdomen and began passing blood in his urine. Only then did he visit a physician. A sonogram found that Greg's kidney was the size of a cantaloupe. He had stage III renal cell carcinoma: kidney cancer that had spread to local lymph and fat tissue. He had surgery to remove the kidney the following week.

Soon after the surgery, he "was nothing but skin and bones," Greg recalls. "We were all concerned about my weight, so I ate everything I could get my hands on—milk shakes, ice cream, and steaks. Little did we know that we were feeding the cancer."

Nine months later Greg found swollen lymph nodes on his neck. He had stage IV metastatic kidney cancer. He was also jaundiced, and his doctor told him it appeared the cancer had spread to his liver. "He told me I should get my affairs in order," Greg recalls, "because I had six months to live." But Greg was unwilling to accept this as a final verdict. With the help of a nurse whose father had come to me with the same disease as Greg and who had survived for over seven years despite having been told that he had only months to live, he found our clinic. As he recalled our first meeting, "You said anything was possible and that you wouldn't give up on me. After hearing you, I felt I could beat it. You were the first doctor who told us there was even a chance."

Kidney cancer, as I mentioned, is an immunogenic cancer, one that the immune system recognizes as composed of alien cells. We immediately started Greg on interferon-alpha, which was then, in 1990, commonly used to treat kidney cancer because it activates the immune system. As part of his Sphere 1 interventions, we also advised him to begin each day with meditation or prayer, to reduce stress hormones that can inhibit the immune system,[62] and spend twenty minutes on a stationary bike to increase the activity of his T cells and natural killer cells.[63] He adopted the Life Over Cancer diet, with an emphasis on reducing unhealthy fats: the typical American diet, with its high fat content, tends to push the immune system toward the pathway that produces infection-fighting Th2 cells rather than cancer-killing Th1 cells. (The whole grains and low-glycemic-index plant proteins in the LOC diet also tend to reduce problems with glycemia, another important terrain factor in kidney cancer.)

Because kidney cancer is immunogenic, I believed Greg's best shot at recovery was supporting his immune system in a way that would complement his interferon treatment. To increase his population of Th1 cells—the ones that destroy cancer cells—it was necessary to prod his system to produce these at the expense of Th2 cells. I therefore put Greg on the traditional Chinese herb astragalus (much later, a 2003 study confirmed that it strengthens Th1 functions) and on immune-supporting mushrooms such as shiitake and maitake. I also recommended additional vitamin C, which a 1993 study showed increases the activity of NK cells.[64.]

The resulting changes in Greg's internal environment may have helped support his interferon therapy. He achieved complete remission from his cancer and went on to build the LOC system into his lifestyle permanently. As I write, it is eighteen years since Greg was told he had six months to live. Where he and his family once raised beef, they now raise organic produce. The eight hundred pounds of red meat Greg had in his freezer just before meeting me went, little by little, to his pet cats.

CHAPTER 17

BLOOD CIRCULATION AND CANCER: THE THICK AND THE THIN

In the early 1990s, when I served as codirector of the cancer center at a local Chicago hospital, I became acutely aware of a problem that often strikes bedridden patients: blood clots. At that time, chemotherapy was mostly an inpatient procedure, so patients would stay in the hospital for the duration of their treatment and receive the infusion while lying in bed.

Even back then I believed that a diagnosis of cancer gave people more reason, not less, to be physically fit. With the other medical staff I had been introducing exercises that our chemo patients could make part of their daily routine, even if they could not get out of bed (see Chapter 9 for exercises you can do even if confined to a bed or wheelchair). I also made sure they received regular massages to improve their circulation. Also, with considerable difficulty, I was slowly nudging the kitchen staff to provide healthier meals—more fruits, vegetables, plant-based proteins, and whole-grains and less high-fat, processed fare.

And then I began noticing something. My patients were experiencing fewer treatment-related side effects and complications than patients of other physicians in the unit. In particular, my patients had fewer dangerous blood clots (thrombi), which usually form in the leg but can break loose and travel to the lungs, lodging in a blood vessel with potentially fatal results. This is called a pulmonary embolism. I attributed this phenomenon to the fact that I had physical therapists come into the unit to help my patients exercise even when bedridden, and also to the healthier diet I was struggling to introduce.

Blood clots are responsible for more than 240,000 deaths in the United States each year, including 10 percent of hospital deaths. Among cancer patients, a significant proportion will develop thrombi because of their tendency toward hypercoagulation—"sticky blood"—as well as bleeding complications as a result of hypocoagulation, or failure to clot. Cancer patients are approximately 25 percent more likely to develop an embolism, three to five times more likely to develop recurrent blood clots, and twice as likely to experience major bleeding while taking standard anticoagulant therapy for preventing thrombi and emboli. In fact, even when on anticoagulants, one in six cancer patients will develop recurrent blood clots.[1]

Bad as that is, coagulation imbalance doesn't stop there. Coagulation abnormalities fuel cancer metastasis and growth.[2] The stickiness of your blood, in other words, is a key component of the biochemical terrain that makes it either hospitable or hostile to cancer cells. This chapter will explain how to make this aspect of your terrain as unfriendly as possible to cancer while reducing your risk of a life-threatening clot.

Coagulation Imbalance and the Challenges of Cancer

When you are healthy, your blood is neither too thin nor too thick. If it becomes too viscous, it is in a state of *hyper*coagulation. This can happen when you have cancer: tumors cause clot-forming platelets to become overactive, and they stimulate production of a protein called fibrin, which knits blood cells together and thus makes the blood "sticky." If your blood becomes too fluid or "thin," on the other hand, it is in a state of *hypo*coagulation. This can happen from a loss of platelets, impairment in liver function, or use of anticoagulants, either pharmaceutical or nutritional. Too few platelets or their loss of "stickiness" can lead to capillary leakage or full-blown hemorrhage. Both hypercoagulation and hypocoagulation are bad news. The first raises the risk of thrombi and embolisms and can promote tumor progression and metastasis. The second can lead to uncontrolled bleeding. These conditions are especially dangerous for cancer patients, because they have an impact on several aspects of your disease.

The crucial players in the dangers of hypercoagulation are your body's platelets. Critical for normal clotting activity, platelets are activated to start the clotting process by biochemicals called pro-coagulants. The ever-wily cancer cells secrete these pro-coagulants and use them to hijack your clotting functions. In cancer patients, activated platelets aggregate around cancer cells, acting as a shield against the activity of natural killer cells.[3] They also drill a path from an existing colony of cancer cells into the lymph system or blood vessels, allowing malignant cells to migrate to distant sites. Activated platelets also allow malignant cells to migrate from the vessel into an organ to begin a new colony. Finally, activated platelets secrete substances that encourage angiogenesis, the development of new blood vessels that nourish growing tumors.[4] Many of the nutritional approaches I will discuss deactivate platelets, which is critical to keeping all this from happening.

Challenge	Link to Imbalanced Coagulation
Reducing tumor growth and spread	Activated platelets pump out growth factors that stimulate tumor growth, angiogenesis, and metastases. They also create pathways by which cancer cells can travel to distant sites. Activated platelets can hinder the body's natural "cleanup" operations that suppress micrometastases during and after conventional therapy.

Reducing tumor bulk and improving treatment response	Hypercoagulability can keep chemotherapy drugs from reaching the tumor site, reducing their effectiveness, and may contribute to multidrug resistance.
Tolerating conventional treatment	If chemotherapy reduces your platelet count below a safe threshold, your risk of bleeding and hemorrhaging will soar, requiring you to stop chemo. Other standard treatments can cause hypercoagulation, putting you at risk for deep vein thrombosis and also requiring you to stop treatment.
Optimizing daily functioning	Hypercoagulability can cause painful deep vein thrombosis, restricting your mobility and threatening tissue damage.
Reducing the risk of life-threatening complications	Hypercoagulability raises the risk of pulmonary embolisms. In rare cases low platelet counts, usually due to treatment-related marrow suppression, can lead to life-threatening bleeding.

▶ Reducing Tumor Growth and Spread

Tumors can cause platelets to become overactive. But the effect runs two ways. Just as tumors increase the activation of platelets, so overactive platelets—which are synonymous with hypercoagulation—seem to make tumors more aggressive. The reason is that activated platelets pump out growth factors including VEGF, the target of the new cancer drug Avastin (bevacizumab); these factors stimulate tumor growth and promote angiogenesis as well as other steps in metastasis. As a result, platelet activation is associated with increased metastases and more aggressive cancers.[5] A 2002 study, for instance, found that blood stickiness strongly predicted three-year survival in patients with several types of advanced cancers; those with the stickiest blood (as measured by fibrin levels) were four times more likely to die of their cancers than those with the least sticky blood (lowest fibrin levels), and patients with active disease had much stickier blood than patients in remission.[6] Another study that year found that breast cancer patients who had stickier blood had a 130-fold increase in the risk of dying from their disease. Conversely, reversing hypercoagulation seems to improve cancer prognosis. As early as the 1960s, researchers observed that a drop in platelet counts—meaning less active platelets—had an anti-metastatic effect. Metastatic breast cancer patients whose tumors were growing most rapidly and who had the shortest survival had higher levels of platelets and fibrin.[7] Because of the increasing understanding of how activated platelets help cancers spread, researchers now view hypercoagulability as a major target in containing cancers.

▶ **Reducing Tumor Bulk and Improving Treatment Response**
Oncologists have known since the 1970s that cancer patients with coagulation problems tend to respond poorly to chemotherapy.[8] Their tumors do not shrink as much, and their survival rates are poorer. A 1995 study, for instance, found that blood stickiness, as measured by fibrinogen, is correlated with reduced response to treatment in patients with lung cancer.[9] Lung cancer patients with high fibrinogen levels prior to chemotherapy had significantly poorer survival and a reduced likelihood of responding to their treatments, according to another study that year. Blood stickiness has been linked to poor response to chemotherapy and survival among leukemia patients as well. The reverse holds, too: decreased blood stickiness has been associated with better response to treatment among patients with ovarian cancer, and with better survival among patients with metastatic melanoma.[10]

On the basis of such studies—and many more reached the same conclusion—mainstream oncology is now investigating drugs that inhibit platelets, in the hope of improving survival. The signs are encouraging. Patients with acute promyelocytic leukemia had higher remission rates when chemo was followed by anticoagulant therapy with the blood-thinning drug heparin; of the patients receiving heparin, 86 percent went into remission compared with 49 percent of other patients. Heparin also improved survival rates among patients with small-cell lung cancer.[11] Like all drugs, however, heparin can have side effects, such as prolonging the time for normal clotting or causing internal bleeding. This chapter will give you completely safe natural methods to lower platelet activation.

▶ **Tolerating Conventional Treatment**
"Thin" blood—a low platelet count—can make you bruise easily or bleed excessively. The latter is a real risk during chemotherapy or surgery. To find out whether you might have thin blood, answer these questions:

- Do you or any close relatives have a history of bleeding problems such as frequent nosebleeds, prolonged menstrual bleeding, or excessive bleeding from former injuries?

- Do you have a history of easy bruising, gastrointestinal hemorrhage (bloody or dark stools), hematuria (blood in your urine), or hemarthrosis (blood in a joint space)?

- Have you been taking medications that have strong blood-thinning effects, such as aspirin, ibuprofen, heparin, or warfarin?

- Have you also been taking nutrient or herbal agents, particularly in high doses, that have blood-thinning effects, such as vitamin E, vitamin C, ginger, garlic, ginkgo, fish oil, or feverfew?

- Did you have excessive bleeding during or after surgery or dental procedures?

If you answered yes to any of these, be sure to tell your doctor before you undergo surgery or chemo. Even if you do not have a personal or family history of low platelet counts, cancer and cancer treatments can cause you to develop this condition. Among them are:

- Surgery
- Chemotherapy

- Deficiency of vitamin K
- Lung cancer
- Gastric cancer
- Leukemia
- Prostate cancer
- Anticoagulant drugs
- Pancreatic cancer
- Blood transfusion reactions
- Liver metastases
- Acute infections and sepsis

You should tell your doctor if you experience any of the following signs of low platelet count and its attendant bleeding:

Symptoms of Thin Blood

Headaches

Bowel movements that are red or black

Unexplained bruising

Nosebleeds

Urine that is cloudy or red

Vaginal bleeding

Severe pain in the back or abdomen, which can be caused by bleeding into that area

Vomiting with blood

Coughing with blood

▶ **Optimizing Daily Functioning**
Abnormal clotting or bleeding can have an adverse impact on your quality of life. If bleeding with resulting blood clots

occurs in your urinary tract, it can cause considerable discomfort. Blood passed in the stool can lead to anemia and fatigue. Sticky blood can cause deep vein thrombosis, an uncomfortable and potentially dangerous condition in which a clot forms deep in one of your leg veins. If the clot breaks loose, it can cause injury and damage where it impacts, resulting in a major setback on your road to recovery. If you experience any of these symptoms of deep vein thrombosis, contact your doctor immediately.

Symptoms of Deep Vein Thrombosis

The foot, calf, back of the knee, leg, or ankle is painful, tender, or swollen (without a recent history of a sprained ankle or fall)

Constant or intermittent pain in leg

Discomfort in calf when flexing foot

Leg is red, tender, or warm to the touch, or unusually firm and hard

A tender vein protrudes prominently from the leg

▶ **Reducing the Risk of Life-Threatening Complications**

When a blood clot lodges in the lungs, it is a pulmonary embolism, which can be fatal and therefore requires immediate medical attention. Symptoms include shortness of breath and chest pain. As a cancer patient, you are at greater risk of an abnormal blood clot; about one in eighty cancer patients develop such a clot.[12] A stroke or cerebral event can occur when a clot travels to and collides with brain tissue. The following cancers are most closely associated with abnormal clotting, thrombosis, and embolisms:

Diagnoses with a High Risk of Thrombosis

Pancreatic cancer

Lung cancer

Ovarian cancer

Endometrial cancer

Brain tumors

Acute promyelocytic leukemia

Myeloproliferative cancers (e.g., chronic myelogenous leukemia)

Once you have had thrombosis, you are at high risk of a recurrence. These are additional risk factors:

Risk Factors for Thrombosis

Surgery, especially in the several days following an operation

Having a chemotherapy infusion port implanted in your chest

The period during chemotherapy

Receiving hormonal treatments, notably tamoxifen

A family history of blood clots

Long periods of inactivity such as plane, train, or car trips, or being bedridden

Being overweight

Being on birth control pills

Prior thrombosis (also called deep vein thrombosis or DVT)

Paralysis of any limb

Someone without cancer may be able to repair coagulation imbalances through lifestyle and dietary changes. Cancer patients face a more difficult challenge. Because cancer treatments can cause coagulation imbalances, such changes will probably not be enough. This is why the LOC strategy also calls for supplementation and terrain modifiers based on your lab results.

SOME WORDS OF CAUTION ABOUT BLOOD-THINNING SUPPLEMENTS

1. If you do anything to intentionally thin the blood during chemotherapy or other conventional treatments (such as taking blood-thinning herbs or medications such as aspirin), you must alert your doctor. If your blood becomes too thin, you run the risk of hemorrhage, prolonged bleeding, or both.[13]

2. If you have any of the risks or symptoms of thin blood listed above, if you are about to undergo surgery, if you are on anticoagulant therapy, or if your platelets drop below 60,000, then herbs or supplements can lead to dangerous blood thinning. Unless you are receiving expert guidance about what you should take and your blood response is being monitored, I advise that you play it safe by *not* taking fish oil, plant-based essential fatty acids, vitamins E and C, garlic, ginkgo, ginger, ginseng, green tea, feverfew, and other supplements that thin the blood. In those situations, also be cautious with anti-inflammatory herbs.

3. Many blood-thinning supplements also interact with anticoagulant drugs such as warfarin and heparin. Though rare, this could become a problem. If you are taking a prescription anticoagulant, consult a knowledgeable dietitian, nutritionist, herbalist, holistic nurse, pharmacist, or integrative doctor before you start any supplementation program for sticky blood or inflammation.[14]

4. Many patients receiving chemotherapy will need to watch out for the risk of developing thrombocytopenia, an abnormally low level of platelets that can impair the

capacity to form normal blood clots in the case of cuts or injury. The medical staff at the Block Center warn chemotherapy patients to temporarily stop taking blood-thinning supplements if their platelet level drops below 60,000 (150,000 to 440,000 is normal). Patients undergoing chemotherapy should have regular platelet counts drawn to make sure their platelets do not become too low and their blood does not become too thin.

5. You should also stop any blood-thinning supplements five to seven days before surgery. If you are scheduled for emergency surgery, tell your surgeon what supplements you have been taking so he or she can be prepared for any possibility of unusual bleeding.[15] You need not worry as long as you inform your surgeon and anesthesiologist, since they can make any needed adjustments.

YOUR SELF-CARE PROGRAM

To begin your self-care program for normalizing coagulation, make sure that you are following the LOC recommendations for diet, fitness, and mind-spirit wellness, including the Healthy Dozen food families. Then add these refinements.

▶ **Eliminate Clotting Offenders**
Cigarette smoke is the major clotting offender. It stimulates platelet aggregation, increases blood clotting, and increases blood levels of fibrinogen, thrombin, and other coagulation factors. The blood of smokers shows an elevated platelet count.[16] If you have cancer, this effect is, to say the least, undesirable: platelets are major sources of tumor-promoting growth factors and angiogenic factors. Do not smoke, and avoid secondhand smoke.

▶ **Fitness Adjustments**
Being sedentary is bad for your clotting system. Exercise increases blood circulation and makes blood more fluid. When

you move around, the contractions of your leg muscles force blood to travel back to the heart, but when you sit still for long periods blood moves much more slowly. For this reason the blood viscosity of trained athletes is typically lower than that of sedentary people.[17] Bed rest is therefore your enemy. Needless to say, there will be times during your recovery from cancer—such as following surgery or other invasive procedures, or during a long hospital stay—when you are likely to be confined to bed. Ideally, hospital personnel will instruct you in techniques for avoiding deep vein thrombosis, such as regular stretching and leg movement, and give you compression garments that help prevent it. If not, do not be bashful about requesting a visit from one of the hospital's physical therapists.

When you are up and about, watch out for "economy class syndrome," in which sitting or lying still in one place for several hours, such as an airplane, raises the risk of deep vein thrombosis (a 2008 review article demonstrated that this problem applies to all types of travel, not just plane travel).[18] If you are in this situation, stand and walk up and down the aisles of the plane or train every one to two hours, or take a break from driving and stretch your legs. When you are sitting or lying down, shift your body position and do leg exercises, such as making circles with your feet and doing small leg lifts. Also, it is helpful to flex and point your toes a few times each hour. Wear loose-fitting clothes, and avoid tight shoes. Do not drink alcohol, which can dehydrate you, and instead drink lots of water or juice.

▶ **Improve Dietary Intake**
Reduce Fat. Total fat intake has a strong effect on blood coagulation, increasing levels of clotting factors. Sticky blood is therefore yet another reason to eat a diet low in total fat, by avoiding food high in saturated fats and cholesterol such as dairy products, meat, butter, egg yolks, margarine, coconut oil, palm kernel oil, shortening, partially hydrogenated fats, hydrogenated fats, cottonseed oil, and lard. Watch the kind of fats you eat, too: omega-3 fats yield anticoagulant compounds when they

are metabolized, while omega-6s tend to yield pro-coagulation chemicals such as thromboxane A2.[19]

Reduce Dairy. High intake of dairy products may cause rapid blood coagulation, possibly because, by raising blood lipids, dairy products sensitize you to clotting factors. As I've said before for other reasons, reduce or avoid dairy and cow's milk products, especially those with high levels of saturated fat such as cream, whole milk, cheese, ice cream, and sour cream.[20]

Avoid High-Protein Diets. Popular high-protein diets can also induce hypercoagulation, apparently by raising levels of fibrinogen. In one study that compared patients on a low-fat, heart-healthy diet with patients on a high-protein diet, the latter showed a worsening of heart health (increased artery blockage) and a 14 percent increase in fibrinogen levels after a year.[21] Follow the Life Over Cancer core diet recommendations on protein intake. The LOC diet can be adjusted to be vegetarian and even vegan, and I do believe this is a healthy approach to eating. However, a vegetarian diet should be designed carefully, and blood clotting is one reason why: if you avoid animal products entirely, you run the risk of becoming deficient in taurine, an amino acid found in animal foods that appears to be crucial to normal blood clotting. Low levels of vitamin B_{12} can increase homocysteine, which also promotes sticky blood. Vegetarians should ensure that their B_{12} levels are normal. If you do adopt a strict vegan diet, supplementation with vitamins and taurine will be helpful to avoid or correct an imbalance in coagulation.[22]

Choose Foods That Reduce Platelet Aggregation. A diet high in whole grains, high-fiber foods, legumes, vegetables, and fruit reduces clotting factors and is associated with reduced platelet aggregation. Many of the phytocompounds in vegetables and herbs have blood-thinning effects. For instance, flavonoids such as the anthocyanins, isoflavones, and catechins thin the blood; and pectin, the soluble fiber in apples and citrus, appears to decrease fibrinogen production. Coumarin inhibits vitamin K, a potent pro-coagulant. Phytocompounds in tomatoes—no one is sure which ones—inhibit platelet aggregation: patients who consumed a cup of tomato juice daily for three weeks had significantly less platelet "stickiness" than the control group. In a 2004 study, people following a diet emphasizing whole grains, legumes, olive oil, fruit, and vegetables had lower blood levels of coagulation factors than people following a standard high-fat, low-fiber diet.[23]

When you are choosing fruits, vegetables, and herbs from the core diet list, if you have sticky blood emphasize ones that are rich in anticoagulant phytochemicals.[24] You can also get these in a green-vegetable-and-fruit drink formula containing the Healthy Dozen powerfoods.

The following are rich in coumarin; try for two or three servings of any of these each day:

Carrots	Parsley
Celery	Onion
Fennel	Tomatoes or tomato products

These foods are rich in pectin or flavonoids, so get one or two servings of any of these each day:

Apples	Raspberries
Citrus fruits	Red grapes
Fresh pineapple	Tart cherries
Pomegranates	

Get one serving a day of one of these sources of omega-3s:

Canola oil	Pecans
Flaxmeal	Pumpkin seeds
Flax oil	Walnut oil

From these platelet-deactivating, coumarin-rich, and flavonoid-rich drinks, get one most days:

Chamomile tea	Purple grape juice
Licorice root herb tea*	Red clover herb tea
Pomegranate juice	Tomato juice

*Don't use every day long-term or if you have high blood pressure or fluid buildup.

And add some of these platelet-deactivating spices and seasonings each day:

Anise	Fenugreek
Asafetida (an Indian spice)	Fresh garlic*
Clove	Ginger
Curry powder	Turmeric
Fennel	

*Crush and let sit ten minutes before using.

If you must take blood thinners, work with your medical team so that your coagulation rate is optimal. Many foods can thin blood. Others, such as leafy greens, contain vitamin K, which counteracts blood thinners (especially Coumadin). A stable diet pattern with balanced and regular intake of different foods will be important for you. Be especially careful with green drinks, which can be very high in vitamin K. Both supplements with blood-thinning properties (see below) and anti-inflammatory supplements have the potential to interact. You can consume greens or green drinks as long as you take them consistently every day and are monitored routinely by your doctor.

Take Supplements. Fish oil (containing EPA and DHA) or marine plant oil (containing DHA) supplements can lower fibrinogen levels. Fish oil can act synergistically with an anticoagulation diet. As is usually the case with supplements, however, it is not a substitute for a healthy diet: a low-fat diet *without* enrichment from fish oil supplements showed only a minor improvement in blood stickiness, and a high-fat diet *with* enrichment from fish oil nullified the beneficial effects of supplementation.[25] Other kinds of healthy fats don't seem to do the trick. In one study that had men take high levels of fish oil (14 grams) or a comparable amount of olive oil, for instance, the latter experienced no change in fibrinogen levels but the former had an average decrease of 13 percent after three weeks. Fibrinogen levels returned to their previous levels three weeks after stopping the fish oil.[26] That's why I recommend making a high-quality fish oil or marine-plant-based omega-3 supplement a regular part of your routine.

Take a daily multiple vitamin, mineral, and co-factor formulation designed for cancer patients. Micronutrients including vitamins B_6, C, and E can inhibit platelet aggregation, reducing the stickiness of blood.[27]

In addition to the above steps, I encourage the use of a combined support supplement that contains micronutrients and plant extracts and low to moderate doses of agents that support normal coagulation. Below are suggested components for a combined support supplement.

Search for a supplement containing a combination of as many as possible of these herbs and phytochemicals for circulatory support or at least take one or two. Be sure to work with your integrative practitioner in selecting agents and dosages and in minimizing the pills you take.

RECOMMENDATIONS FOR A COMBINATION CIRCULATORY SUPPORT SUPPLEMENT

Nutraceutical and Dose	Effect on Sticky Blood
Red wine extract (95% polyphenols): 50–100 mg	The polyphenol gallic acid suppresses platelet activation[28]
Grape seed extract (oligomeric procyanidins): 50–100 mg	Lowers the interaction of platelets with fibrinogen and lowers platelet aggregation[29]

Green tea catechins: 250–750 mg	EGCG inhibits platelet aggregation caused by thrombin[30]
Ginko biloba extract: 80–120 mg	Lowers platelet aggregation[31]
Gingerroot: standardized, 1,000–1,500 mg	Inhibits platelet aggregation[32]
Garlic extract standardized to allicin potential: 11,000–15,000 mcg allicin potential	Inhibits platelet aggregation through multiple biochemical pathways[33]
Mixed tocotrienols: 200–400 mg	Reduces lipids (fats) in the blood[34]
Resveratrol: 20–40 mg	Inhibits platelet aggregation even in patients for whom aspirin does not work[35]

MEDICAL PARTNERSHIP

Once you have laid the self-care foundation, the next step is to acquire information about the coagulation status of your biochemical terrain. Lab tests can assess your initial level of blood stickiness and then monitor those levels as you take steps to rein it in.

▶ **Measuring Coagulatory Disruption**
At the Block Center, we run tests for conditions related to blood stickiness to help us determine problem areas for our patients. With continual monitoring, this enables us to provide the right supplements and adjust doses. (If lab testing is not possible, return to Chapter 13 and review the section "Determining Your Terrain Disruption.") Among the tests for blood coagulation you should ask your medical partner about are:

1. **Prothrombin fragments 1.2,** a generalized and early marker for hypercoagulability. The normal range is 0.4 to 1.6 nmol/L, depending on gender.

2. **Fibrinogen,** which produces fibrin and promotes platelet aggregation. The normal range is 200–400 mg/dL.

3. **Homocysteine,** which can increase coagulation. There is no firm agreement on a "healthy" homocysteine range. Although an upper limit of 12–16 µmol/L has been used, some evidence suggests that this is less than optimal. I prefer 4–10 µmol/L, with lower numbers being optimal.

If these tests indicate that your blood coagulation is fine and you have no prior history, you can go to the next aspect of your terrain that you identified in Chapter 13. Otherwise, if your tests are not improving, your next step is to adopt terrain modifiers.

▶ **Terrain Modifiers**
Once you know from these tests which (if any) measures of coagulation are abnormal, you can address the problem more precisely and include the right terrain modifier. Below is an abbreviated version of food and supplement recommendations suitable for terrain modification. Your medical partner should be using appropriate caution to screen these for negative drug interactions among patients taking medications. On the next page are a few examples of how we match supplements to specific lab results.

COAGULATION TERRAIN MODIFIERS

Lab Test Result	Consider
Elevated fibrogen	*Supplements:* garlic extract,[36] bromelain,[37] vitamin C[38]
Elevated TXA2	*Supplements:* ginger extract,[39] curcumin[40]
Elevated homocysteine	*Supplements:* folic acid,[41] vitamin B_{12},[42] betaine (trimethylglycine, TMG)[43] (may raise LDL cholesterol levels), vitamin B_6[44]
Prostacyclin (PGI2)	*Supplements:* Ginger extract,[45] magnesium,[46] oligomeric proanthocyanidins (OPCs—grape seed extract or pine bark extract)[47]
Elevated prothrombin fragment 1.2	*Supplements:* Nattokinase, bromelain, papain, combination enzyme products

After you have been taking the relevant terrain modifiers for about three months, have blood tests repeated. If test results have normalized, then you can continue with your basic support, including a cancer-specific multiple, concentrated fish oil, a green-vegetable-and-fruit drink containing the Healthy Dozen food families, and a broad-spectrum supplement that supports the entire terrain, but drop the specific terrain modifiers. Get retested approximately every three months to see if your coagulation status remains normal.

▶ **Pharmaceutical Therapy**
If dietary supplements do not right your coagulation disruption, you should discuss with your physician whether you might increase your dosage of your circulation support supplement and

terrain modifier, or whether prescription medications might help. ReoPro (abciximab), for instance, is a new monoclonal antibody blood-thinning drug. It inhibits platelet aggregation and, in animal and cell culture experiments, blocks angiogenesis and metastasis.[48] Coumadin (warfarin), one of the oldest anticoagulants, slows progression in patients with small-cell lung cancer, probably due to effects on metastasis. Coumadin is commonly and safely used to combat deep vein thrombosis and has been shown to prolong survival in this cancer.[49] Lovenox (enoxaparin), a newer form of heparin, also lowers the risk of deep vein thrombosis, has less risk for bleeds, and it too reduces the progression of lung cancer, according to a 2003 study.[50] If these measures do not correct hypercoagulation, you and your medical partner will also have to determine if there are underlying causes of blood stickiness. These can include persistent inflammation or oxidative stress, which you can have assessed through tests explained in the medical partnership sections of the previous two chapters. Insulin resistance, high levels of lipoprotein(a), disrupted cortisol and/or adrenaline, and even periodontal disease can increase platelet aggregation, and can be easily assessed.

As noted above, there is a fine balance between sticky blood and blood that is too thin. Anticoagulant therapy, if improperly managed, can lead to excessive bleeding, which is of special concern in patients with thrombocytopenia (low platelet count), brain cancer, or recent surgery or other invasive procedures.[51] For this reason I prefer natural alternatives such as fish oil, garlic, and vitamin E.

Shannon: A Second Problem

In Chapter 15 I discussed how we managed Shannon's inflammatory terrain. She also experienced a problem with blood clotting. Shortly after beginning her initial chemotherapy treatments, Shannon began to experience discomfort in her chest and shortness of breath. She had a pulmonary embolism, a potentially fatal blockage of a blood vessel due to a clot that formed elsewhere and lodged in a lung. This occurred at a time when her markers of inflammation had begun to fall but had not yet reached normal levels. She was also just starting chemo, which increases clot risks. Given the link between inflammation and hypercoagulation, I believe Shannon would not have thrown this clot if we had had more time to cool down her inflammation. Because she had had her other lung surgically removed, a problem in her remaining lung was especially dangerous. We admitted her to the hospital immediately and she received clot-busting and blood-thinning medications. She pulled out of the crisis quickly. She had no further clots; while clinical research would be needed to confirm this, her later normal clotting patterns may have been supported by her supplement program.

Bill: A Sticky Case

Bill was a fifty-year-old engineering superintendent when his doctor found that he had a PSA level of 8.12 ng/ml; a normal reading is below 4.1. A needle biopsy confirmed that Bill had prostate cancer, and showed signs that the malignancy extended beyond the prostate, an indication of more advanced disease. Bill refused surgery and other conventional treatments, and instead started searching for alternatives.

He came to the Block Center in June 2003. Although we counseled him to reconsider his refusal to undergo conventional treatment, Bill insisted on first seeing if he could manage his disease with diet and lifestyle changes. Since he fully understood the options and the potential consequences of his choice, we agreed to this strategy. The first priority, we told him, was to bolster his anti-cancer defenses and shift his biochemistry to one that was hostile to cancer. We reviewed a comprehensive plan that included a therapeutic diet, supplemental herbs and nutrients, and a program of exercise and mind-body techniques including emotional and social support. I explained the importance of careful laboratory as well as clinical monitoring, and pointed out the importance of staying open to the need for more

aggressive and even invasive treatment if his cancer did not respond to this alternative strategy.

Step one was to assess Bill's nutritional status. Even though
Bill had always been active—lifting weights, biking, walking,
camping, and scuba-diving—he was overweight. His total cholesterol was normal, but his HDL "good" cholesterol was low.
Bill had recently adopted an overly restrictive macrobiotic diet
after his cancer diagnosis, so I had my dietitians help him make
adjustments so that his protein and calorie intake was more
medically sound. I recommended he follow the LOC nutrition
program, and started him on a supplement program of concentrated fish oil to boost omega-3 intake, a multiple to augment
his powerfood intake, and a concentrated green vegetable drink
rich in phytochemicals, equivalent to consuming twelve servings or about 1½ pounds of vegetables daily.

An assessment of his terrain revealed disruption in oxidation, inflammation, and coagulation. His levels of oxidized
LDL and fibrinogen were at the highest end of the normal
range (where "normal" applies to healthy people and is, I believe, too high for cancer patients). One of his markers for
hypercoagulation, called prothrombin fragments 1.2, was sky-
high at 30.3 nmol/L, compared with a normal level for adult
men of less than 1.1. To address these terrain problems, I had
Bill begin taking a broad-spectrum antioxidant (a high-potency
enzyme formulation that helps to support normal coagulation)
and, later, Celebrex (the anti-inflammatory COX-2 inhibitor).
Finally, I recommended a standardized extract containing
immune-supporting ganoderma mushroom, and high-dose antioxidant green tea extract. Bill also took a tomato concentrate
for its high content of lycopene. Lycopene appears to contribute to normal platelet function and prostate health.

Two months after his first visit, Bill's prothrombin fragments
dropped to 1.5, which is near normal. His PSA had also
dropped from 8.12 to a near-normal 4.2, suggesting that his
prostate cancer was coming under better control. With few
exceptions, his frequent PSA checks have remained just a fraction above normal ever since. Armed with his aggressive diet,

supplement, and lifestyle program, Bill has so far fought his cancer on his own terms. No "watchful waiting," as the non-surgical, non-radiation, non-chemo approach to prostate cancer is called; this was total war against prostate cancer, what I call "active participating." I would not recommend this low-invasive approach for a man who had signs of advancing disease and whose PSA level was very high (it can climb well into the high double and even triple digits), but this active less invasive approach has been Bill's choice and, to date, has worked.

CHAPTER 18

GLYCEMIA: BREAKING CANCER'S SUGAR ADDICTION

Tumors are gluttons for glucose. They consume this blood sugar at a rate ten to fifty times higher than normal tissues. PET scans, which detect glucose consumption, have shown that the higher the rate of glucose accumulation in cancer cells, the more aggressive the tumor—that is, the more invasive and likely to metastasize it is.[1] Could it be, then, that having high levels of blood glucose, as diabetics do, makes you more susceptible to cancer in the first place and leads to a worse outcome if you develop cancer?

For several cancers, the answer is yes. Diabetics are more prone to cancers of the colon, breast, prostate, liver, and pancreas. In one study, for instance, the risk of developing fatal pancreatic cancer was five times higher in diabetic men than in non-diabetic men.[2] And when it comes to existing disease, the picture is even more disturbing. Diabetics with stage II and III colon cancer survived only 6 years compared with 11.3 years for non-diabetics with the same cancer. But diabetes is not the only blood sugar disorder that increases cancer risk, promotes tumor growth, and impacts survival. Patients who have what's called prediabetes (blood sugar levels that are high but not high enough to be diabetes) or metabolic syndrome (a precursor to type 2 diabetes, or what used to be called adult-onset diabetes) have abnormally high blood sugar. They also tend to have elevated levels of insulin because of what is called "insulin resistance." Insulin is the molecule that transports glucose into muscle, brain, and other tissue. In insulin resistance, cells block the entry of glucose. When this happens, blood levels of both insulin and glucose increase in a futile attempt to overcome this resistance. Insulin, unfortunately, promotes cancer growth: women with early breast cancer who had the highest insulin levels were twice as likely to have their tumor metastasize and three times as likely to die of breast cancer as women with the lowest insulin levels, a 2002 study found. And in patients with prostate cancer, high insulin levels and metabolic syndrome are linked to earlier deaths, found a 2005 study in the *European Journal of Cancer.*[3]

These human studies are strongly supported by animal research, where it is often easier to establish cause and effect. When mice that were injected with an aggressive mammary tumor were placed on either of three different diets—producing low, medium, or high levels of blood glucose—after two months animals with low or normal blood sugar had half the death rate of mice with high blood sugar. Comparing the two extreme groups, mice with the highest blood sugar had twelve times the mortality rate of mice with low blood sugar—67 percent compared with 5 percent.[4]

Blood Sugar Imbalance and the Challenges of Cancer

If you have diabetes, whether type 1 (the kind that results from destruction of the pancreatic cells that make insulin) or type 2 (in which the body's cells are resistant to insulin, causing blood levels of glucose to build up), you already know the importance of controlling your blood sugar. Even without diabetes, small elevations in glucose or insulin can wreak havoc on your health and fuel malignancy. But because unstable blood glucose, insulin resistance, and the incidence of prediabetes and type 2 diabetes are soaring, and because these conditions are often symptomless, many cancer patients do not even know they have one of these problems. This can be a dangerous form of ignorance.

Challenge	Consequence of Imbalanced Blood Sugar
Reducing tumor growth and spread	High insulin and blood sugar levels stimulate growth of many cancers.
Reducing tumor bulk and improving treatment response	Insulin-like growth factor I partially blocks effects of tamoxifen and may help cancer cells resist radiation and chemo.
Tolerating conventional treatment	Diabetic patients and those with elevated blood glucose, but not at a diabetic level, are at higher risk of surgical complications and toxicity from particular chemotherapy agents.
Optimizing daily functioning	Excess blood sugar can worsen depression.
Reducing the risk of life-threatening complications	The muscles of cachectic patients resist the activity of insulin and consequently cannot access their usual energy source—one of the reasons for muscle wasting.

▶ **Reducing Tumor Growth and Spread**

Cancer cells depend on blood sugar to a far greater extent than normal cells. The more rapid their proliferation, the more glucose cancer cells consume. This insatiable sweet tooth is strongly correlated with increased invasiveness. In addition, there is now evidence that high levels of blood sugar can activate molecular targets associated with tumor progression (they are called PKC, NF-kappaB, and *ras* oncogene).[5] These effects may explain not only the link between high blood glucose and worse outcomes in breast cancer, lung cancer, and leukemia, as mentioned above, but also the association between high blood glucose and a higher rate of death from prostate cancer: in a 2001 study, researchers found that men who had high blood sugar levels after a glucose challenge test were more likely to die from their disease than men with a normal glucose level.[6] A 2008 study observed that diabetic colon cancer patients whose blood glucose was well controlled with medications had less advanced and less aggressive tumors than those whose blood glucose was poorly controlled.[7]

In addition to fueling the growth and spread of tumors directly, high glucose levels also trigger the production of insulin and its close relative, insulin-like growth factor 1, or IGF-1.[8] Insulin is an especially powerful growth stimulant for breast, prostate, and colon cancers, as I mentioned above. And overweight women with breast cancer have long been known to have a worse prognosis than slim women; scientists now suspect that high levels of insulin and IGF-1 are the reason. IGF-1 seems to feed even more types of tumors than insulin does. It stimulates the growth of prostate, colon, lung, pancreatic, and breast cancers, promoting angiogenesis and metastasis as well.[9]

▶ **Reducing Tumor Bulk and Improving Treatment Response**
High levels of insulin and IGF-1 seem to impede the activity of some anti-cancer medications, in particular those that act by inducing apoptosis, or programmed cell death. IGF-1 has also been observed to help cancer (especially breast cancer) cells resist the otherwise lethal effects of chemotherapy drugs and radiation.[10]

Let's look at the effect on chemotherapy in more detail. Breast cancer cells that contain estrogen receptors (and whose growth is therefore stimulated by estrogen) can also be stimulated by IGF-1. Nolvadex (tamoxifen), one of the hormonal therapies for breast cancer, suppresses estrogen's growth effects. This can cause the tumor to shrink or at least stabilize. There is one group of breast cancer patients who do not respond well to tamoxifen, however: postmenopausal diabetic women with high levels of insulin and IGF-1. This suggests that insulin and IGF-1 might somehow overcome or compensate for tamoxifen's anti-cancer effects. That is, although tamoxifen keeps estrogen from fueling the growth of breast cancer, insulin and IGF-1 more than make up for it.[11] Perhaps even more worrisome, given the hope that the new targeted molecular therapies have brought to cancer patients, in some cases IGF-1 interferes with the activity of Herceptin (trastuzumab), according to a 2001 study in the *Journal of the National Cancer Institute*.[12] Clearly, breast cancer patients who want to optimize their response to conventional treatments would do themselves a big favor by keeping their blood sugar, insulin, and IGF-1 levels within a healthy range. Initial research suggests that this will help in other cancers, too.

▶ **Tolerating Conventional Treatment**

Many cancer patients undergo repeated surgeries. That can be a major problem for diabetic patients: one of the effects of constant high blood sugar levels is an abnormal vascular system. These abnormalities in the blood circulation can complicate surgery. During surgery, blood sugar can temporarily spike even in nondiabetics, which increases infections and causes difficulty in recovery from surgery. (This sugar spike seems to result from high levels of inflammatory biochemicals and stress chemicals caused by surgery, a vivid demonstration of the interconnectedness of your terrain factors.)[13] Another problem for diabetics is an apparent higher risk of side effects from certain chemotherapy drugs: patients with diabetes and other risk factors for heart disease were more likely to develop cardiac toxicity when they received the drugs Ellence (epirubicin—an Adriamycin relative) and Taxol for metastatic breast cancer.[14]

▶ **Optimizing Daily Functioning**

Excess sugar in the diet can worsen depression, and depressed individuals are often insulin-resistant. Although the evidence is still preliminary, and although the conventional medical community scoffed for years at the thought that sugar and

depression could be linked, this is where the evidence is point-
ing. For instance, the correlation between the rates of major
depression with per capita sugar consumption in six countries
is almost perfect, a 2002 study in the journal *Depression and
Anxiety* reported, and a number of investigators have found
links between depression and insulin resistance. A 2006 study
in *Molecular Psychiatry* found that young men in Finland who
had insulin resistance were three times as likely to have depression as those with normal insulin levels. Moreover, successful
treatment of depression seems to improve insulin resistance.[15]
Does it work the other way? That is, can treatment of insulin
resistance alleviate depression? There is intriguing evidence
that normalizing insulin may normalize the brain's use of the
neurotransmitter serotonin, which plays a central role in mental and emotional health. As discussed in the mind-spirit section, it is not unreasonable for someone with cancer to suffer
from depression.[16] However, if you do suffer from depression,
besides approaching this from a mind-spirit perspective, I suggest you have tests to determine whether you are insulin-
resistant and take the steps outlined in this chapter to get your
blood sugar under control.

▶ Reducing the Risk of Life-Threatening Complications

Insulin resistance is one of the hallmarks of cachexia, the muscle-
wasting syndrome prominent in gastrointestinal and lung cancer.
Even when cachectic patients manage to eat (they often don't,
since cachexia tends to be associated with low appetite), they
don't gain weight, partly because muscle cells won't let insulin
exert its activity.[17] One possible way to foster weight gain in cancer patients with cachexia (in addition to controlling the underlying inflammation, as discussed in Chapter 16) is therefore to
control this potentially lethal form of insulin resistance.

The Life Over Cancer strategies for controlling your blood
sugar, insulin, and IGF-1 and decreasing any insulin resistance
you may have are similar to those for making your other terrain
factors hostile to cancer, starting with diet, lifestyle modifications, and a broad-spectrum supplement, then moving on to terrain support supplementation.

YOUR SELF-CARE PROGRAM

Make sure you are following the LOC recommendations for diet, fitness, and mind-spirit wellness, including making the Healthy Dozen powerfoods or a green-vegetable-and-fruit drink containing them a part of your daily regimen before adding the steps below. A word of caution: if you are already diabetic and taking medication to control your blood sugar, consult with your medical partner as you begin both the self-care program and additional supplementation, since these could alter your needs for medication or cause hypoglycemic reactions if not monitored carefully.

▶ **Eliminate Glycemic Offenders**
Blood sugar spikes, insulin resistance, excess insulin, and IGF-1 production are typically the result of lifestyle and nutritional factors.

Glycemic Offenders

Overweight and obesity

Infrequent, large meals

Poor sleep

Psychological stress

Inactivity

High-glycemic-index foods

An inflammation-producing diet

Eat Frequent, Smaller Meals. Instead of three large meals, frequent smaller ones will keep your glucose levels steadier, since large meals lead to rapidly increased output of glucose and insulin. Also, since obesity makes you prone to blood glucose imbalances and insulin resistance, eat the right quantity of food for your target weight.[18] Overeating will increase blood sugar in the short run and, by increasing fat tissue, further disrupt blood sugar regulation in the long run. You can refer back to Chapter 5 for advice on healthy portion sizes. And don't skip breakfast. People who do are 35 percent to 50 percent more likely to develop insulin resistance and obesity due to a biological compensation or possibly because they allow their blood sugar level to plunge, which makes them ravenous; when they overeat, blood sugar skyrockets.

Improve Sleep. Sleep deprivation is associated with increased insulin resistance and diabetes. A 2008 study in the journal *Sleep,* for instance, found that men who got less than five hours of sleep a night were 50 percent more likely to develop diabetes than those with an average sleep time of seven to eight hours. (Those who slept more than nine hours also were more likely to develop diabetes.)[19] After inadequate sleep, the body produces higher levels of cortisol and inflammatory biochemicals called cytokines, some of which appear to be responsible for causing insulin resistance.[20]

Reduce Psychological Stress. Stress, by raising cortisol levels, provokes insulin resistance and thereby elevates blood sugar. It can also prompt your body to accumulate abdominal fat, a strong risk factor for insulin resistance.[21] If you are one of those people who reach for cookies or donuts when stressed, be aware that refined carbohydrates contribute to insulin resistance. To combat this stress-insulin connection, implement the recommendations of the LOC mind-spirit program in Chapter 11.

▶ **Fitness Adjustments**
Being inactive makes you more prone to insulin resistance and blood sugar imbalances. So does being overweight.[22] If you are overweight, follow the diet outlined in Chapter 5 and the fitness regimen in Chapter 9, and attempt to normalize your weight. Since a sedentary lifestyle is a major cause of insulin resistance, engage in the mild to moderate aerobic exercises I recommend

to improve your blood sugar control and insulin sensitivity, thus lowering your level of insulin over time. Thirty minutes a day is a necessary goal.

▶ **Improving Dietary Intake**
Avoid Refined Carbohydrates. Substitute high-fiber, low-glycemic-index foods for refined carbohydrates. High-fiber diets have been shown to reduce blood insulin levels and may prevent, if not reverse, insulin resistance. In fact, a 2004 study in the journal *Diabetes Care* found that people who consumed lots of whole grains had a lower likelihood of developing insulin resistance.[23] Stick to the LOC diet, which reduces or excludes foods that make glucose spike or increase insulin production or IGF-1 levels, such as foods containing refined flours and sugars (commercial baked goods, sugary desserts, soda, honey, cane sugar, maple syrup, and excessive fruit juice).[24] There is a reason why hungry office workers who need a quick sugar hit during the midafternoon doldrums reach for a candy bar, cookie, pastry, or sugary drink: they pack a glucose wallop, sending blood glucose levels soaring. This may energize you temporarily, but it wreaks havoc on your efforts to keep your glucose levels on an even keel and stave off insulin resistance. The more intense and prolonged the glucose spike, the happier your glucose-devouring cancer. Even some complex carbohydrates can cause blood glucose to spike; these include white rice, potatoes, and bananas. The glycemic index, and a related variable, the glycemic load, are measures of the tendency of food to make your blood glucose spike. Although you can find lists of the glycemic index of foods on the Internet (see, for example, www.mendosa.com/gilists.htm), they should be used with caution, since many low-glycemic-index foods, such as whole milk, are problematic for battling cancer. Additionally, the LOC diet combines foods in a manner to control the glycemic index.

Although dietary fat does not immediately raise levels of blood glucose or insulin the way simple carbohydrates do, over the long term a diet high in fat (especially saturated fats) increases your risk of developing insulin resistance. A study first released in 2007 showed that macrophages, a type of immune cell, trigger insulin resistance when they reside in pro-inflammatory environments.[25] Diets in which omega-6s predominate over omega-3s also seem to promote insulin resistance even over the short term, probably because they increase your production of the inflammatory biochemicals that trigger insulin resistance.[26] You should therefore avoid or at least reduce your intake of animal products high in arachidonic acid and saturated fat, including beef, chicken, pork, lard, lamb, milk, cheese, ice cream, and egg yolks; vegetable oils that are high in saturated fats, such as coconut oil, palm oil, and shortening; and vegetable oils that are high in linoleic acid, such as soy, corn, and mixed "vegetable oil."

A diet high in monounsaturated fats, such as olive oil, generally improves insulin sensitivity.[27] Follow the dietary recommendations in Chapter 5 for guidelines on daily servings and good ways to get monounsaturates.

Prepare Food Healthfully. Preparation methods can influence a food's glycemic effect. Whole apples cause the smallest glucose spike, apple puree a moderate spike, and apple juice the greatest spike. Similarly, unground grain has a lower glycemic ranking than cracked grain, followed by coarse flour and fine flour. So emphasize whole foods that have undergone the least processing (which also reduces a food's fiber content and thus raises its glycemic index), and pair carbohydrates with a protein or high-fiber food, which can prevent a blood sugar and insulin surge.

Spice Up Your Meals. Use spices and herbs that have been shown to lower blood sugar: cinnamon, fenugreek, onions, garlic, chives, leeks, bay leaf, and cloves (buy whole-leaf herbs or unground spices for maximum activity).[28]

▶ Take Supplements
If these steps do not reduce blood glucose and improve insulin sensitivity, I recommend adding a supplement that targets insulin resistance, high glucose levels, and IGF-1 through several pathways. The support supplement should contain micronutrients and plant extracts in low to moderate doses.[29] Here are

suggested components similar to what we use in the clinic for a combined support supplement.

RECOMMENDATIONS FOR A COMBINATION GLYCEMIC SUPPORT SUPPLEMENT

Nutraceutical	Effect on Glycemic Pathways
Cinnamon (a standardized water-soluble extract): 200–400 mg	Reduces blood sugar levels[30]
Coffeeberry extract: 50–100 mg (standardized)	Improves glucose tolerance[31]
Berberine complex: 200–400 mg (from any combination of the following: barberry, Oregon grape, goldenseal)	Reduces blood sugar levels[32]
Holy basil: 400–800 mg	Decreases blood sugar levels and cortisol levels[33]
Lycopene: 5–10 mg	Reduces IGF-I levels in patients with colon cancer[34]
Retinol (preformed vitamin A): 3,000 IU	Inhibits the activity of IGF-I[35]
Vitamin D: 600–800 IU	Inhibits the activity of IGF-I[36]

Search for a supplement containing a combination of as many as possible of these herbs and phytochemicals for glycemic support, or at least take one or two. You should locate a cinnamon supplement that has been through clinical testing, as taking ordinary cinnamon in the long term can trigger mouth irritation in some people.[37] Be sure to work with your integrative practitioner in selecting agents and dosages and in minimizing the pills you take.

MEDICAL PARTNERSHIP

Once you've laid the self-care foundation, the next step is to determine which specific aspects of glucose metabolism and insulin use may be out of kilter. Lab tests can assess your initial level of glycemia, and then monitor those levels as you take steps to rein it in. Again, if you are already taking diabetes medicines, work closely with your medical partner in using blood-sugar-lowering supplements, to prevent hypoglycemic episodes.

▶ **Measuring Glycemic Disruption**
At the Block Center, we run a panel of glycemic markers to help us determine which ones are elevated in our patients. With continual monitoring and reevaluation, this enables us to provide the right supplements and adjust doses. (If lab testing is not possible, return to Chapter 13 and review the section "Determining Your Terrain Disruption.") Among the tests for glycemic disruption you should ask your medical partner about are:

1. **Fasting blood sugar** measures glucose levels when you have not eaten for at least eight hours or, preferably, overnight. You want levels between 79 and 99 mg/dL after an overnight fast (if you have not fasted, acceptable levels are 70–125 mg/dL). Levels of 100–125 mg/dL after an overnight fast indicate impaired fasting glucose (pre-diabetes). Levels over 125 mg/dL on more than one screening indicate diabetes.

2. **The oral glucose tolerance test** measures blood glucose before and after drinking a solution containing 75 g of glucose. Levels are measured one hour and then two hours after drinking. Levels below 200 mg/dL are considered normal at one hour. At two hours, a level below 140 mg/dL is normal; 140–200 mg/dL constitutes impaired glucose tolerance, and over 200 mg/dL is diabetes.

3. **Fasting insulin levels** can be used as an index of insulin resistance. After an overnight fast, levels should be 5–20 microunits/mL, though these levels may differ between laboratories.

4. **Serum IGF-1 levels** depend on age and gender; your medical partner will explain your lab results to you.

The results of these tests will help you evaluate whether glycemic disruption is indeed a terrain factor you need to focus on. If not, then proceed to the next factor you identified in Chapter 13. If one or more of your glycemic function tests are abnormal, however, you should proceed with taking a relevant terrain modifier.

▶ **Terrain Modifiers**
Once you know from these tests which (if any) measures of glycemic function are abnormal, you can address the problem more precisely and include the right terrain modifier. Below is an abbreviated version of food and supplement recommendations suitable for terrain modification. Your medical partner should be using appropriate caution to screen these for negative drug interactions among patients taking medications.

GLYCEMIA TERRAIN MODIFIERS	
Lab Test Result	Consider
Elevated fasting blood sugar or oral glucose tolerance	Supplements: American ginseng,[38] coffeeberry extract, holy basil extract, bitter melon extract[39]
Elevated fasting insulin	Supplements: bioactive chromium,[40] fish oil (EPA/DHA)[41]
Elevated IGF-I	Supplements: lycopene, retinol (preformed vitamin A), vitamin D[42]

After you have been taking the relevant terrain modifiers for about three months, have blood tests done again. If test results have normalized, then you can continue with your basic support, including a cancer-specific multiple, concentrated fish oil, a green-vegetable-and-fruit drink containing the Healthy Dozen powerfoods, and a broad-spectrum supplement that supports the entire terrain, but drop the specific terrain modifiers. Get retested approximately every three months to see if your glycemic status remains normal. Because supplements are not as well researched as drugs, we can't predict their effects as easily. Continued testing—and careful monitoring for those already on anti-diabetes drugs—is advisable. You can also ask your physician to test for elevated cortisol, which can increase both insulin resistance and blood sugar levels. Lack of antioxidants in the diet can aggravate the harmful effects of disrupted glycemic status.

▶ **Pharmaceutical Therapy**
If dietary supplements do not right your glycemic imbalance, you should discuss with your physician whether you might increase the dosage of your glycemic support supplement and terrain modifier or whether prescription drugs might help. Glucophage (metformin), which is approved for insulin resistance,[43] reduces the liver's ability to release glucose and so may be helpful for patients whose glucose imbalance results from this mechanism. The diabetes drugs Actos (pioglitazone) and Avandia (rosiglitazone), besides controlling blood sugar, show preliminary evidence of anti-cancer activity. Note that these drugs also increase your chances of congestive heart failure and heart attacks, and have received "black box" warning labels from the FDA for patients at risk of heart disease.[44] Among the drugs that can lower IGF-1 are Evista (raloxifene), which is approved for treatment of osteoporosis and also inhibits tumor growth, and possibly the synthetic vitamin A called fenretinide.[45] Again, these should all be discussed with your physician.

Joe: The Case for Blood Sugar Control

Joe Horcher, whom I introduced in Chapter 5, first came to my office in October 1987, shortly after being diagnosed with inoperable prostate cancer. He was told his cancer had broken through the capsule of the gland and appeared to have invaded both the lymph and bones. Joe was a carpenter, age sixty-three, and happily married. When I first met Joe he was quite overweight and suffered from high blood pressure. He told me he had eaten a standard American diet—high in fat and sugar— throughout his life. I reviewed Joe's options with him. The first was surgical castration, which decreases the production of the sex hormone testosterone, which fuels the growth of prostate cancer. Like many men, Joe found this option unacceptable. The second option was hormonal therapy, also to cut off the tumor's testosterone fuel, but he did not want to endure the side effects (especially hot flashes, muscle loss, and impaired sexual functioning) and their impact on his quality of life. Joe raised a third option, watchful waiting. I explained that this was more often advised with earlier-stage disease, and I was not fully comfortable with it. Nonetheless, this was Joe's choice. He knew that I felt there was much that could be done to try to delay further spread, and he understood that by refusing other therapy he could very well lose the possibility of containing the disease. However, Joe elected this route and accepted the risks.

I explained to Joe how an integrative strategy would both offer him an active role in his care and, I hoped, impact his outcome. Blood tests to assess his condition and his terrain revealed that two terrain factors were out of balance: he had chronic low-grade inflammation and poor regulation of blood sugar, with a blood glucose level above 210—he was diabetic. We pursued dietary, supplement, and lifestyle changes to first calm the fires of Joe's inflammation. I explained to him the importance of keeping blood sugar under control, especially for men with prostate cancer: type 2 diabetes shortens survival.[46] Since Joe was intent on less invasive treatment, I wanted him to chuck the "watchful waiting" mind-set and follow what I call "active participating." Joe therefore adopted the LOC integrative plan for reducing stress, improving his fitness, losing weight and body fat while building lean muscle, shifting his diet to emphasize whole foods, and using support supplements. All of these measures were designed to improve his blood sugar levels and thus his diabetes in addition to his ongoing inflammation.

Joe stuck to the plan to the letter. As I mentioned in Chapter 5, he went home after the appointment and found his wife cooking a temptingly greasy roast dinner. Instead of starting the program the next day, Joe walked right into his kitchen and exclaimed to his wife, "Honey, throw out the roast! We're going vegetarian!" Over the next several weeks, Joe's previously diabetic blood sugar level of over 210 fell into the normal range. He lost forty pounds. For the next four years, Joe followed our program diligently and his general condition improved, though his prostate, while stable, was still of considerable concern.

By 1991, with Joe now sixty-seven years old, his PSA had more than doubled, to 681, and a bone scan showed malignancy in his hip and spine. Knowing that the median survival of patients with metastatic prostate cancer is about two and a half years, Joe agreed to begin monthly shots of Lupron (leuprolide), which blocks the production of cancer-promoting testosterone.[47] Many patients in Joe's circumstances would have started treatment earlier. Joe told me that he refused to look back. Once he began Lupron, he responded well; within ten months his spinal lesion had disappeared, and by 1995 all his bone scans were completely clear. Unlike many prostate cancers, Joe's has not become resistant to hormones; his response to treatment has been extraordinary. (We have kept Joe on several therapies intended to reduce his chances of becoming hormonally resistant. Anti-resistance therapies will be discussed in Chapter 24.)

Joe's challenges didn't end there. Though he had managed his diabetes and thrived with our integrative program for ten years, by 1997 Joe had begun slipping and put on about ten pounds. Due to his increased body fat, to just plain getting older, and possibly to Lupron (a 2006 study found it can decrease insulin sensitivity), Joe's glucose levels had returned to the diabetic range. I felt that lowering his blood glucose and insulin levels would be critical for the long-term control of his prostate cancer, so I revised Joe's strategic plan and started him on an oral anti-diabetes drug. I also adjusted his LOC diet plan, adding the supplements alpha-lipoic acid, chromium, and carnosine,[48] to support healthy regulation of carbohydrate metabolism. We were again able to normalize Joe's blood sugar, and soon he had reestablished control over his diabetes. While it was certainly not the only factor responsible for his excellent outcome, I am convinced that Joe's success in controlling his blood sugar with the LOC diet, our individualized supplement plan, his diet and lifestyle changes, and the use of medication were key reasons why he continues to outlive the grim prognosis of metastatic prostate cancer. Joe Horcher celebrated his eighty-fourth birthday in 2008, twenty-one years after being diagnosed with inoperable prostate cancer, and seventeen years after being diagnosed with bone metastases—very impressive for a patient with a disease that even with hormonal therapies has at best an approximate 25 percent survival rate at ten years![49] The years since Joe's diagnosis with inoperable prostate cancer are obviously more than just a biological victory for Joe. They've been years filled with a lot of good living and precious time with his family and his network of close friends.

CHAPTER 19

STRESS CHEMISTRY: CREATING HEALTHIER BIORHYTHMS

You have many more internal resources than you may have ever imagined, and you can harness them. The chapters on mind-spirit techniques explained how to reduce stressors in your life. But because the body's biochemistry can still generate a stress response even after the original stressors are removed, sometimes your stress biology needs stronger medicine.

The body responds to stressors—chemical, physical, nutritional, or psychological—by secreting stress hormones. These enabled our ancestors to respond quickly to predators or other threats by producing an immediate surge of energy, which also comes in handy in modern times when, say, a car swerves into our path or a barking dog jumps out at us. Once the danger has passed, our stress hormones return to normal levels. At least they're supposed to. But when the stress is chronic, so is the response.

Chronically elevated stress hormones produce a terrain that is worrisomely hospitable to cancer cells. With your stress machinery stuck on high, continued exposure to stress hormones can severely damage your body and disturb your vital reserves of nutrients, enzymes, hormones, antibodies, and immune cells,

all of which are essential to your recovery. For instance, chronically elevated levels of the stress hormone adrenaline increase
levels of blood glucose and clotting factors, which, as you
learned in the previous chapters, are conducive to the growth
and spread of cancer.[1] And a blood clot colliding with the lungs
or brain can be fatal. Chronically high levels of another stress
hormone, cortisol, make it difficult for insulin to ferry blood
glucose into your tissues; this is tantamount to the insulin resistance, which, as you read, can stimulate tumor growth.[2]
Cortisol also suppresses some immune system activity and can
increase biochemicals that support the growth and spread of tumors. In general, high levels of cortisol and adrenaline contribute to faster disease progression, quicker relapse, poorer
natural killer cell function, and decreased survival.[3]

Levels of hormones rise and fall throughout the day. Cortisol
levels normally rise early in the morning and remain elevated
for a few hours, giving you the "oomph" you need to start your
day, then they drop in the late morning, declining to about half
of their morning high by 4:30 P.M. Levels of melatonin, a hormone that helps control some consequences of chronic stress,
are almost the mirror image of cortisol's, rising in the early
evening, then dropping as daylight returns. They are normally
low first thing in the morning, peaking just before bedtime.
Levels of the hormone DHEA (dehydroepiandrosterone), which
is sometimes called a "mother hormone" because it is a building block for other hormones, follow their own cycle. DHEA
improves sleep, mood, memory, energy levels, and stress resilience by, scientists believe, curbing excessive production of
the stress hormones adrenaline and noradrenaline.[4]

Advanced cancer patients, unfortunately, frequently have
low levels of both DHEA and melatonin, and high levels of cortisol.[5] But it is not only the absolute levels of these hormones
that affect your biochemical terrain: it is also their intricate circadian dance. The twenty-four-hour circadian cycles of rising
and falling hormone levels can be disrupted by a number of factors, producing abnormal or imbalanced production of these
hormones. Among the culprits are poor diet, low activity levels,
poor sleep patterns, persistent emotional distress, cancer, and

conventional cancer treatments (which alter the body's stress response machinery). If these hormone cycles are disrupted, so will be your sleep-wake cycle. And that disruption is correlated with poorer response to standard cancer treatment, longer surgical recovery time, and slow wound healing. It can also trigger fatigue, depression, insomnia, poor memory, and shorter attention span, and affect other aspects of your internal terrain. For instance, if you are chronically sleep-deprived, your body loses its ability to regulate blood sugar levels.[6] What is so frustrating about these maladaptive patterns is that, although they are triggered by chronic stress, even when the stressor is removed the biochemical residue can remain.

This chapter will help you identify maladapted stress patterns and keep your stress hormone cycles healthy and your sleep-wake cycle in good working order.

Stress Hormone and Biorhythm Malfunction and the Challenges of Cancer

No one enjoys insomnia or fatigue, but for cancer patients they are more than unpleasant: they can be warning signs of disrupted stress hormone cycles that can affect the response to chemotherapy and adversely impact survival. The reverse is also true: reestablishing regular biorhythms of rest and activity can improve your prognosis. Indeed, the terrain disruption that results from chronic stress and sleep disruption affects every one of the five cancer challenges.

Challenge	Consequence of Stress Disorder
Reducing tumor growth and spread	Altered stress chemicals (high cortisol and low melatonin at night) and disrupted sleep/activity rhythms may contribute to increased disease progression, quicker relapse, poorer function of natural killer cells, and poorer survival odds.

Reducing tumor bulk and improving treatment response	Disrupted sleep/activity rhythms are correlated with poorer response to treatment.
Tolerating conventional treatment	Abnormal cortisol levels and disrupted sleep/activity rhythms may increase surgical recovery time, slow wound healing, and diminish treatment tolerance.
Optimizing daily functioning	A maladapted stress pattern can produce fatigue, depression, insomnia, poor memory and attention span, bowel irregularities, and a weakened ability to respond to stressors. This cascade can erode your determination and spirit.
Reducing the risk of life-threatening complications	A pattern of depleted stress hormones and disrupted daily rhythms can intensify a vicious cycle of insomnia and inactivity that is not only debilitating but also increases the risk of potentially fatal complications such as pneumonia, sepsis, and embolisms.

▶ ## Reducing Tumor Growth and Spread

As far back as 1982, animal studies showed that a rise in blood cortisol in response to stress could accelerate tumor growth.[7] As I thought about how this might apply to my patients, I realized that cortisol exerts a number of ill effects, any one of which could explain the animal results and apply to people as well. Cortisol suppresses immunity, which, as you learned in Chapter 16, is crucial to mopping up malignant cells that remain after surgery, chemo, or radiation. Cortisol and adrenaline together increase blood glucose levels; as you recall, many tumors live on glucose. Cortisol also promotes insulin resistance, causing glucose levels to increase through yet another pathway. It also appears to stimulate the growth and metastatic potential of some tumor cells.[8]

These effects on cancer cells and the biochemical terrain, studies began to show, translate into cancer prognosis and survival rates. Among the findings:

• Breast cancer patients who lacked normal cortisol rhythms had significantly reduced activity of natural killer cells and shorter survival times than patients with normal rhythms, according to a 2000 study in the *Journal of the National Cancer Institute.*[9]

• Low nighttime production of melatonin has been linked with more aggressive cancers, while cancer patients with high melatonin levels tend to have better outcomes.[10]

• Metastatic colon cancer patients who had a restful sleep between 11:00 P.M. and 7:00 A.M. showed superior responses to treatment, better overall functioning, fewer disease symptoms, and dramatically prolonged survival, while those with the most abnormal sleep/activity rhythms—for example, being out of bed most of the night—were five times more likely to die within two years of their diagnosis.[11]

• Five-year survival rates for colorectal cancer patients with normal sleep-activity rhythms were as much as 50 percent higher than for patients with abnormal rhythms, as demonstrated in a 2003 study in *Biomedical Pharmacotherapy.*[12]

• Metastatic colon cancer patients with the poorest sleep-activity rhythms had the highest levels of circulating tumor growth factors.[13]

• Norepinephrine, one of the stress hormones, along with cortisol, increases the invasiveness of ovarian cancer cells in lab tests; it also increases their secretion of enzymes important in angiogenesis and metastasis.[14]

As I evaluated each new piece of research, I became even more convinced that rhythmic variations of cortisol may be critical to surviving cancer.[15]

▶ Reducing Tumor Bulk and Improving Treatment Response

One of the simplest yet most powerful ways to improve the response to chemotherapy is to administer chemo drugs in concert with daily sleep/activity rhythms. In this technique, called chrono-chemotherapy, special pumps are programmed to deliver the largest drug doses at a time when cancer cells are most susceptible and normal cells are least vulnerable. This is how we often administer chemotherapy at the Block Center. Numerous, large randomized trials have demonstrated that it improves survival, as a 2002 study in *Chronobiology International* and a 2003 study in *Integrative Cancer Therapies* documented.[16] For chrono-chemotherapy to work, obviously, your sleep-activity and hormone rhythms need to be working properly. A 2008 study observed thirty metastatic lung cancer patients and rated their psychospiritual health and daily cortisol rhythm. Patients who had low psychospiritual scores were more likely to have abnormal daily rhythms and less likely to receive benefit from their chemotherapy. This suggests that mind-body health, biorhythms, and stress hormones are intimately linked with the possibility of recovery for cancer patients.[17] Chapter 23 will review chronotherapy in more detail. Supplemental melatonin has also been found in several controlled studies to improve response to treatment.[18]

▶ **Tolerating Conventional Treatment**
Early in my career, I observed that patients who felt helpless or hopeless were more likely to develop infections, recovered more slowly from treatments, and had poorer sleep quality and greater fatigue. In addition, I noticed that my older and less robust patients generally had high cortisol levels, especially after surgery and other treatments. Anecdotes are not data, as scientists are fond of saying, but in this case my observations were borne out by rigorous studies: high cortisol levels and disrupted sleep-wake cycles are indeed associated with slower healing and recovery from surgery, greater fatigue, more pain, and diminished appetite.[19] Disrupted sleep, a sign of disrupted stress-hormone rhythms, can intensify chemo side effects, whereas good-quality sleep and normal rhythms can minimize them.

▶ **Optimizing Daily Functioning**
Chronically high levels of stress hormones can aggravate the mental anguish many cancer patients experience, amplifying

anxiety and depression. Each hormone has its own unpleasant specialty. High epinephrine levels are associated with anxiety, while high cortisol levels are linked with depression and feelings of helplessness or hopelessness.[20] Just as emotional distress can raise cortisol levels, so elevated cortisol levels can bring on more distress. They can also impair your attention and memory, limiting your ability to reason through problems and decisions—which, as you know all too well, cancer patients face in abundance.[21] And it will not surprise you to learn that patients with poor sleep quality tended to also have worse quality of life.[22] It takes energy, resilience, and hope to stick with the often grueling treatments necessary to overcome cancer; don't let elevated cortisol and disrupted stress hormone rhythms rob you of one of your greatest allies in your battle.

▶ **Reducing the Risk of Life-Threatening Complications**
Fatigue, anxiety, poor sleep, and even depression may seem like small potatoes compared with having cancer, but they can cascade into life-threatening problems.[23] To be sure, this is rare, so please do not jump to the conclusion that your chronic insomnia will kill you. But I feel obliged to note that elevated cortisol—the usual culprit behind these "small potatoes"—suppresses the immune system, increasing the risk of life-threatening infections, and also increases insulin resistance. It has also been associated with poorer prognosis among breast cancer patients. In addition, insomnia and disrupted sleep rhythms can launch you into a vicious cycle in which daytime sleepiness leads to reduced physical activity, which leads to muscle deconditioning and loss of muscle mass. Combined with other aspects of advancing cancer such as cachexia, appetite loss, and weakened immunity, this can bring on sepsis or pneumonia.[24] As I have noted before, most cancer patients do not die of their disease; they die of its complications, including this pernicious pair.

But don't despair. I have observed again and again that patients who adopt the Life Over Cancer diet, fitness, and mind-spirit regimens escape their maladaptive stress hormone rhythms and get their cortisol and melatonin rhythms back to health.

Jeff: Beating the "Monster"

Jeff Roth was twenty-seven when he was diagnosed with the most lethal kind of brain tumor, a glioblastoma multiforme. Median survival time after such a diagnosis is seven to fifteen months. Yet Jeff always believed he would "beat this monster," as his father later told me, and so embarked on a journey through the world of conventional and experimental drugs, alternative nutritional formulations, and brain cancer specialists.

Two months after his diagnosis, Jeff came to the Block Center. Surgery to remove his tumor, followed by high-dose whole-brain radiation, had left him with no peripheral vision on the right side and serious cognitive problems. His short-term memory was impaired, as was his ability to understand written and verbal communication and to focus. And he still had some residual cancer. The first thing I, Dr. Mark Renneker (a close colleague at the University of California, San Francisco), and Dr. Henry Friedman (a leading brain cancer specialist from Duke University Medical Center) helped Jeff with was choosing chemotherapy. After several consultations, Jeff elected to receive Temodar (temozolomide), CCNU, Camptosar (irinotecan), and Vepesid (etoposide). After a year of chemo, during which he followed our recommendations for the Life Over Cancer diet, fitness, and mind-spirit regimens, Jeff's residual tumor had not grown. We recommended hyperbaric oxygen therapy, which resulted in a full recovery of Jeff's memory, cognitive function, and communication. This was obviously great news. Jeff was well enough to get married in front of three hundred ecstatic family members and friends ten months after he began treatment at our center.

Jeff's cortisol rhythm was measured at the time he initially came to the Block Center, drained from the trauma of diagnosis, surgery, and radiation. Cortisol is typically high first thing in the morning and then declines through the day and into the evening. Jeff's cortisol levels, however, were "flatlined"—low all day long, as well as at night. His level of the cortisol precursor DHEA was also low. I therefore prescribed the mushroom cordyceps, which can improve vitality and energy,[25] in addition to the LOC Sphere 1 program. Nine months later, when Jeff began complaining of daytime fatigue and disrupted sleep, tests showed that his cortisol levels were normal during the early morning and evening but low at midday. His melatonin levels, though, were extremely low. These abnormalities necessitated adjusting Jeff's Life Over Cancer program. I counseled him to include more daytime activity with sun exposure in his schedule, and recommended melatonin at bedtime. I also suggested that, while continuing to take cordyceps supplementation, he also take pantothenic acid;[26] the Chinese herb *Rehmannia glutinosa,* which is used in Chinese medicine to support adrenal function;[27] and a Chinese herbal formula (Minor Bupleurum) containing the herbs bupleurum, Asian ginseng, and licorice to support a normal stress response.[28] Five months later, Jeff's bedtime levels of melatonin were still a bit low, but his cortisol levels had normalized. He was no longer so sluggish, and was able to walk and maintain a workout routine.

I hope that, if you have read this far, you have gotten my message of hope and possibility. It would be misleading to suggest that every patient defeats his cancer, however. My experience is that the LOC integrative therapies extend survival and quality of life, as they did with Jeff, but sometimes even they are not enough. It was deeply saddening to all of us when Jeff's residual glioblastoma recurred, and at age thirty-one he lost his heroic battle against cancer. He had lived nearly five years after his diagnosis, two and a half years beyond medical expectations, and most of it was—thanks to interventions that restored his energy and strength—quality time. Jeff's father, Dennis, worked actively with the Brain Tumor Society, and with Jeff's entire family launched the nonprofit Have a Chance Foundation, organizing successful fund-raising walks to support the search for better treatments for this dread disease.

YOUR SELF-CARE PROGRAM

To begin the self-care program for stress chemistry and circadian rhythm, you should make sure that you are following the

LOC recommendations for diet, fitness, and mind-spirit balance. Now you can add specific refinements to restore your circadian rhythms and return your stress hormones to normal.

Eliminate Stress Hormone and Biorhythm Offenders

Remember, of course, that you are not trying to eliminate all cortisol production. Cortisol is a critical element in your ability to navigate the normal stresses of the day. The problem is excess cortisol, or poor timing of its production, and imbalances in its circadian cycling. The list below summarizes the offenders that can cause excess cortisol production or throw off your normal rhythms of sleep.

Stress Offenders

Caffeine

Alcohol

Overwork and schedule disruption

Sleep disruption

Timing of snacks and drinks

Inactivity

Extreme exercise

Low-carb, high-fat diet

Low-carb, high-protein diet

High ratio of omega-6s to omega-3s

Overeating

Reduce Caffeine and Other Stimulants. High consumption of coffee, caffeinated tea, chocolate, ginseng, and bitter orange peel can disrupt your sleep cycle, intensify your stress reaction, and keep you on edge. If you are feeling uneasy or jittery, try to gradually wean yourself from caffeine. But ease off slowly, since going cold turkey can cause withdrawal symptoms, including headaches. Ginseng, which many cancer patients take for fatigue, can cause tension and insomnia if taken in excess. Bitter orange peel contains compounds similar to the stimulant ephedrine and can make you feel jittery.[29]

Avoid Excessive Alcohol Consumption. People will sometimes take an alcoholic drink as a nightcap to relax. But alcohol tends to disrupt your melatonin production. If you have too much, you may fall asleep, but you are likely to wake up repeatedly during the night.

Avoid Overwork. Overwork can upset stress chemistry rhythms because it can cause anxiety and dial up adrenaline and cortisol production, and because it can discourage regular bedtimes. Your health is far more critical than any work projects or deadlines. Although I encourage patients to continue normal activity during cancer treatments, there are times when taking a leave of absence, trimming hours to part-time, or going on disability makes sense.

Improve Sleep Hygiene. Do you need an alarm clock to get up? Is it a struggle to get out of bed in the morning? Do you frequently fall asleep while watching TV or in a boring meeting? Do you often feel drowsy when you drive? If you answered yes to two or more of these questions, you are probably sleep-deprived. You should answer the questions on page 165 and evaluate your level of sleep disruption. You can then review the sleep hygiene program outlined in Chapter 8 and implement suggestions that are relevant to you. If you have been sleeping poorly for only a week or so, it could be a temporary stress reaction; in that case, focus on addressing the stressful situation and then work on getting back on your regular sleep schedule after the stress ends. If you have trouble with implementing the sleep hygiene program, psychologists and therapists who have expertise in sleep care can diagnose your sleep problem and find a way to solve it.[30]

Let me add a few tips on sleep hygiene that are more specific to the issue of stress chemistry. First, remember that anything that disrupts your sleep cycle or causes you to have poor-quality sleep is a stress trigger. For this reason, you should avoid disruptions in your natural melatonin rhythms, which, as you recall, should peak just before bedtime. Your pineal gland (which produces melatonin) is highly sensitive to natural light-dark cycles. By going to bed at the same time regularly, sleeping in complete darkness, and getting exposure to sunlight or full-spectrum light during the day, especially early in the day, you will produce melatonin on schedule and sleep well. Early morning light helps get melatonin secretion rhythms coordinated with the dark-light schedule. I also recommend relaxed abdominal breathing before bedtime to help you unwind.

Properly Time Snacks and Drinks. If you need a late-night snack, keep it light so it doesn't add much to your caloric intake. Your snack should consist of protein and/or whole grains, which contain tryptophan, an amino acid that is used in the synthesis of the calming neurochemical serotonin. You shouldn't eat during the last hour before you go to sleep, especially if you experience heartburn at night or have gastrointestinal reflux disease. And if you find that you are frequently waking at night to use the bathroom, consume more fluids early in the day, but limit your fluid intake after 8:00 P.M. If spicy foods disturb your digestion, eliminate them, especially at night.

▶ **Fitness Adjustments**
Particularly among older people, researchers have found that sleep and circadian rhythms are improved by exercise. Tai chi and moderate exercise have been found to improve sleep in older people and discourage early evening sleeping, which tends to shift sleep times out of their normal rhythm.[31] Practice aerobic and strength training during the late afternoon or early evening (at least five to six hours before bedtime) to synchronize your workout with circadian rhythms. Set aside a little time in the evening for a calming and meditative exercise such as yoga. (In a 2004 study in the journal *Cancer,* Tibetan

yoga was found to improve the sleep quality of lymphoma patients.[32])

When you exercise too hard for too long, however, you exhaust your body, your muscles become weakened, and, significantly, your cortisol levels rise. Exercise in moderation, as Chapters 7, 8, and 9 recommend; you simply do not need the excess cortisol in your system that overtraining brings.[33]

▶ **Improving Dietary Intake**

NEGATIVE IMPACT OF DIET ON EMOTIONAL WELL-BEING	
Diet	Physiological Change and Effect
Low-carbohydrate, high-fat, high-protein diet	Increased cortisol levels raise tension and anxiety
Low-carbohydrate, high-protein diet	Excessive drop in brain serotonin, low melatonin production, leading to reduced resilience to stressful situations, poor sleep
High-fat diet	Increased red cell aggregation, low oxygen transport leading to increased fatigue, lethargy, boredom
High omega-6/ omega-3 ratio	Reduced fluidity of cell membranes leading to depressed mood
Overeating	Melatonin deficits leading to poor sleep

Avoid Excessive Animal Protein. A diet high in protein and low in complex carbohydrates—even a meal high in animal protein—

has been associated with high cortisol levels along with depression.[34] Protein *quality* also matters: casein (from cow's milk) raised cortisol in people who are prone to stress reactions, and increased depressive moods, while whey protein did the opposite, according to a 2000 study.[35]

Watch Carbohydrate Consumption. Carbohydrates are crucial in the synthesis of serotonin, a natural mood-enhancing neurotransmitter, so diets low in carbohydrates may predispose you to anxiety and depression, which in turn raise cortisol levels. Focus on complex carbohydrates.[36]

Ensure a High Ratio of Omega-3s to Omega-6s. Because saturated fats make cell membranes more rigid, while unsaturated fats make them more flexible, neurotransmitters pass into and out of neurons more easily with a diet containing more unsaturated fats. The most unsaturated are omega-3s, which may have the most beneficial effect on brain function, mood, and stress coping.[37] A high ratio of omega-6s to omega-3s may increase the risk of depression; according to several studies, the lower the omega-3 level the more severe the depression.[38] The specific role of omega-3 supplements in depression is not yet clear.

▶ **Take Supplements**
Sometimes stress chemistry and biorhythms cannot be completely corrected by diet, fitness, and mind-body techniques. I encourage the use of a combined stress hormone support supplement in addition to systematically including the Healthy Dozen food families in your diet or taking a green-vegetable-and-fruit drink, using a concentrated fish oil supplement, and taking a cancer-specific multiple. The support supplement should contain micronutrients and plant extracts in low to moderate doses of agents that support normal stress hormone balance. Here are suggested components for a combined support supplement:

RECOMMENDATIONS FOR A COMBINATION STRESS HORMONE SUPPORT SUPPLEMENT

Nutraceutical	Effect on Stress Chemistry
Pantothenic acid (vitamin B_5): 5–20 mg	Important in the production of cortisol[39]
Vitamin C: 500 mg	Reduces stress-induced cortisol levels[40]
Chinese herbs *Magnolia officinalis* (Magnolia bark) and *Phellodendron amurense* (Amur cork tree) (we encourage use of a standardized, proprietary blend of the two plant extracts): 250–500 mg	Normalize cortisol, improve DHEA levels, and reduce stress-induced symptoms of anxiety, depression, irritability, and emotional lability[41]
5-HTP (5-hydroxy-L-tryptophan): 25–50 mg	During daylight and activity, increases the level of serotonin, which is metabolized to melatonin during sleep[42]
Siberian ginseng (eleuthero or eleutherococcus): 100–200 mg	Improves the body's ability to handle stress[43]
L-theanine: 50–100 mg	Has a calming effect on brain chemistry while helping to maintain alertness[44]
Rhodiola rosea: 50–200 mg	Improves resistance to a variety of physical, chemical, and biological stressors[45]

Magnesium: 300–350 mg	Associated with muscle relaxation and pain relief; also improves the body's ability to tolerate exercise[46]
Mimosa tree bark (*Cortex albizziae*): 500–1,000 mg of a solid extract at a 5:1 concentration ratio	Dubbed the "happiness herb" in traditional Chinese herbology because of its long history of calming body and mind[47]

Search for a supplement containing a combination of as many as possible of these herbs and phytochemicals for stress hormone support, or at least take one or two. Be sure to work with your integrative practitioner in selecting agents and dosages and in minimizing the pills you take.

MEDICAL PARTNERSHIP

Once you have laid the self-care foundation, the next step is to acquire information about your biorhythm and stress hormone status. Lab tests can assess your initial level of stress hormone imbalances, and then monitor those levels as you take steps to rein it in.

▶ **Measuring Stress Hormone and Circadian Rhythm Disruption**
At the Block Center, we run a panel of stress hormone tests to help us determine which ones are elevated in our patients. With continual monitoring and reevaluation, this enables us to provide the right supplements and adjust doses. (If lab testing is not possible, return to Chapter 13 and review the section "Determining Your Terrain Disruption.") Among the tests for stress hormones and circadian rhythms you should ask your medical partner about are:

1. **Actigraphy.** A motion detector worn as a wristband or armband measures rest and activity patterns. Actigraphy is the most

general and nonspecific assessment of a disruption of your stress chemistry.[48] If you are overly active from about 11:00 P.M. to 8:00 A.M. and resting for too long when you should be awake and active, that is a sign of disrupted circadian rhythms. By pinpointing which hormones—cortisol, melatonin, or DHEA—are disrupted, your medical partner can determine your particular pattern of disruption and make supplement and lifestyle recommendations.

2. **Cortisol measurement.** Probably the best single measure of stress, cortisol levels can be obtained with a cheap and simple saliva test. Cortisol is typically measured two to four times a day to detect whether its rhythm of secretion is normal. Morning cortisol levels are normally 13–23 nmol/L, while evening levels are 1–3 nmol/L.

3. **Melatonin.** Melatonin is usually measured at 8:00 A.M., when it should be low, and 9:00 P.M., when it should be high. In people with advanced cancer, these measurements can be reversed. Stress, too, can alter melatonin rhythms, as can alcohol and tobacco. The morning reading should be 1.1–3.2 pg/mL, the evening reading 3.8–21.6 pg/mL.

4. **DHEA.** Also measured in saliva, DHEA levels tend to decrease as cortisol levels rise. DHEA is usually measured in the morning. A healthy morning level is 14–277 pg/mL. A normal ratio of DHEA to morning cortisol ranges from 35 to 435.

▶ **Terrain Modifiers**
By pinpointing which hormone systems are disrupted, your medical partner can recommend targeted supplements and correct dosages, monitor your progress, and make adjustments as you enter new phases of treatment and recovery. The tests will also reveal whether you fall into one of the three common disrupted patterns:

• The **hyperadapted** or high-stress pattern is marked by prolonged elevated cortisol, usually as a result of hypersensitivity to stressful events. The result is a delay in the normal afternoon drop in cortisol levels. Although usually temporary, this pattern can lead to a blunting of the normal evening peak of melatonin and a disruption in sleep, followed by a shift into the inverted pattern.

• The **inverted** pattern, in which daily timing of cortisol and melatonin pattern reverse, is marked by overproduction of cortisol, which remains elevated in the evening and pushes the normal peak of melatonin from evening to morning. The elevated cortisol may keep you from feeling fatigued even when you do not sleep the optimal eight hours. Catecholamine output is also stuck in "high," with DHEA and melatonin blunted.

• The **non-adapted** pattern, in which hormone levels are low and have lost their circadian rhythm is marked by a flatlining of cortisol levels at either high or depleted levels, with melatonin flatlining at low levels. Normal rises and falls of these hormones stop. The result is usually exhaustion, low energy, and weakness. Generally, levels of DHEA are low.

Maladapted Pattern	Consider
Hyperadapted	Siberian ginseng, ascorbate, pantothenic acid, L-theanine, *Rhodiola rosea* extract
Inverted	Phosphatidylserine,[49] L-theanine, melatonin (at bedtime, dosed by lab results)[50]
Non-adapted	Ginseng, pantothenic acid, licorice, *Rehmannia glutinosa*, bupleurum, ashwagandha, DHEA

If tests indicate that you have a hyperadapted pattern of stress-hormone activity, focus first on cortisol-reducing measures such as social support, stress management, music therapy, and massage.[51, 52] L-theanine and calming herbs such as valerian, hops, lavender, lemon balm, chamomile, and passionflower can also be helpful (these come in different forms, including herb capsules, liquids, and standardized extracts, with appropriate dosages listed on packaging).[53]

If tests indicate that you have an inverted pattern of stress-hormone activity, I recommend minimizing your intake of animal protein, which tends to raise cortisol. To normalize melatonin, be sure to exercise during the day as outlined above, and get early morning exposure to sun or full spectrum light. Placing a full-spectrum light box or lamp a few feet from you for thirty minutes each morning will also help.

If you have a non-adaptive pattern of stress-hormone activity, you are probably suffering from exhaustion, and your first priority is to get truly restorative rest.[54] Implement all the sleep strategies above. If those do not help, investigate a mindfulness-based program. (See www.lifeovercancer.com.) You can also ask your medical partner to recommend biofeedback or hypnotherapy, or to refer you to a sleep clinic.[55] As an antidote to physiological and psychological tension, choose a calming exercise system such as yoga, tai chi, or qi gong. Continue to avoid red meat, fatty foods, refined carbohydrates, caffeine, and alcohol.

The importance of circadian rhythms does not end here. As I mentioned above, one of the most promising advances in cancer treatment has been the discovery that administering chemotherapy drugs at specific times can favorably impact effect and toxicity, an approach called chrono-chemotherapy. In addition, some studies suggest that timing radiation and surgery in concert with biological cycles may enhance their effectiveness and result in a notable improvement in survival.

▶ **Pharmaceutical Therapy**
Between the stress-reducing therapies of the LOC mind-spirit program and the natural therapies outlined in this chapter, you have a wide variety of ways to manage stress without drug therapy. But sometimes these therapies are simply not enough. I have had patients who strongly resisted any kind of medical intervention for stress or depression as a sign of psychological instability. This feeling about medications is fairly common among people interested in natural therapies, but it can result in

needless emotional suffering, which then manifests itself as elevated levels of stress hormones. If your efforts at natural approaches to stress and emotional disturbance do not bring enough relief, please do not hesitate to talk to your doctor about exploring conventional medications. Keep in mind, as well, that we need more research on natural supplements in order to fully understand how best to use them.

Antidepressants, tranquilizers, and even stimulant medications can assist cancer patients in many situations. Your physician will need to work with you to determine which type of medication will be helpful for you, and which medications will not interact with chemotherapy agents you may be taking. Tranquilizers can intensify the sedating effects of some of the medications that are given along with chemotherapy. Your medical team will probably be alert to these possibilities, but you will also need to be sure they have the full list of supplements you are taking as well. St. John's wort, for instance, can have a harmful interaction with conventional antidepressant drugs.

Lani: Overcoming Cortisol and Insomnia

Lani, a homemaker and breast cancer patient, struggled for years with sleep problems, fatigue, and depression. She was first diagnosed in 1986 and had a mastectomy. Thirteen years later, another tumor developed in the remaining breast. Lani came to see me at the Block Center in 1999. She complained of chest and rib pain; a bone scan revealed a suspicious spot in her spine. Lani underwent four cycles of Cytoxan (cyclophosphamide) and Adriamycin (doxorubicin), standard chemotherapy drugs for metastatic breast cancer, to shrink her tumor to a manageable size, and then four cycles of Taxol (paclitaxel) to kill the remaining cancer cells. She also underwent radiation therapy. She tolerated her treatments well, and several months later another bone scan and other tests showed no evidence of disease.

While undergoing treatment, Lani started on the Life Over Cancer core diet and supplement regimen. She had already been taking melatonin, but since she still had difficulty falling asleep and staying asleep throughout the night, I recommended a higher dose, 12–15 mg before bedtime. Even that helped only somewhat, so Lani began taking a prescription antidepressant and sleep medication. Still, her sleep problems persisted and even worsened. I ordered a full set of lab tests.

The results were eye-opening. Her morning melatonin was extremely high and her morning cortisol was very low, the opposite of what is healthy. Also, her evening melatonin was low and her evening cortisol was high, a prescription for insomnia. Lani's stress-hormone rhythms were completely inverted.

At this point, I advised Lani to discontinue melatonin, which clearly wasn't helping, and start a full integrative program to rebalance her stress chemistry. I emphasized the importance of her adhering to the rest and activity cycles I covered in the LOC circadian fitness program (Chapter 8). This involved early morning exposure to sunlight to switch off her body's abnormal morning production of melatonin and a brisk morning walk to help reset her biological clock. She continued with her sleep medications. Four months later, Lani's morning and evening melatonin and cortisol levels had both returned to normal. Her evening cortisol, in fact, was at the low end of normal, suggesting considerable improvement in her ability to manage stress and her stress hormones. She was no longer taking melatonin, and she was taking only a very small and infrequent dose of sleep medication. Lani's insomnia and fatigue improved dramatically, and at the time of this writing she remains cancer-free.

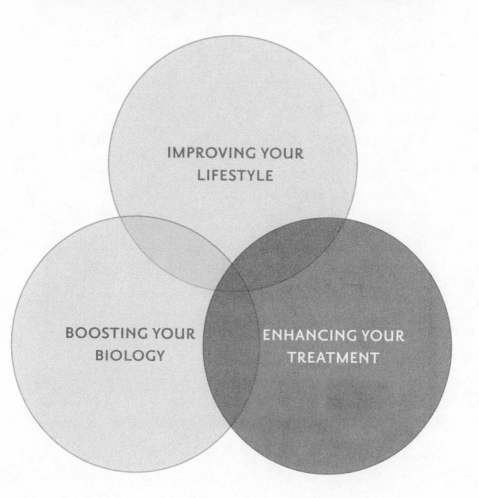

SPHERE 3

IMPROVING YOUR
LIFESTYLE

BOOSTING YOUR
BIOLOGY

ENHANCING YOUR
TREATMENT

CHAPTER 20

THE THREE PHASES OF CANCER TREATMENT: HITTING CANCER WHERE—AND WHEN— IT COUNTS

Much as I wish it were otherwise, the interventions outlined so far—diet, fitness, and mind-spirit regimens that will help you battle cancer, and specific steps that will make your biochemical terrain hostile to lingering malignant cells—are essential but seldom enough to eliminate an *established* cancer. As you noticed, those recommendations assumed that you were either planning for or had already undergone surgery, radiation, or chemotherapy to remove or shrink your tumor. If you are reading this book before or during such treatment, then this is the section where you want to start.

Having addressed your *biography* through what you eat and how you care for yourself in Sphere 1, and your *biology* through correcting any biochemical disruptions that can promote cancer in Sphere 2, Sphere 3 will focus on attacking your *pathology*, the existence of detectable tumors. The goal is to combat your disease, improve response and survival, and do it all with as few debilitating side effects as possible. Besides

improving your quality of life and your tolerance of and response to treatment, the Life Over Cancer strategies will help
control the growth of any leftover malignant cells while changing the conditions that allowed them to develop in the first place.

As dedicated as I am to the benefits of diet, lifestyle, mind-
spirit medicine, and natural medicines, I'm equally dedicated to
making sure you get the best cutting-edge anti-tumor therapies
available from medical oncology. You'll need these interventions to help eradicate both the visible tumor and the invisible
cancer cells. This will happen in three phases of care. First is an
attack phase built around surgery, radiation, chemotherapy,
and targeted molecular therapies. Then comes a containment or
growth control phase to stabilize or restrain cancer growth, especially the growth of any remaining tumor cells. Finally, once
you achieve a full remission, the remission maintenance phase is
intended to reduce the risk of recurrence, largely by strengthening your natural defenses with a range of integrative cancer
therapies. (These steps can also contain disease in the event that
you do not achieve a full remission. I will discuss this in Chapter
28.) A possible fourth phase, the crisis phase, may occur temporarily when you encounter a medical emergency or psychological setback. It is discussed in Chapter 21. In Chapter 27, I
also explain what to do when illness or prior treatment have left
you so depleted that you cannot take your next recommended
treatment.

The most effective way to gain control of a systemic disease is
to confront it simultaneously at every one of its vulnerable
points. If the systemic disorder that allowed cancer to take hold
and grow is not eliminated, the cancer may reappear, and with
greater resilience than initially. That is what happened to a patient who came to see me after he had been diagnosed with kidney cancer, which his surgeon had removed with a new
technique called radiofrequency ablation (discussed in Chapter
25). Following the procedure, the physician spoke those wonderful words, "You are cancer-free!" You can imagine this
man's shock, then, when he was later diagnosed with metastatic
kidney cancer that had spread to his lungs. His doctor's enthusiasm had left him completely unprepared for the recurrence.

My patient felt that he had lost valuable time; assuming his cancer was behind him, he'd never looked into further treatment options. But it was the lack of any attempt to reduce his very real risks of a recurrence that bothered him the most.

That is why Block Center staff members advise patients that even with successful surgery, radiotherapy, or chemotherapy, you deserve and need a follow-up plan and a remission maintenance program to reduce your risk of recurrence. While I believe in the psychological and physical benefits of optimism, I don't want optimism to get in the way of preparedness. I don't want you to let down your guard. Although mainstream oncology is excellent at reducing the bulk of visible disease, that is only one part of the battle. Cancer only infrequently disappears after surgery, radiotherapy, or chemotherapy. Because some malignant cells are usually left behind, I believe that telling patients they are "cancer-free," implying that they are through with care, can be detrimental to a full recovery.

This is not to suggest you shouldn't be relieved and enthusiastic after being pronounced in remission. You certainly should. But you also need to use the period immediately following treatment, when visible disease has been eliminated, to begin a program aimed at mopping up any remaining invisible cells and reducing your odds of ever seeing cancer again.

Just as today no cardiac surgeon would think of sending a patient off after bypass surgery without a referral to a program that teaches diet and exercise, so you should not be sent off after cancer therapy without something to do to help you stay in remission.

Mapping Tumor Growth: The Dynamics of Cancer's Life Cycle

The three major phases of cancer treatment are shown in the figure below.

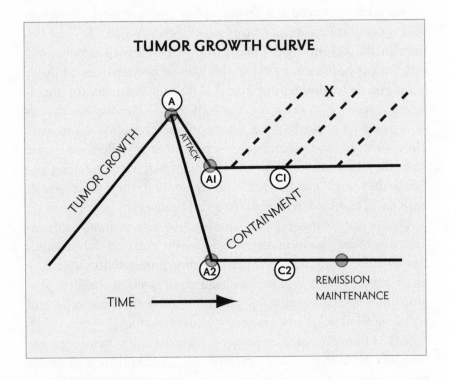

Most cancers are diagnosed where the growth curve peaks, marked A, or just before. By this point, the tumor has been growing and active for quite some time. This is when your physician will implement the attack phase of treatment, which uses some combination of conventional therapies such as surgery, chemotherapy, radiation, and molecular target therapies to reduce or eliminate the tumor. Known as cytoreduction (*cyto-* means *cell*), this process is intended to vanquish both the observable tumor and the microscopic individual malignant cells. The result is a steep drop in the tumor growth curve. An effective attack phase brings about either partial remission, shown at point A1 on the chart, or a complete remission, shown at point A2. In a partial remission, evidence of cancer is still visible in scans, X-rays, or MRIs. In a complete remission, there is no visible cancer, although residual cancer cells may lie invisible in the body.

As long as any residual cells remain dormant (whether you have visible disease or not), you can help yourself remain free of clinical disease by utilizing therapies that help control growth. This containment phase is represented by either of the flat lines C1 and C2 in the figure above. Although visible disease may exist (C1) or residual cells may remain (C2), strategies can be implemented to help curb further disease growth or proliferation of leftover residual cells. The containment phase focuses on containing and controlling the growth of these cells with a vigorous application of natural and conventional therapies to provide you with a survivor's edge.

For those of you in complete remission, congratulations! You will commence on path C2, using the strategies of the containment phase to consolidate your gains and keep any invisible cancer cells from proliferating. However, a word of caution: with some exceptions, even complete remission is rarely synonymous with *cure*. Returning to your old lifestyle, which may have contributed to your cancer, could also contribute to its return. After being on path C2 for about a year (the exact time depends on your specific circumstances), you can transition from the containment phase to the remission maintenance phase, which uses strategies that are closer to those of cancer prevention. For those of you with a partial remission, my goal is to keep you on path C1, with the hope that you will move toward complete remission, either when our rehabilitation program enables you to return to cytoreductive therapies or when new conventional therapies become available.

It is important to recognize that, as happened to my patient with metastatic kidney cancer, a seemingly successful attack phase may not be a permanent cure. Eliminating the primary tumor may have little or no impact on rogue malignant cells or micrometastases that may have escaped and are setting up camp near the original tumor, in nearby lymph nodes, or in distant organs. These cells have not succumbed to chemo or radiation, usually because they have undergone extreme genetic makeovers that make them resistant to treatment; they can therefore be more aggressive and harder to vanquish than the original tumor. These renegade cells can rear their heads months or even years later, as shown in the upper right quadrant of the figure, the area labeled X. Although the figure shows repopulation occurring after partial remission, it can also occur even years after a complete remission.

It is impossible to know with certainty whether residual cells will sit quiescent in the body until the patient dies of old age or whether they will come roaring back. That's why I believe in playing it safe, blending conventional oncology, innovative approaches to conventional care, experimental treatments (including immunotherapies and gene therapies), off-label use of medicines, nutrition, supplements, targeted therapies, and lifestyle and mind-spirit approaches to keep residual cells in check.

Attack

The goal of attack, or cytoreduction, is to shrink and debulk the tumor and flatten the tumor growth curve with the least amount of toxicity. Our aim is to come as close as possible to eliminating all visible disease. From the perspective of integrative oncology, this is a time when conventional treatments can work synergistically with natural therapies that pack an anticancer wallop. These natural therapies, including complementary nutrition and supplementation, increase the power of conventional therapies while making them safer and less draining so you can tolerate more of a toxic drug with fewer side effects. Skipping doses or lowering dosage, the commonest responses to chemo drug toxicity, means less tumor shrinkage or cancer cell killing. So by including nutrition and supplementation, you can reduce treatment-related toxicity, and improve tumor response and overall survival. By mitigating side effects, you can complete the full course of treatment and thus improve your chance of putting your cancer into remission. Blending mainstream and complementary therapies may lead to results like those I described in Chapter 1: our patients with metastatic breast and prostate cancer used the same radiation, hormones, and chemotherapy drugs as other patients but had median survivals over twice as long as would generally be expected.[1] Our results showed a 38-month median survival—an additional eighteen months' survival—for the breast cancer study, and a 60-month median survival—an additional thirty months—for the prostate cancer group. (Consider that some new drugs are approved on the basis of their lengthening survival by only two to three months.)

The attack phase needs to be carried out in close collaboration with a supportive medical team. At this point your relationship with your treating physician is extremely important; make sure it is one that makes you feel confident and comfortable.

Containment

The goal of the containment phase is to keep the tumor growth curve as flat as possible for as long as possible. Whether you have visible disease or not, containing and controlling cell growth will help you hold the gains you achieved during the attack phase. This is a time to be particularly aggressive, using diet, nutritional therapy, and other integrative therapies. I have seen these strategies work even with patients who had been too debilitated to tolerate further conventional treatment: through an aggressive rehabilitation program, we have been able to assist many of them in getting well enough to return to treatment. These strategies can also help patients whose cancers have resisted conventional treatments: through experimental and off-label drugs, aggressive nutritional therapies, and natural medicines, we have been able to help many patients contain the cancer enough that the patient can live with it as a chronic illness for many years.

Remission Maintenance

If you have achieved complete remission, celebrate! But don't assume you are out of the woods. Because rogue, resistant cancer cells often remain in the body, you need a long-term program that fights the regrowth of any leftover cells. The longer you are in remission, the better your chances are of beating it back once again if it does recur. If nothing else, the longer you hang in there the more medical breakthroughs you will be able to take advantage of. That is why, in contrast to a focus on just shrinking a tumor, I also put a premium on keeping rogue cells in check. By following a program of remission maintenance, you can improve your odds and reduce the worry that a few cancer cells may remain.

Doug: Life Is Different Now

I know the integrative approach can be a lot to manage when you're already stressed to the hilt. Unfortunately, in the absence of true cancer cures, we're forced to confront cancer on its own terms. This wily, multifaceted adversary requires equally wily, multifaceted modes of healing. And your response to cancer needs to be both thorough and lifelong.

In September 1995, in his third week of marriage, twenty-nine-year-old Doug was hit with the awful news that he had a brain tumor, and probably had only six months to live. But he and his wife had a can-do spirit and worked with our center through a grueling road of treatments. Early in his illness, at a routine follow-up meeting, I was explaining to Doug that he needed to make permanent adjustments in the way he was going to live his life. At that point, he looked me in the face, nose to nose, and started shouting and crying, "I want my life back!"

"I know you do," I replied.

That made him start shrieking even louder. "I don't think you understand—I want my *life back*!"

I told him calmly but with certainty that regardless of whether or not he was able to overcome his disease, he would never have his old life back the way it was, but it was possible to have a new life.

That's when Doug said it hit him like a ton of bricks: he and his wife had been viewing his ordeal as if he were training for the Olympics, feeling that once he was victoriously in remission, with his gold medal in hand, the event would be over. Then they looked at each other and acknowledged instantly that life was never going to be the same as it once was. Life was just different now, and the efforts to keep cancer at bay would have to be lifelong. As of the writing of this book, Doug does continue to thrive and remain cancer-free fourteen years after his original diagnosis.

Putting the Pieces Together: Your Healing Timeline

Sphere 3 is organized by where you are in your treatment and recovery, or what I call your healing timeline. That timeline reflects the tumor growth curve. In my experience, the most successful treatments are matched to whether you are in the attack, growth containment, or remission maintenance phase of your recovery. To get the most out of these chapters, use the table below to find where you are on the healing timeline, and turn to the corresponding chapter first.

If, for instance, you are coming to this book only after you have undergone surgery, it is not urgent that you read Chapter 22, which deals with preparing for surgery and the immediate aftermath. Please do keep in mind the importance of maintaining healthy habits of diet, fitness, and mind-spirit balance, as described in Chapters 4 to 12, as well as keeping your internal biochemistry as hostile as possible to cancer, as described in Chapters 13 to 19: you do not want the attacks you mount on cancer to be subverted by features of the biochemical terrain—from inflammatory factors to blood sugar—that promote the

YOUR HEALING TIMELINE

Clinical Situation	Goal	Phase of Treatment and Recovery	Starting Point
Medical emergency		**Crisis**	Chapter 21
Undergoing surgery	Prep for surgery; rebuild and recover post-op	**Attack**	Chapter 22
Undergoing chemotherapy	Improve tolerance to treatment; rebuild and recover post-chemotherapy	**Attack**	Chapter 23
Undergoing chemotherapy	Optimize tumor and cellular reduction	**Attack**	Chapter 24
Undergoing radiotherapy	Optimize tumor and cellular reduction; improve tolerance; recover post–radiation therapy	**Attack**	Chapter 25
During or after treatment when suffering from cancer side effects/ symptoms	Manage symptoms using natural agents and strategies	**Attack, Containment**	Chapters 23, 25, 26
First year after conventional treatment	Thwart tumor and residual cell regrowth	**Containment**	Chapter 26

Unable to tolerate further conventional treatment even though you still have visible disease	Restore your strength so you can tolerate further treatment. (Rehabilitation)	**Containment**	Chapter 27
No further conventional treatments are available, yet you want other options	Find experimental and off-label drugs and other alternative therapies to contain the cancer and to live with it as a chronic illness and await a medical breakthrough (No Stone Unturned program)	**Containment**	Chapter 28
One year or more after completing treatment; no visible disease remaining	Enact a repair and detox program to help recover from treatments and reduce the risk that cancer will recur (Repair and Detox program)	**Remission maintenance**	Chapter 29

growth of malignant cells. Directly targeting your tumor, as described in the following chapters, while maintaining a biochemical terrain hostile to cancer buys you better odds for long-term survival.

CHAPTER 21

CRISIS: WHEN TO CALL YOUR DOCTOR AND GO TO THE EMERGENCY ROOM

Among the saddest experiences our staff has had in caring for patients is when a patient has done all he or she could to battle cancer, only to be threatened by something that isn't cancer at all. But as I've noted, cancer patients usually do not die from their cancers. They die from the *consequences* of cancer and its treatment—cachexia, pneumonia, sepsis, embolism, and organ failure. For this reason certain emergencies take priority over everything else, even over continuing treatments meant to beat back your cancer or keep it in remission. The story of Shannon's pulmonary embolism on page 387 is an example of such a crisis, with a successful resolution after appropriate medical care.

There are two types of crisis during cancer: psychological and medical. Psychological crises, or critical stresses, can arise at any time but are most likely soon after initial diagnosis as shock, anger, or depression sets in, or during the late stages when you are confronting the results of a new scan or a setback in your prognosis. A confrontation with mortality can spur a spiritual crisis. I discuss these psychological and spiritual stresses in Chapter 12. Medical crises are based on serious complications that occur as a consequence of disease or treatment.

Often there are telltale signs that a crisis is looming. When you have cancer, symptoms that you might once have left to resolve themselves must be addressed immediately in order to keep them from escalating. High fever, for instance, might reflect sepsis (blood infection), weight loss might lead to marked and rapid wasting, and shortness of breath might indicate a blood clot has traveled to the lung. Paying attention to these warning signs can prevent an otherwise life-threatening event.

I list the most common crisis situations below. These crises are not limited to the late stages of cancer; some can occur when you are newly diagnosed and can even be what leads to a diagnosis. For instance, a bowel obstruction requiring emergency surgery can reveal colorectal cancer. If you experience any of these symptoms, you should definitely not try to manage them with the LOC diet or lifestyle interventions or with supplements. You should also not hesitate or feel at all bashful about contacting your doctor or going to the emergency room. Your doctor will want to know about these symptoms, and the earlier you inform him or her, the better.

Medical Emergencies for People with Cancer

▶ **Symptom: Fever of 101°F or higher, or fever with chills**

Possible Causes: Infection, particularly if you recently received chemotherapy

What to Do: Contact your doctor if a fever between 101° and 103° persists for more than a day, particularly following chemotherapy. (Drink fluids and stay hydrated when you have a fever.) If it climbs over 103°, go to the nearest hospital and seek medical help immediately.

▶ **Symptom: Shortness of breath with high or persistent fever with cough and yellow-green sputum**

Possible Causes: Pneumonia; lung tumor may be blocking major airway, causing infection in part of lung behind the blockage

What to Do: Seek medical help. Do not wait until breathing is so difficult that you cannot speak or there is blueness around the lips. In these cases, go to the emergency room at once.

▶ **Symptom: Marked shortness of breath, persistent cough; sometimes pain in the side that gets worse when you breathe in**

Possible Causes: Pleural effusion (fluid buildup in the chest around the lungs)

What to Do: Call doctor immediately unless you have already been assessed as having pleural effusion and are certain of the cause and are being treated. Do not wait until breathing is so difficult that you cannot speak or there is blueness around the lips. In these cases, go to the ER at once.

▶ **Symptom: Leg pain, warmth or reddening of affected area, swelling or fluid buildup**

Possible Causes: Deep vein thrombosis

What to Do: Call doctor or go to the ER.

▶ **Symptom: Sudden shortness of breath or other change in respiration when at rest; chest pain, leg pain (possibly with swelling, coughing, or spitting up blood), irregular heartbeat or pounding heart**

Possible Causes: Pulmonary embolism

What to Do: Call doctor and go to the ER.

▶ **Symptom: Rapid weight loss (more than two pounds a week or five pounds per month), often accompanied by poor appetite and severe weakness**

Possible Causes: Cachexia, chronic inflammation due to the cancer and secondarily to nutritional imbalances; anorexia due to treatment

What to Do: Seek expert help and aggressive nutritional and pharmacologic interventions: high-dose fish oil and other anti-inflammatories; greatly increased calorie and protein intake; Megace, Marinol, and Oxandrin; resistance training.

▶ **Symptom: Back pain followed by weakness or loss of sensation**

Possible Causes: Spinal cord compression by tumor

What to Do: Call doctor.

▶ **Symptom: Coughing up blood**

Possible Causes: Blood clot, infection, or tumor

What to Do: Go to the emergency room if blood loss is profuse; if not, call doctor.

▶ **Symptom: Vomiting material that looks like coffee grounds**

Possible Causes: Bleeding from the stomach, esophagus, or duodenum

What to Do: Call doctor immediately or go to the ER. If you feel dizzy or faint, go to the ER at once.

▶ **Symptom: Passing jet-black, tarry stools**

Possible Causes: Bleeding from the lower bowel

What to Do: Call doctor or go to the ER. If you feel dizzy or faint, go to the ER at once.

▶ **Symptom: Large bruises or purple spots on the skin**

Possible Causes: Bleeding in the skin—may be due to low platelets, particularly after chemotherapy or if there is excessive marrow toxicity

What to Do: Call doctor. If you feel dizzy or faint, go to the ER at once.

▶ **Symptom: Bleeding from the nose or mouth**

Possible Causes: Low platelets, particularly after chemotherapy or if there is excessive marrow toxicity

What to Do: Call doctor. If you feel dizzy or faint, go to the ER at once.

▶ **Symptom: Inability to urinate, or extreme difficulty with urination; may be accompanied by inability to walk**

Possible Causes: Sudden problem in the spinal cord, kidneys, or pelvis

What to Do: Call doctor immediately. If you have numbness or weakness in the legs or buttocks, go to the ER at once.

▶ **Symptom: Sudden swelling of the face, arms, or upper chest**

Possible Causes: Problem in the mediastinum (in the upper chest cavity) that is causing obstruction to large veins there

What to Do: Contact doctor. If you also have shortness of breath, go to the ER immediately unless your doctor is familiar with your condition and you can contact him or her right away.

▶ **Symptom: Chest pain of rapid onset, especially with difficulty breathing, decreased exercise tolerance, dizziness, or lightheadedness**

Possible Causes: Possible pericardial malignancy (cancer near the heart) or pericardial effusion (fluid in sac around heart)

What to Do: Go to the ER immediately.

▶ **Symptom: Severe, persistent abdominal pain lasting hours; constipation or inability to pass gas for three days**

Possible Causes: Obstruction of the bowel, possibly due to tumor

What to Do: If moderate to severe, call your doctor. If you can't reach the doctor, go to the ER.

▶ **Symptom: Protracted vomiting or diarrhea resulting in dehydration (marked by muscle weakness or lethargy, decreased urination or dark urine, sunken eyes, dry or sticky feeling in mouth, loss of skin elasticity)**

Possible Causes: Effect of chemotherapy, bowel obstruction, or high calcium levels in the blood

What to Do: Call doctor. If vomiting or diarrhea persists and limited liquid intake lasts for more than twenty-four hours, contact your medical team or go to the ER.

▶ **Symptom: Pain in a new region, incessant or unrelieved pain, change in pain intensity**

Possible Causes: Progression of tumor or recurrence

What to Do: Call doctor.

▶ **Symptom: Sudden paralysis of one side**

Possible Causes: Stroke or tumor affecting the central nervous system

What to Do: Call doctor.

▶ **Symptom: Confusion, grogginess, disorientation, difficulty waking**

Possible Causes: Brain metastases

What to Do: Call doctor.

▶ **Symptom: Seizures**

Possible Causes: Problem in brain or with blood salts

What to Do: If this is your first seizure, call doctor and go to the ER. If seizure is a single convulsion and you're on anticonvulsant medication, wait to recover. Call doctor and go to ER if seizures are recurrent.

▶ Symptom: Sudden loss of consciousness

Possible Causes: Problem in the brain or central nervous system; analgesic drug overuse; excessive calcium in the blood; marked change in fluid volume (dehydration)

What to Do: Go to the ER immediately.

Often there are telltale signs that a crisis is looming. When you have cancer, symptoms that you might once have left to resolve themselves must be addressed immediately in order to keep them from escalating. High fever, for instance, might reflect sepsis (blood infection), weight loss might become marked and rapid wasting, and shortness of breath might indicate a blood clot traveling to the lung. Paying attention to these warning signs can prevent an otherwise life-threatening event.

Experiencing these symptoms does not always indicate a grave situation. But I would rather you err on the side of caution than miss an opportunity to prevent or control a crisis. You should take with you to the emergency room a full list of the medications and supplements you are taking, including doses. This should be prepared in advance—ideally, when you start taking medications or supplements—and updated as needed.

During a time of crisis, you may have to temporarily put aside specific components of your integrative treatment regimen. For example, you may need to stop taking blood thinners to treat clots if you experience sudden bleeding or severe thrombocytosis (markedly low platelets). Crisis treatment will usually last only a short time; once the problem is gone or stabilized, you should be able to return to your prior treatment. If you had to stop any aspect of your Sphere 1 and Sphere 2 programs, such as exercise or botanicals with blood-thinning or anti-inflammatory effects, this would be the time to restart them. After such a crisis, reevaluate which aspects of your terrain need particular attention. If you have suffered an embolism, for instance, go back to Chapter 17, on blood clotting. If you had a serious infection, refer back to Chapter 16, on the immune system, and ramp up your efforts to strengthen routine immune surveillance. If you experienced a pain crisis, revisit Chapter 15 on overcoming inflammation. Improving your terrain can reduce the risk of future crises and help you better confront life-threatening complications. Prevention is infinitely better than treatment.

CHAPTER 22

THE SURGICAL
SUPPORT PROGRAM

In the attack phase of cancer treatment, the goal is to eliminate as much cancer as possible. This is the heart of mainstream oncology and is called debulking. If it is not technically
possible to remove all of your tumor or tumors, the goal is to remove as much tumor as possible. This is called optimal debulking. Sometimes that really does mean that the surgeon removed
all visible cancer and got the invisible (microscopic) cancer as
well. However, in many cases even optimal debulking leaves behind some cancer cells. That is why cancer patients who have
undergone successful surgery often are advised to undergo subsequent radiation or chemotherapy. These postsurgical strategies are called adjuvant therapies, and their purpose is to keep
the disease from returning by ridding the body of not only visible disease, but invisible tumor cells as well.

Effective cytoreduction is absolutely critical. Unfortunately,
some alternative approaches reject these mainstream treatments. We have had heartbreaking experiences with patients
who have come to the Block Center seeking medical validation
of their determination to avoid surgery, chemo, or radiation.
For instance, two women with breast cancer came to me while
receiving dietary-only treatment from alternative practitioners;
they had shunned all conventional intervention. In both cases

the tumors grew so large they tore through the skin and had formed extensive and distant metastases. Sadly, their conditions were so far advanced that they did not respond to treatment.

But the story can have a happier ending. Another woman, with a huge fifteen-centimeter breast tumor, came to me after refusing the advice of six different surgeons to have the tumor removed. Though I, too, thought she needed surgery, I avoided discussing it during our initial visit. I instead explained that despite the value of certain complementary therapies, I had strong doubts that these alone would shrink, let alone eliminate, her massive tumor. After four weekly visits I felt I had gained her trust, and so at that point I conveyed my serious concern that her tumor would soon rupture and that her cancer had probably metastasized. I explained what I thought surgery could accomplish, and assured her that an integrative approach could help fight her cancer, reduce side effects, and possibly even improve treatment. After some coaxing, she agreed to have surgery, which went well. Scans confirmed my hunch that she had developed lung metastases. After considerable discussion, she agreed to chemotherapy, and with aggressive integrative treatment was able to get through it with ease. She remained in remission for six years before suffering a recurrence and eventually dying from her cancer. Still, after repeatedly refusing any new conventional treatments she lived three times as long after being diagnosed with lung metastases as a typical metastatic breast cancer patient.

Historically, complementary (as distinguished from alternative) therapies have left the debulking to surgeons or oncologists while focusing on stimulating the body's natural anti-cancer defenses and preserving well-being. No longer. Today, an integrative approach to cancer treatment, as we practice it at the Block Center, eradicates these false distinctions between complementary and conventional medicine, recognizing only good medicine or faulty medicine. When the attack phase involves an *integrative* attack on cancer, rather than only a conventional attack, it can be far more effective, longer-lasting, and gentler. How? By incorporating approaches that enhance the power of mainstream therapies to kill cancer cells, while also shielding normal cells. This allows integrative doctors to moderate side effects while maintaining crucial cytoreduction.

Surgery is the first therapy for most cancer patients. In some early cancers—including those of the cervix, breast, prostate, colon, and lung—surgery can be curative. Although few physicians discuss this, there are ways you can get in shape nutritionally, emotionally, and physically so as to improve your outcome and shorten your recovery time. This is especially important if you face repeated surgeries, such as those for removing metastases. Also, surgery can offer benefits beyond tumor debulking, as I discuss below. I first offer steps you can take before surgery to get the most out of it, and then turn to what you can do after the operation to minimize complications and put yourself on a trajectory to recovery.

Plotting Your Strategy Before Surgery

▶ **Banking Tumor Tissue**
The first thing to consider before surgery is whether you want to have samples of your tumor tissue kept. There are three reasons for doing this: having the tissue tested to determine which chemotherapy agents are most lethal to it, having it tested to determine which molecular targets are its Achilles' heel, and preserving it so it can be used to create an autologous cancer vaccine. In some cancers, tissue samples are taken routinely. All surgeons take samples of breast tumor tissue, for instance, to send to the pathology lab to test it for standard markers such as estrogen receptors. This enables them to determine whether the tumor is estrogen-sensitive, in which case using estrogen-blocking drugs such as tamoxifen or an aromatase inhibitor makes sense, or whether it is studded with molecules called HER2/neu, in which case you are an excellent candidate for the targeted molecular therapy Herceptin.

Since I believe that information is power and more is better than less, I often recommend that my patients ask their surgeon to obtain fresh samples from the operation or biopsy (you will need to plan in advance so the tissue is collected properly, particularly for chemosensitivity testing and an autologous cancer vaccine). If you are being treated at a comprehensive cancer center, the chances are good that its laboratories will be able to test for molecular markers associated with your type of cancer. If your hospital does not have the necessary facilities and expertise, you can request that an outside lab be used.

Fresh Tissue from Surgery for Chemosensitivity Testing. I will discuss the rationale for chemosensitivity testing, or determining which chemotherapy agents are most likely to be effective, in Chapter 24. However, you will need to decide before your surgery whether to request this, and make the proper arrangements. Chemosensitivity testing is not yet routine and generally requires fresh tissue. I find this testing particularly useful when you have surgery for recurrence, when knowing which agents are more likely to be lethal to your specific type of tumor helps with choosing among protocols. Chemo protocols for initial treatments are generally more widely accepted, though chemosensitivity testing can be helpful here as well. As I write, insurers are not always willing to cover this procedure, but that is beginning to change. In addition, a test for early-stage breast cancer patients has recently become available that predicts the potential benefits from having chemotherapy, on the basis of an analysis of twenty-one genetic markers on tumor cells; this test is covered by many insurance companies.[1]

To store tumor tissue for chemosensitivity testing, have the chemosensitivity testing lab send you or your surgeon a tumor-preservation kit, which will need to be sent back overnight with the fresh sample after your surgery. Only a few labs are equipped to perform chemosensitivity testing; you can check www.lifeovercancer.com for the latest list. Your surgeon or oncologist may be skeptical about the value of some types of chemosensitivity testing, probably because early assays showed few clinical benefits. However, not all tumor tissue assays are the same. You will want to investigate further before deciding which type of testing you wish to use. I favor apoptotic assays

over prolifererative ones. Other new assays are also showing
promise.[2] The LOC website will explain this further.

Samples for Targeted Molecular Testing. This is an area that is
developing quickly, and you will need to discuss with your oncologist before your scheduled surgery the status of targeted
therapies that are appropriate for your tumor, and the procedures that will need to be used in obtaining a sample.
Realistically, most oncologists are unlikely to order tests for
markers for which there are not yet approved treatments. But as
long as you have arranged to have a sample of your tumor preserved (the standard procedure performed by the hospital's
pathologist where your surgery was performed is to preserve it
in so-called paraffin tumor blocks), you will be ready with crucial information to discover whether an experimental or newly
approved therapy might be right for you. This will even help
you in considering whether you wish to enroll in a clinical trial.
You will need to know which trial is the appropriate one—that
is, the one that is felt to target the molecules or pathways that
drive the growth of your tumor. Test results can also be helpful
when deciding which nutraceutical or nutritional supplement to
use. Tell your oncologist or surgeon that you would like to have
this tissue preserved for future testing. If you forget, or if you
are reading this after your surgery, don't worry: as long as tumor tissue is preserved in tumor blocks, which pathologists in
most hospitals do routinely, you can have these tests run at any
time, even months or years later.

Tissue for an Autologous Cancer Vaccine. Autologous cancer
vaccines are vaccines composed of your own cancer cells or
components of them (antigens, protein "bar codes" found on
the outside of cells). The idea is that injecting these cells or cell
fragments will provoke an immune response intended to wipe
out remaining malignant cells, and thus will prevent or treat a
recurrence. Autologous cancer vaccines are being studied and
tested and can already be received in several overseas clinics.[3] I
will discuss vaccines further in Chapter 29, but for now let me
say that to date I believe their most promising role is either for

stabilizing and containing cancer or for targeting and mopping up any leftover microscopic (invisible) cells that might remain after surgery, radiation, or chemotherapy, though new vaccine research may soon change this by developing an ability to affect bulky disease.

To keep this option open, you will need samples of your original tumor to produce the custom-made vaccine. This requires taking a sample of fresh tissue that has been removed during surgery and properly preserving it for immediate shipping to a cryopreservation facility (though some hospitals can do this in-house). The size of the required sample and the transport solutions and kits differ from one banking facility to the next and from one cancer to the next. Unfortunately, many hospitals lack the needed equipment for properly freezing tissue for later use in vaccines, but I suspect the practice will become more common as cancer vaccines prove their value. You can check the LOC website for cryopreservation facilities, which will give you ⓘ instructions to pass on to your surgeon.

▶ Timing of Surgery

A growing body of research shows, and my own experience confirms, that novel methods of integrative oncology can help during the attack phase, too. One example is surgical timing for breast cancer, where the operation date affects results. There is good evidence that timing surgery according to the phase of the menstrual cycle may reduce recurrences.[4] Women who are pre-menopausal and who undergo mastectomy during the second half of the menstrual cycle (counting the first day of bleeding as day 1, this is typically days 15 through 28) appear to have a lower risk of recurrence and better survival than women who have surgery during the first half of their cycle. Taken together, studies from major cancer centers show a 15 percent increase in ten-year survival for women operated on during the second half of their cycle. This makes biological sense. During the first half of the cycle levels of hormones and growth factors that might speed the progression of breast cancer are present at high levels in the blood. Surgery to remove the tumor can release malignant cells into the blood, where the hormones may spur them to proliferate. In contrast, these growth-promoting hormones are at lower levels during the second half of the monthly cycle. As an added benefit, new studies show that biochemicals that promote angiogenesis, the growth of blood vessels that feed tumors, are also at higher levels during the first half of the cycle, while ones that discourage angiogenesis are higher during the second half.[5]

Whether you should request surgery during the second half of your cycle hinges on several factors. If your situation is urgent, if the tumor is large or growing at an accelerated pace, it is important to review this research with your doctor. Otherwise, and if scheduling surgery during the second half of the cycle means waiting only a few days longer, I advise patients that there is likely a benefit to waiting. Specifically, if the tumor is small (less than one centimeter) and shows no signs of growing rapidly (a grade 1 tumor with low Ki-67, low S-phase fraction, or low number of necrotic cells), it may be advantageous to schedule surgery during the second half of your cycle. Look for updates on this rapidly evolving field on the LOC website.

▶ **Physical, Emotional, and Mental Prepping**
Most cancer patients are in good enough physical condition to get through surgery when they are first diagnosed. But getting through is not enough. If you prepare properly, you can not only make a possibly difficult experience easier but also reduce the risks of surgery and shorten your recovery time. Even more important, if you need multiple surgeries, being in optimal shape going into each operation will help you avoid the debilitating consequences of these procedures and make recovery easier.

To prepare physically for surgery, it is important to improve your nutritional condition. See Chapter 6 for treatment preparation and adjustments in your LOC diet program, using the High-Intensity Nutritional Support diet if you are nutritionally in poor condition. Even if you have only a week or two before your operation, you can benefit from following the advice on LOC physical care. In addition, improving your resilience and physical fitness can reduce your risk of complications and speed your recovery time. You can find guidance on physical fitness in Chapter 9.

To prepare mentally for surgery, be willing to ask for the emotional support you need from family, friends, doctors, nurses, and the surgeon before, during, and after the operation. Don't hesitate to ask your surgeon to explain what will happen at each step, from the moment you enter the hospital until you are discharged. Knowing what to expect can ease your anxiety. It will also allow you to visualize each step; by imaging the procedures going well beforehand, when you actually experience them your anxiety is likely to be much less. I recommend relaxation techniques, meditation, hypnosis, or imagery to calm yourself prior to your operation, starting a few days before. You can use relaxation, hypnosis, or imagery recordings, or therapists at clinics such as ours can help you with preparation and imagery; see www.lifeovercancer.com for suggestions. At the Block Center, we commonly customize CDs for our patients before they undergo a procedure. There is some evidence that you can hear and process sounds while under anesthesia, with beneficial physiologic effects. That is, not only will you feel better, but your outcome may be better.[6] In an analysis of more than 100 studies of mind-body interventions administered prior to surgery, researchers found that patients experienced across-the-board improvements in outcomes, including fewer days in the hospital, fewer medical complications, and less need for pain medication.

▶ Boosting Immune Surveillance and Immune Priming

It is also a good idea to prepare immunologically for surgery. If your immune surveillance system is functioning optimally before surgery, you are less likely to develop a postoperative infection. And you are more likely to keep any malignant cells that may be loosened or shed during surgery from migrating to distant sites in your body and seeding metastases. As a first step, follow the basic Life Over Cancer nutrition program, as described in Chapter 5, for as long as possible before your operation; in particular, emphasize anti-inflammatories and the steps in Chapter 16, which will stimulate the activity of natural killer cells and other infection-fighting cells so they are active during and immediately following surgery. It is important to avoid formulations that act as anticoagulants, or you may suffer excessive bleeding. Keep in mind, if you are taking anticoagulant supplements such as vitamin E, vitamin C, garlic, or anti-inflammatory herbs and need emergency surgery, tell your doctor.

It may also be possible to take advantage of surgery to prime your immune system to better recognize cancer cells. For priming to occur, dendritic cells, which direct the activity of other immune cells, must be exposed to the proteins on the surface of cancer cells.[7] The dendritic cells then take this information and pass it on to cancer-fighting cells, letting them recognize the malignant enemy and mount an attack. A number of natural agents can activate dendritic cells preoperatively, including beta-glucans (starch-like compounds derived from yeast, grains, or medicinal mushrooms such as shiitake, maitake, and reishi),[8] Asian ginseng (a possible anticoagulant), and aloe vera. The drug Leukine (GM-CSF) may also activate dendritic cells. Discuss the use of these agents or other herbal immune boosters before surgery with your integrative or medical partner to decide which might be the most suitable approach for you.

▶ **Anti-Inflammatory Steps**
A common postoperative problem is swelling and inflammation. But better than treating inflammation is preventing or minimizing it in the first place. I therefore advise following the steps in Chapters 5 and 15 on diet, fitness, and supplement use to lower your inflammatory potential. Since most anti-inflammatories, whether pharmaceutical (such as COX-2 inhibitors or aspirin) or nutritionally based, have some anticoagulant properties, I advise starting them two weeks before surgery, then stopping one week before. Fish oil consumed even a few weeks before surgery can change the fatty acids in the membranes of your cells and thus reduce post-op swelling and inflammation.[9]

▶ **Angiogenic Inhibition**

One of the ironies of cancer is that when you have a primary tumor, for many years you will typically not develop metastatic cancer. The reason is that the primary tumor produces compounds that inhibit the growth of blood vessels in micro-metastases. But surgery removes your primary tumor. This removes the check on micro-metastases, allowing them to grow the blood vessels they need to survive. However, to date, surgery is still considered a better option than leaving the primary tumor in place. I therefore recommend that our patients take the following anti-angiogenesis agents before surgery. Work with your integrative practitioner to select agents and doses from the following table.

RECOMMENDATIONS FOR ANGIOGENESIS-INHIBITING HERBS AND SUPPLEMENTS

Natural Agent	Effect
Soy genistein (300–600 mg a day)	Numerous cell and animal tests find anti-angiogenic effects from genistein and a soy-based diet.[10] Because the data on genistein and estrogen-dependent cancers, while looking favorable, are not clear, we would not suggest this for patients with breast, ovarian, or endometrial cancers that carry estrogen receptors. However, there is no indication that moderate consumption of soy foods, such as tofu and tempeh, poses problems for these patients.
Polysaccharides from *Coriolus versicolor* (500–3,000 mg a day)	Reduce formation of new blood vessels and reduce tumor secretion of angiogenesis-promoting VEGF in mice.[11]

Natural Agent	Effect
Luteolin (usually extracted from perilla leaf, but parsley, celery, peppers are good sources) 2–4 mg	Reduces the size of tumors implanted in mice by 50 percent; blocks operation of VEGF.[12]
EGCG (350–700 mg a day) *or* 500–1,000 mg decaffeinated green tea extract	Suppresses angiogenesis in mouse models.[13]
Inositol hexaphosphate (IP6). Start with ½ gram a day and increase as tolerated. Studies have used up to 18 g per day.	In lab animals, reduces the growth of blood vessels and tumor secretion of VEGF.[14]

▶ **Avoiding Adverse Interactions**

Herbs and supplements that have anticoagulant effects do not mix well with surgery and so should be stopped five to seven days prior to surgery.[15] You should also stop using any herbs or supplements that help you sleep or to remain calm, since they can magnify the effects of anesthesia.[16] These supplements include valerian, kava (which you should not be using in any case, because there is some indication it may cause liver failure), passionflower, hops, skullcap, chamomile, inositol, GABA, 5-HTP, and melatonin. Stimulants such as ginseng may oppose the effects of anesthesia, so you should stop them a week before surgery, too. If you have been using anticoagulant or sedative herbs or supplements and suddenly face emergency surgery, don't panic. Simply tell your doctors what you have been using so they can make appropriate adjustments. People using prescription or over-the-counter medications that have anticoagulant or sedative properties face emergency surgery every day; doctors are accustomed to handling possible interactions.

Plotting Your Strategy After Surgery

▶ **Improving Wound Healing**

To improve postsurgical wound healing, as soon as you are able to eat, consume adequate protein in the days after your surgery. One way to do this is to follow the Treatment Support diet (or even the High-Intensity Nutritional Support diet if you have unintentionally lost weight) described in Chapter 6. In addition, a variety of supplements may improve wound healing and reduce wound swelling, including pancreatic and plant enzymes such as bromelain (2–3 capsules two or three times a day, one hour before or two hours after meals; this should supply 4,000–6,000 GDU or 6,000–9,000 MCU of total enzyme activity units daily) and curcumin (1,000–1,400 mg daily), which your integrative practitioner can help you with.[17] Follow the pre-op strategy for anti-inflammation as well. This will aid healing and reduce the swelling and chronic inflammation that can occur postoperatively.

▶ **Reducing Nausea and Vomiting; Improving Bowel Function**

After an operation, it is common to suffer nausea and vomiting. There is not much you can do to prevent this, but after the operation acupuncture can help: stimulating the wrist acupuncture point significantly reduces postsurgical nausea. At the Block Center we also find that auricular acupuncture performed with tiny needles to the ear can be quite effective, as well as an acupuncture point on your wrist (called P6).[18] Surgery can also impair bowel function; your doctor will not discharge you from the hospital until your gastrointestinal tract has returned to normal. The bowel typically takes days to wake up and recover from surgery, and you will not be permitted to eat until it does. While there are limitations to what you can do in the way of diet and lifestyle if you are recovering in the hospital, you may speed things up by drinking lots of fluids (at least six 8-ounce glasses of water every day) and getting up and walking around. Ginger capsules (500 mg every four to six hours) can relieve nausea, though there is some possibility that they may increase bleeding.[19] Ask your medical team if this might be right for you.

▶ **Pain Management**

Pain medications are a must after surgery. The usual choice is morphine. Recent research indicates that Ultram (tramadol) is also effective, and it seems to lack the immune-suppressing properties of morphine, although it does tend to increase nausea (morphine causes constipation).[20] Your medical team can help you balance these risks and benefits to find a pain medication that is right for you. Do not be concerned about becoming addicted to postoperative pain medication; this is simply not a problem. The potential difficulties due to unrelieved pain, however, can be significant.

CHAPTER 23

THE CHEMOTHERAPY SUPPORT PROGRAM: REDUCING TOXICITY AND SIDE EFFECTS

In this chapter I'll outline several approaches for reducing the toxicity of chemotherapy. Some emerge from conventional medicine, while others use natural agents. If you are about to undergo chemo, you should also follow the advice in Chapter 6 on diet-based ways to manage common symptoms, the advice in Chapter 9 on using physical care to ameliorate these symptoms, and the steps in Chapter 12 on mind-spirit techniques that improve tolerance of and reduce the side effects of chemo.

Gerry: "I Couldn't Believe How Good I Felt"

Gerry Jilka was forty-nine when he was diagnosed with colon cancer in December 2002. Three years later, having endured two surgeries and twelve cycles of chemo, he was in remission, but his joy at this news was short-lived. In January 2006, his oncologist told Gerry that he had stage IV metastatic colon cancer, which has an average life expectancy of between six months and two years. Gerry rejected this prognosis, determined that it would not apply to him and that, with the right doctor, he could find a treatment plan that would help him beat his cancer. He found our center.

Though enthusiastic about our philosophy of care, Gerry was reluctant to begin chemotherapy again. The progression of his disease had left him extremely weak, and he expressed concern about the effects of chemo. When I assured him that we would design a program intended to enhance his treatment tolerance, reduce the toxicity of his treatment, and boost its effectiveness (testing had identified the "molecular fingerprint" of Gerry's cancer), he agreed to give it a try. His program included therapeutic nutrition to boost stamina, counter fatigue, and reduce chemo's side effects; mind-spirit interventions to reduce stress; and exercise to build up his strength and fitness. Crucially, we administered the chemo through chronotherapy via an FDA-approved portable pump, small enough to fit in a fanny pack, which delivered supplemental intravenous nutrients at the same time as the chemo drug.

"I couldn't believe how good I felt throughout my chronotherapy treatments," Gerry told me later. "Because the pump was portable, I was able to remain active. Having been confined to a hospital room for my previous chemotherapy, this freedom was invigorating." With each of his scans, Gerry showed improvement. Because he reported no troubling side effects and tolerated his chronotherapy treatments so well, there was no need to reduce the dose. After seven chronotherapy sessions (five fewer than he received of conventional chemotherapy), Gerry showed no evidence of disease, and today in 2009, seven years following his original diagnosis, he is in complete remission and back at work.

Innovative Approaches from Conventional Medicine

Chronotherapy. Timing chemotherapy can increase survival. The reason is that cancer cells are more sensitive to treatment at specific times of night or day.[1] Most chemotherapy drugs work best when cancer cells are active and dividing, which makes them most vulnerable to chemo, and are least toxic when healthy cells are at rest. Ideally, then, you would time chemo for this period. Why does chronotherapy lead to fewer side effects than untimed chemo?[2] Chemo drugs target dividing cells, because malignant cells are demons of division. But the drugs cannot tell a healthy dividing cell from an aberrantly dividing one, so the former are often also killed. Among the normal cells that are fast-dividing are gastrointestinal cells (whose death by chemo leads to nausea, mouth sores, ulcers, vomiting, and other gastrointestinal effects), bone marrow cells (whose death by chemo leads to dangerous drops in red and white blood cells), and hair follicle cells (whose death leads to balding). But these normal cells divide rapidly only at certain times of day; they all have a resting phase. With chronotherapy, you can receive toxic drugs when cancer cells are actively dividing but normal cells are resting and therefore less likely to be targeted. As you know, if toxic effects get bad enough, your oncologist may be forced to interrupt your treatment, reduce dosing, or stop the treatment altogether, allowing your tumor just the respite it needs to start growing back. That's not what you want. This is probably one of the reasons why cancer patients getting chronotherapy tolerate treatment better and survive longer than patients getting standard schedules of drug delivery: spared toxic side effects, they can receive the full chemo regimen.[3]

Another reason is that each timed dose of chemotherapy can be more potent than the identical dose of the identical chemo drug given without regard to timing.[4] That's because each cell type and each drug has a period of peak sensitivity. For instance, normal rectal cells divide more often during the day and less at night, so by giving chemotherapy for colon cancer at night we can avoid damaging the normal rectal cells but kill more malignant cells.

Chronotherapy has significantly increased patients' survival. One 1999 study reported that it increased the five-year survival of patients with advanced ovarian and bladder cancers fourfold, and a multicenter trial in Europe found that patients with advanced metastatic colorectal cancer receiving the chemotherapy drug 5-FU (5-fluorouracil) via chronotherapy had a 50 percent greater median survival time than patients receiving the same drug on a conventional schedule.[5] In a 2001 study of chronotherapy for advanced ovarian cancer (stages III and IV), the chronotherapy group had half as many adverse side effects as patients receiving standard chemotherapy; the latter had to have their drug dosages reduced or chemo treatment delayed due to side effects four times as often as the chronotherapy group. This is undoubtedly part of the reason why 44 percent of the chronotherapy group survived for five years compared with 11 percent of the control group.[6]

A major benefit of chronotherapy is that patients can rechallenge their cancer by using the same drugs in a chronotherapy regimen that they had previously been unable to tolerate with standard dosing. In 2005, the Block Center conducted a study of twenty-six of our colon cancer patients. Six were in stage III and twenty in stage IV; the majority of the stage IV patients received chronotherapy after initial therapy with conventional timing had proved ineffective or intolerable (due to side effects such as mucositis, nausea, and diarrhea severe enough to require treatment in the intensive care unit). But when we gave the patients the same drugs using chronotherapy, none suffered serious toxicity. (In patients like this receiving the same drugs but through standard chemo, the rate of severe toxicity ranges from 24 percent to 65 percent.) What's more, our twenty stage IV patients had a median survival of twenty-seven months, an excellent record in a disease with a median survival of twelve to eighteen months.[7] Let me underline this: if you suffer few to no severe toxic side effects that necessitate stopping or delaying your chemo, you have a better chance at long-term survival.[8]

Chronotherapy is optimally given over several hours, ratcheting from a minimal dose to a peak dose, and then back down. It is possible to deliver optimally timed chemotherapy in a hospital, so that if your peak sensitivity to a specific drug is, say, 4 A.M. you can receive your peak dose of chemo then. But it is much more convenient to use specialized portable pumps that can be programmed to deliver a drug whenever cancer cells are most susceptible to the drug and normal cells are least vulnerable to its toxicity, as I did with Gerry.

I have used chronotherapy since the 1990s, but as I write there is only one other cancer center in the United States that offers chronotherapy, that run by a pioneer of this field, William Hrushesky, at the Veterans Administration Hospital in Columbia, South Carolina. Europe has at least forty large cancer centers offering chronotherapy. Multiple randomized studies, especially in advanced cancers, have favored chronotherapy over routine infusions, so you may consider receiving treatment using this technique, especially if you have trouble with chemo side effects.[9]

▶ **Fractionated Dose Therapy**
Traditionally, chemotherapy is given in a single large dose, often as high as a patient can tolerate. This sort of chemo is called bolus dosing. But a number of recent studies show that fractionated or continuous infusion, in which a drug is administered in small doses over the course of a day or several days, is better tolerated and possibly more effective. Although additional clinical studies are needed to confirm this, the better tolerance might improve survival, just as it does with chronotherapy. Ask your oncologists if they have adopted this approach.

▶ **Amifostine**
We once had a patient with non-small-cell lung carcinoma who came for care at the center but who could no longer receive a chemotherapy drug, cisplatin, that was making his tumor shrink: it was also causing his kidneys to fail. We put him on the full LOC program, as well as the conventional drug Ethyol (amifostine), which protects against the renal toxicity associated with cisplatin. Amifostine, which is given by injection, works because it is a potent antioxidant and thus can protect normal tissue from the damaging effects of free radicals, which is how radiation and some chemo drugs exert their cell-killing effects.[10]

We proceeded with chemotherapy and Ethyol, and he had an excellent response. His kidney function also returned to near normal.

Amifostine is usually used with radiation patients, but while there is controversy around its value, I believe it deserves further study and wider use. It protects a broad range of normal tissues, including bone marrow, the lining of the gastrointestinal tract, and the mouth, kidneys, heart, lungs, and salivary glands.[11] As a result, it has been shown to reduce chemo-induced toxicity to the heart, muscles, blood cells, kidney, and nerves (including hearing loss and peripheral neuropathy). It is especially effective in fighting bone marrow toxicity from cisplatin or carboplatin (commonly used in lung cancer treatment).[12] Of nineteen recent studies that paired amifostine with chemotherapy in 1,300 patients, nine found decreases in toxicity. Ten found no benefit or questionable benefit. None found that amifostine protected tumors from or interfered with the effects of therapy.[13] However, a recent review of amifostine in radiotherapy suggested there is a 2 percent chance that treatment might fail because of interference from amifostine. In the past, amifostine was given intravenously, which caused side effects including low blood pressure, nausea, and vomiting. But subcutaneous injection has eliminated most of these side effects. Again, if you have experienced debilitating side effects of chemo or radiation, ask your medical team if amifostine might help you, including discussion of the small failure risk.

▶ **Neupogen, Neulasta**
The drugs Neupogen (filgrastim) and Neulasta (pegfilgrastim) reduce risk of sepsis from low white counts after chemo—thus preventing treatment delays.

▶ **Erythropoetin Alpha**
Erythropoetin alpha, sold as Epogen or Procrit or the longer-acting Aranesp (darbepoetin alfa), helps red blood cells recover between chemo cycles. Recent data on these medications indicate that excessive use may make patients susceptible to cardiovascular complications and may in some circumstances shorten

survival. If your doctor prescribes these drugs for you, he or she will carefully monitor your hemoglobin to make sure it does not rise to excessive levels.

▶ **Preserving Fertility**
The prospect of losing your fertility can be one of the most upsetting aspects of cancer treatment. Men, of course, can bank sperm, and there has been progress in cryopreservation (freezing) of ovarian tissues, eggs, or embryos. Doctors in Israel have recently found that Trelstar Depot (triptorelin) fools the body into thinking it has not yet reached puberty, with the result that menstrual cycles may resume after chemo or radiation and lead to successful pregnancies.[14] Another option for a woman undergoing radiation treatment of her lungs or abdomen is to have her ovaries surgically moved to a different location in the body, away from the radiation field.[15] If you are interested in any of these techniques, talk to your oncologist about what options may be available.

Approaches from Natural Medicine

In the mid-1980s, I began searching for agents that could diminish the harshness and toxicity of chemotherapy. Even though mainstream medicine has yet to embrace the idea of pairing natural compounds and pharmaceuticals, a range of studies—from test-tube experiments and animal studies to human studies—suggests that this may be effective. After years of research, I found studies suggesting that matching specific natural agents with specific drugs can reduce toxicity and therefore such side effects as nausea, fatigue, insomnia, headaches, bowel discomfort, nerve damage, heart muscle injury, and urinary tract infections. I call this *logical coupling*. By *logical*, I mean that the natural compounds and other agents paired with conventional treatments should have a specific rationale and purpose—in this case, preventing or minimizing the specific side effects of conventional chemotherapy and radiation, making them more tolerable and less risky, and thereby leading to a significantly better outcome for patients. Otherwise, integrative cancer care is just a kitchen-sink approach in which supplements and other alternative medicines are mixed together willy-nilly. The natural compounds that make chemo more tolerable are sometimes called *cytoprotectants,* since they protect normal cells from toxic damage. *Coupling* is one of the most important strategies in integrative cancer treatment, and a major focus of the cancer care at the Block Center.

In this section, I focus on natural strategies that may improve your chances of beating cancer by mitigating the toxic side effects of chemo that make many terrified of it—in some cases, so terrified that they refuse to undergo life-extending or even lifesaving treatment. I will be as specific as possible, pairing a particular agent or technique with a specific conventional treatment whose toxic effects could be ameliorated or prevented, or with a side effect it could counter. For example, L-carnitine is a natural antioxidant found in food and produced within the body; it's essential to energy metabolism. Taken as a supplement, it has been observed to reduce fatigue in chemo patients, and protect against heart toxicity caused by Adriamycin, other anthracyclines, and the biotherapy drug interleukin-2.[16] Similarly, alpha-lipoic acid given intravenously has been found to reduce the painful tingling in the hands and feet (peripheral neuropathy) caused by the potent chemotherapy drugs Eloxatin (oxaliplatin), Taxol (paclitaxel), Platin (cisplatinum), and related drugs. In the United States, alpha-lipoic acid, which is given for diabetic neuropathy, is available only in oral form. I have observed the oral form also to reduce neuropathy or prevent it altogether.[17]

▶ **Mitigating Toxicity**
A traditional Chinese herbal formula called Shi Quan Da Bu Tang (Ten Significant Tonic Decoction) is often used in cancer treatment. Chinese research reports that these herbs reverse fatigue, protect immune functions, and reduce the adverse side effects of many chemotherapy drugs.[18] This is one of a number of different supplements you could consider. The ingredients below can be taken once in the morning and once before bed. You

should be working with your integrative practitioner to refine agents and dosages for your situation.

- 1,500–2,300 mg Ten Significant Tonic Decoction (see the discussion of supplement quality on the LOC website for ⓘ comments on imported herbal formulas)

- 250–900 mg alpha-lipoic acid

- 500–1,250 mg L-carnitine

- 150–300 mg *Rhodiola rosea* (standardized extract)

There are specific logical couplers that mitigate the side effects of particular chemo drugs.[19] All are based on scientific studies, though not on the extensive human trials required for FDA approval—an extremely expensive process that is truly not suitable for most uses of herbs and supplements, which are difficult to patent and thus would be unable to recoup the expenses of the approval process for their manufacturers. For this reason, I am willing to give serious consideration to solid scientific evidence that does not emerge from a randomized control trial. This is in order to help patients who may otherwise have to delay or stop chemotherapy due to toxic side effects. There are too many logical couplers to list them all, and ideally your integrative medical partner would determine the one most likely to help you. Here are examples of couplers for chemotherapy drugs which are supported by clinical studies.

- **Platin (Cisplatinum).** Vitamin E appears to reduce the risk of nerve, kidney, and inner-ear damage resulting from cisplatin without diminishing its tumor-killing effects. In one 2006 clinical trial, of thirty patients undergoing six cycles of cisplatin, sixteen patients were randomly assigned to take 300 mg of vitamin E twice a day. Of these, 21 percent developed neurotoxicity, compared to 68 percent who did not take vitamin E.[20] If you are undergoing radiochemotherapy (simultaneous administration of radiation and chemotherapy) with cisplatin and 5-FU, glutamine supplements (as much as 30 g/day) may prevent the reduction in the immune cells called lymphocytes and reduce gastrointestinal symptoms.[21]

• **Taxol (paclitaxel).** Alpha-lipoic acid has been reported to minimize the neuropathy associated with Taxol, as mentioned above. Glutamine, acetyl-L-carnitine, and vitamin B_6 may reduce weakness and numbness due to peripheral neuropathy.[22]

• **Adriamycin (doxorubicin).** An antioxidant called coenzyme Q_{10} (200–600 mg per day), which often becomes depleted as a result of cancer and its treatments, may help protect the heart against damage from this drug; L-carnitine may also help (2–4 g per day).[23]

• **Eloxatin (oxaliplatin).** Intravenous calcium and magnesium (1 g) before oxaliplatin may reduce the risk of neurotoxicity common with this drug. Alpha-lipoic acid and glutamine, as well as vitamin B_6 and acetyl-L-carnitine, may also assist in managing oxaliplatin neuropathy.[24]

• **Bone marrow transplantation.** Glutamine may reduce the mucositis that is a common side effect of the very high doses of chemo that precede marrow transplantation. Children with various pediatric cancers given 2–4 g of oral glutamine twice a day, and women with breast cancer who took "swish and swallow" glutamine mouthwash every four hours round the clock for a total of 24 g/day, had less mucositis than controls.[25]

• **5-FU (5-fluorouracil).** This chemo drug can also cause mucositis, as well as intestinal toxicity. In this case, simply sucking on ice chips for five minutes before, during, and after drug infusion can reduce mucositis. Besides mucositis, glutamine, typically 18 g, was observed to reduce intestinal toxicity and therefore diarrhea.[26] The medication Gelclair may also help.

• **Liver damage from chemotherapy.** Taxol and Taxotere, Adriamycin, and the CMF chemotherapy regimen may cause liver damage. Silymarin, an extract from milk thistle given at a dose of 140–210 mg daily, may help prevent it.[27]

In addition to considering these couplers, be sure to check the nutritional tips for managing chemotherapy side effects in Chapter 6.

- **Urinary symptoms.** Drink cranberry juice (blended with other natural juices instead of sugar to improve taste) or take concentrated cranberry tablets to prevent urinary tract infections. The herb uva ursi (*Arctostaphylos*) (500–1,500 mg leaf per day) can also treat bladder infections, but only if the urine is alkalinized by consuming a diet very high in fruits and vegetables or taking 6–8 g sodium bicarbonate each day.

- **Respiratory difficulties.** If exertion suddenly leaves you short of breath or causes breathing difficulties, consult your internist, pulmonologist, or oncologist. If the condition is mild and chronic, and possibly due to anxiety, try the abdominal breathing techniques in Chapter 11. Yoga, Pilates, and qu gong instructors can also recommend specific techniques. For some respiratory difficulties, acupressure and acupuncture may help.

- **Fatigue.** Siberian ginseng (eleuthero), 2–4 g per day; L-carnitine (free form/USP, 1–4 grams per day); and *Rhodiola rosea* (300 mg per day) have all been used for fatigue. If your doctor determines that anemia is causing your fatigue, he or she will treat you according to the type and cause of the anemia. Also, review Chapters 14 and 19, on oxidation and stress chemistry, for ways to restore your energy level.

- **Malaise.** You can address a general ill feeling, often accompanied by fatigue, through the LOC diet and fitness plan. Fu Zheng formulas from Chinese tonic herbs can also help; you should consult your integrative practitioner or an herbalist educated on Chinese medicine for this (making sure they know you are on chemotherapy).[28] Keep in mind that emotional distress can cause fatigue.

- **Joint or muscle pain (myalgia).** Glutamine (10–20 g) may help with muscle pain due to treatment with Taxol (paclitaxel), although results of studies have been mixed. Tart cherry juice concentrate may relieve muscle pain.

- **Upper respiratory tract infections.** Chemotherapy patients may find that they are prone to colds because of a compromised immune system. Herbs that are commonly taken at the first sign of a cold include the Chinese herb kan jang (*Andrographis paniculata*); echinacea or a combination of echinacea, wild indigo, and baptisia; *Pelargonium graveolens* (a South African herb called umcka); and elderberry (*Sambucus nigra*). Follow the dosing directions on the package. Soups containing garlic and hot pepper can help relieve congestion, and gargling with salt water helps relieve a sore throat. If you have severe muscle aches and a fever, you may have a viral infection like influenza or, if you have green sputum, a bacterial infection. You can take these herbal remedies for symptom relief, but if you have persistent symptoms (particularly with a fever), or if you have lung cancer, metastases to the lungs, or an advanced cancer, call your doctor, have your white blood cells checked, and possibly get your sputum cultured. With a cough, particularly one that is chronic, see your physician about a chest X-ray.

• **The antioxidant controversy.** Using antioxidant supplements during chemo has been controversial because of concerns that they might interfere with the oxidizing free radicals generated by chemo drugs to kill cancer cells. Recent research, however, has shown that most chemo drugs use multiple mechanisms, beyond oxidizing free radicals, for their effects. In the past two years, I have published two formal studies that systematically searched and retrieved all randomized controlled clinical trials in which antioxidants were given at the same time as chemotherapy.[29] In one study, we examined whether antioxidants might impact chemotherapy effectiveness; in the other, whether antioxidants ameliorated side effects. Although the analysis indicated that larger trials would be needed to fully resolve this controversy, we found that in none of the trials did the antioxidants decrease the effectiveness of chemotherapy; in fact the antioxidant groups usually had better survival or tumor shrinkage. We also found that antioxidant use was associated with lower risks for neuropathy, low blood counts, kidney damage, and other side effects. These studies suggest that antioxidants do not appear to interfere with chemotherapy. Based on the results of these reviews and on favorable outcomes from studies we have done with patients, including our metastatic breast cancer study, our clinical approach has been to use antioxidants with chemotherapy. But further research is needed to confirm this. If you or your physician wish to take a more cautious approach, a conservative strategy would be to reduce antioxidant use when giving potentially curative treatment with well-tolerated chemotherapy. However, in patients with metastatic disease, in which the ability to tolerate a full course of treatment improves effectiveness and outcome, combining antioxidants with chemotherapy would be reasonable in order to reduce toxicity, improve tolerance, and possibly extend survival.

▶ **Combinations to Avoid**

That is not to say that there is nothing to worry about when you pair natural compounds with drugs. Some natural compounds affect the enzyme systems that break down or activate chemotherapy drugs; this could cause patients to be exposed to either too little drug (which might compromise anti-cancer effectiveness) or too much (which could lead to more severe side effects).[30] These are the more common natural products that can interfere with cancer treatments and should therefore be avoided during treatment:

• St. John's Wort, widely used as an antidepressant, increases the activity of an enzyme (CYP_{450} 3A4) that plays a key role in breaking down or activating roughly half of all prescription drugs, including some chemo drugs. It can therefore alter the efficacy or toxicity of these drugs, in particular Camptosar (irinotecan), Tykerb (lapatinib), etoposide (called Vepesid, Etopophos, Eposin, or VP-16), and Gleevec (imatinib mesylate). My advice: if you are undergoing chemotherapy, avoid St. John's wort.[31]

• Grapefruit and grapefruit juice contain powerful compounds that influence enzymes involved in the metabolism of drugs taken by mouth, resulting either in increased or reduced absorption of the drugs. For instance, grapefruit may cause side effects by increasing blood levels of cyclosporine, the immune-suppressing drug used to prevent rejection in patients receiving transplants, including bone marrow transplants. Other fruit juices may affect drugs also. If you can't get a specific consultation on these interactions, you should avoid grapefruit juice with drugs taken by mouth for the duration of your treatment.[32]

• Vitamin E, ginger, garlic, ginkgo, ginseng, vitamin C, and fish oils have blood-thinning effects. This is a problem only if your platelet counts drop to a low level (less than 60,000 cells per microliter) due to chemotherapy or you are also taking pharmaceutical blood thinners such as Coumadin (warfarin), heparin, or aspirin. The combination may cause too much blood thinning, leading to bleeding disorders. If your doctor has prescribed a blood thinner, discuss your diet and supplements with him or her to be sure you do not overdo it.[33] Be especially sure not to take these within one week of surgery, or you may suffer excess bleeding. If you do have to undergo urgent surgery, simply tell your doctor what herbs you have been taking, and he or she will adjust your surgical medications.[34] On the flip side, the vitamin K in leafy green vegetables and green drinks can block the blood-thinning action of Coumadin (warfarin), and American ginseng can reduce its blood-thinning effects.[35]

• Copper can promote new vascular supply to a malignant lesion, called angiogenesis.[36] If you are taking an angiogenesis inhibitor such as Avastin, you do not want to counteract its beneficial effects by ingesting too much copper. You can generally get any needed copper by consuming a healthy diet, so avoid supplements that contain copper. A list of foods high in copper can be found on the LOC website.

• Folic acid can reduce the effectiveness of the cancer drug methotrexate. If you are receiving this drug, be sure that you are not taking any supplement or multiple containing more than 150–200 mcg folic acid unless it is recommended by your oncologist.[37]

• Artemisinin, an herbal medicine, may cause toxicity when combined with oxidative chemotherapies or radiation.[38] Until we have more research, I advise not taking this herbal while you are undergoing conventional treatment.

• Herbs or supplements that help you sleep or remain calm may magnify the effects of anesthesia. Stop taking valerian, kava (which you should not be using in any case due to the risk of liver failure), passionflower, hops, skullcap, inositol, GABA, 5-HTP, and melatonin five to seven days before surgery.[39] If you face emergency surgery, though, it is not a serious problem; simply tell your doctors so they can make appropriate adjustments.

My purpose is not to cause you undue alarm about nutrient-drug or herb-drug interactions, because they are relatively rare, as we found in 2007 when we surveyed what medications and supplements patients of ours were taking at the time they first arrived at our clinic, and as other researchers have observed.[40] But because new interactions might be discovered—especially as new chemotherapy drugs are introduced—it is important to discuss with your oncologist any supplements you are taking or thinking of taking.[41] If your oncologist is not familiar with nutrient-drug interactions, find an expert in integrative care, a pharmacist, a naturopath, or a nutritionist who is. Two books, *The PDR for Herbal Medicines* and *The PDR of Nutritional Supplements*, provide detailed information on interactions between natural medicines and conventional medicines, as do the subscription databases Natural Standard and Natural Medicines Comprehensive Data-base. The Block Center offers professional consultations to assess and screen patients for drug-supplement interactions. We also search for and recommend combinations with favorable synergisms. In order to fully individualize our support for patients on chemotherapy, we take into account a patient's tumor characteristics, individual biochemistry, laboratory results, chemotherapy protocols, dietary history, and other factors. I hope the above gives you some ideas, and urge you to consult an integrative pharmacist or integrative medical expert.

CHAPTER 24

THE CHEMOTHERAPY SUPPORT PROGRAM: ENHANCING EFFECTIVENESS

In the preceding chapter I discussed ways to make chemotherapy more tolerable. Now I want to give you ways to make it more lethal—to your malignant cells. You may find some, but not all, available at your local cancer center. Discuss them with your medical partner or integrative practitioner.

Diane: Cancer as a Chronic Illness

It was February 2004 when Diane Klenke, forty-six, visited her doctor because of persistent stomach distress. A series of tests showed that she had stage IV pancreatic cancer that had metastasized to her liver. Her doctor told her to "go home and get your affairs in order—you might have three months to live."

Numb and in shock, Diane delivered the devastating news to her husband. "He cried for days," Diane later told me, "but I dried my eyes and got busy." Her first call was to a relative who happened to be the head of radiology at one of this country's leading hospitals. Within a week, Diane found herself in a consultation room, surrounded by cancer specialists evaluating the battery of tests she had just taken. They not only confirmed Diane's earlier diagnosis but offered no real treatment options, telling her the cancer was inoperable and they were not hopeful with chemotherapy. Refusing to give up, Diane came to the Block Center, where, she later told us, she knew right away that she had found the doctors and the philosophy of care she was looking for. I explained to Diane my life-affirming philosophy: that you can approach your cancer like any other chronic illness. We don't necessarily have to cure it for you to live with it. As I have stated previously, *most patients die not from their cancer but from the consequences of the cancer.* Most of these consequences—pneumonia, cachexia, an embolism—can be slowed or prevented altogether with the steps I describe in the fitness, diet, and mind-spirit chapters.[1]

We started by ordering a series of tests to identify the "molecular fingerprint" of Diane's cancer and assess her biochemical terrain. She began a regimen of supplements tailored to her individual biological and medical needs. We modified her diet, started her on an aerobic fitness plan to rebuild her muscle strength and endurance, and tailored mind-spirit work for her. Soon afterward we began her chemotherapy treatments. After six months, scans showed a 20 percent reduction of the tumors in Diane's pancreas and liver. We then began giving Diane chronotherapy, timing the administration of her chemotherapy by using a pump programmed to her specific regimen, which let her maintain her full-time job and active family life. Within two months, Diane's liver scans showed no evidence of disease, and after a year on chronotherapy the pancreatic tumor had shrunk by over 60 percent. At this point we stopped the chemo. The mass in her pancreas continued to shrink and her liver is disease-free. Years after she was told she had perhaps three months to live, Diane is enjoying every day of her life. She danced at her daughter's wedding and recently welcomed her second grandchild into the world. She is living proof that you can live with cancer as a chronic illness, being monitored regularly and adhering to the Life Over Cancer program.

Innovative Tactics for Enhancing Chemotherapy

▶ **Chronotherapy**

As I discussed in the preceding chapter, timing chemotherapy to reduce its effects on healthy tissue can reduce its side effects. It can also be more lethal to cancer cells, hitting them during the time of day when they are most vulnerable and therefore improving your outcome. As I mentioned, few cancer centers in the United States offer chronotherapy, but as new ones begin to do so I will list them on the LOC website.

▶ **Continuous Infusion, Metronomic Chemo, and Related Therapies**

Traditionally, chemotherapy drugs are given in a single large "bolus" dose, often as high as a patient can tolerate. But just as delivering chemotherapy in small frequent doses, or even continuously using a portable pump, can reduce toxic side effects, so can it improve the effectiveness of chemo. The reason is that continuous dosing takes advantage of one of the peculiarities of chemo's cytotoxic mechanism, namely, killing cells that are dividing rather than the cells that are resting. Cancers cells divide much more rapidly than other cells, which is why they are more susceptible to the cytotoxic effects of chemo. But cancer cells do not all divide at the same precise time—say, 2:00 P.M. on the Tuesday afternoon when you are scheduled for your chemo infusion. Giving a drug continuously throughout a day, or over a few days, logically will catch more cancer cells in the act of dividing. Studies show that continuous infusion of some chemo drugs, such as 5-FU in colon cancer, improves outcome.[2] Ask your doctor if your chemo drug has been shown to be more effective or less toxic if given continuously.

In metronomic chemotherapy, the chemo drugs are given every week, or in some regimens every day, in low doses, rather than the typical every three to four weeks in high doses. It appears that blood vessels that feed tumors grow back between standard chemotherapy sessions. But metronomic dosing can kill the fast-growing endothelial cells that make up blood vessels while giving them less time to grow back. Clinicians are still exploring the potentials of metronomic therapy, but we already know that it can work in metastatic breast cancer. Again, ask if this dosing might be right for your cancer.[3]

Pharmaceutical companies, recognizing the benefit of fractionated dosing, have begun revamping older chemotherapies so they can be encapsulated in microscopic liposomal membranes. These are fat-based membranes that allow the drug to be infused all at once but to leach out of the membrane over the course of several days. It's sort of like time-release capsules for a stuffy nose. Because the drug seeps out of the membrane and remains active over the course of several days, it is much more likely to catch malignant cells in the act of dividing than a single big dose. Doxorubicin is available in a liposomal form (Doxil), and liposomal vincristine and cisplatin are in clinical trials. This is a fast-moving field, but your doctor should be able to tell you what's available, and which form offers the possibility of greater effectiveness, for your cancer.[4]

▶ **Combining Chemotherapy and Anti-Angiogenesis**
This has been the biggest recent breakthrough in conventional oncology. Anti-angiogenesis drugs prevent tumors from growing the blood vessels they need to survive. As I write, Avastin (bevacizumab), Sutent (sunitinib), and Nexavar (sorafenib) are anti-angiogenesis drugs that have received FDA approval. None is perfect. Just as tumors can switch to a second growth pathway if their primary pathway is blocked by a chemotherapy drug, so tumors can switch to a backup pathway for growing blood vessels when the first pathway is blocked by an anti-angiogenesis drug. As a result, Avastin (which is approved for use in cancers of the colon, breast, or lung after a regimen of standard chemotherapy) extended survival for only about two months in a recent breast cancer trial.[5] But angiogenesis remains one of the hottest areas of research in oncology, with better drugs coming down the pike. I urge you to ask your physician whether adding an angiogenic inhibitor is right for you. One caveat: Avastin's side effects include life-threatening hemorrhage, especially in patients with brain and ovarian cancer, something you should discuss with your doctor. As I will

discuss in Chapter 27, there are also natural compounds that act as angiogenic inhibitors. It is unlikely that they have anywhere near the potency of drugs, but they may play a valuable role with considerably less risk.

▶ **Chemotherapy Sensitivity Testing**
In Chapter 22, I advised asking your surgeon to save a sample of tumor so you can have it analyzed to determine which drugs it is sensitive to. This reflects one of the greatest frustrations of chemotherapy: it works brilliantly for a few patients, pretty well for some, and poorly or not at all for others. This holds true even for people with the same stage of the same cancer. Every cancer is unique; breast cancer is not a single disease, nor is colon cancer or pancreatic cancer or any other kind of cancer. The trick is to determine, through chemotherapy sensitivity assays, and through testing genetic and molecular characteristics, what is the best match to particular chemo and targeted molecular drugs. Among the labs that conduct this testing is the one we have used at the Block Center for over twenty years, Rational Therapeutics of Long Beach, California. (For other labs, see www.lifeovercancer.com.)

(i)

Patricia: **The Power of Chemosensitivity Testing**

In 2001, surgeons removed an eleven-centimeter tumor from one of Patricia's ovaries. Over the next four years she suffered two recurrences, for which she underwent chemotherapy with seven different drugs, including Doxil and Gemzar. But by 2005, her cancer had developed resistance to all of these, and when she arrived at the Block Center that summer she had multiple metastases and a CA-125 tumor marker of over 2,700. (CA-125 is for ovarian cancer what the PSA test is for prostate cancer: a marker giving clues to the size and extent of the tumor.) Clearly she needed a new strategy.

The first thing we did was arrange for her to have a tumor biopsy at a local hospital. We sent the tissue sample to Dr. Robert Nagourney at Rational Therapeutics. His results: on the basis of her tumor's chemotherapeutic susceptibility, it would respond to a combination of Doxil and Gemzar—even though her cancer had proved resistant to each of these when they were given individually. We verified that the drug combination was safe (it was being given in a clinical trial) and started her on it. In the meantime, her CA-125 had risen to a dizzying 3,255.

Within two months, it had dropped to 540, and her disease had stabilized. Without the tumor analysis, we would not necessarily have chosen this drug combination. We were astounded and elated at the accuracy of the chemosensitivity testing, as was the patient.

Although older sensitivity tests had poor predictive value, research on newer methods shows improved odds. Instead of determining which drugs inhibit cancer cell proliferation, some of the newer tests determine which drugs promote apoptosis, or programmed cell death. Though it was once thought that the way to kill cancer was to stop proliferation, we now understand that encouraging and speeding up a malignant cell's death cycle is frequently more effective. Early results show that chemosensitivity testing does improve the odds of predicting which chemotherapy agents will do the best job of killing cancer cells. In one study of a hundred patients, most of whom had already received several different chemos, choosing a chemo drug by sensitivity testing led to substantial tumor shrinkage or disappearance in 57 percent of patients. In another study, chemotherapy response was compared in ovarian cancer patients who received chemo drugs to which they were sensitive and others who received the same chemo drugs, but whose sensitivity testing showed they were resistant to the drugs. Of those whose assays showed they were sensitive to the drug, 90 percent responded to chemo, while only 29 percent of the patients whose assays showed resistance had responses.[6] Especially with several new methods in development, chemosensitivity testing may give you an edge over choosing protocols through other methods, especially if your cancer cells become resistant to or do not respond well to the first-line chemotherapy, if you experience a recurrence, or if you are undergoing second- or later-line treatment. Be sure to discuss this possibility with your oncologist.

Logical Couplers May Improve the Effectiveness of Cell-Killing Therapy

The effectiveness of chemotherapy and radiation is reduced in two basic ways: first, when a certain portion of the cancer cells have an inherent resistance to the cell-killing effects of the drugs or radiation, and second, when cancer cells acquire that resistance. Many common solid tumors show a good initial response to a cytotoxic agent, with the result that the tumor shrinks, only to recur in a resistant form. What has happened is that tumor cells that were vulnerable to the chemotherapy or radiation were killed by the treatment, but a tiny number of resistant cells survived; with the vulnerable cells eliminated, resistant cells have a clear field to proliferate, making billions of clones of themselves—all of which are also resistant. This is often how cancer recurs, and why cancer recurrence is more difficult to treat. Acquired drug resistance remains one of the biggest barriers to a true cancer cure.

What I call *treatment couplers* are agents that are intended to strengthen the effectiveness of conventional treatments, often by making malignant cells more sensitive to the effects of treatments. *Resistance fighters* reduce resistance to it. Both may lead to a significantly better outcome for patients and, I believe, help explain why so many of our patients respond well to chemotherapy protocols that had previously failed to help them. Here is a sample of natural treatment couplers my colleagues and I at Block Center find most effective.

• **Astragalus.** A Chinese herb with antioxidant and immune-boosting properties, astragalus is often added to chemotherapy drugs such as cisplatin or carboplatin. A 2006 analysis of thirty-four clinical trials of herbal formulas containing astragalus found a 34 percent improvement in the response to chemotherapy and a 33 percent reduction in the risk of death among patients receiving astragalus.[7]

• **Vitamin C.** Most studies of vitamin C and cancer focused on the use of vitamin C as an alternative to chemotherapy, rather than as a logical coupler. I would not suggest using vitamin C as a substitute for proven chemotherapy, but pairing vitamin C with conventional treatment offers real promise. In a clinical trial of thirty patients with advanced breast cancer, those who received vitamin C during chemotherapy had twice the response of patients who did not, with more tumor shrinkage.[8]

• **Docosahexaenoic acid.** DHA, found in fish oil, may help overcome cancer cells' resistance to chemo. In one study, breast cancer patients who had higher levels of DHA in their breast tissue had a better rate of response to chemotherapy than those with lower levels. A 2008 review, and previous research, has shown that DHA can overcome drug resistance through several possible mechanisms, including possibly by allowing drugs to enter cancer cells more easily. Researchers are now studying a new drug in which DHA is attached to the paclitaxel molecule; a preliminary trial of the drug was reported in 2008.[9]

• **L-theanine.** An animal study found that giving theanine (a component of black and green tea) to mice slowed the growth of implanted ovarian tumors that were treated with Adriamycin (doxorubicin), apparently because theanine inhibited the breakdown of doxorubicin in the tumor cells. It did not, however, increase the concentration of chemo drugs in normal cells. Theanine also appears to have a calming and possibly blood-pressure-lowering effect.[10]

• **Black currant oil.** Several lab studies have shown that combining gamma-linolenic acid, a constituent of black currant oil, may improve the effects of chemotherapy. It increased the cancer-killing activity of Taxotere (docetaxel), possibly in part because it suppresses the HER2/neu protein (the target of Herceptin).[11]

• **Silymarin.** Extracted from milk thistle, silymarin contains at least two compounds that may counteract drug resistance. Lab tests show that silybinin can reduce chemoresistance to doxorubicin and cisplatin, two commonly used drugs for gynecological tumors. Silybin, another component of silymarin, enhanced the anti-proliferative effect of cisplatin in cisplatin-resistant ovarian cancer cells and of doxorubicin in doxorubicin-resistant breast cancer cells. A 2008 study observed silibinin's ability to restore sensitivity to Taxol (paclitaxel) in ovarian cancer cells.[12]

• **Quercetin.** Quercetin appears to make Adriamycin (doxorubicin) more lethal to multidrug-resistant breast cancer cells. It may also make cancer cells more sensitive to the anti-cancer drugs Hycamtin (topotecan) and Gemzar (gemcitabine).[13]

• **Melatonin.** The best-studied natural treatment booster, the sleep-inducing hormone melatonin, produced in the pineal gland, is also a potent antioxidant, which accounts in part for its anti-cancer properties. In a series of studies by scientists in Italy of advanced cancer patients, pairing melatonin with standard chemotherapy or radiation dramatically improved survival. For instance, patients with metastatic stage IV lung cancer who received standard chemotherapy plus melatonin (20 mg given orally at bedtime) had significantly higher rates of tumor regression and overall survival than patients who received standard chemo alone. None of the latter patients was alive two years into the study, but close to 40 percent of the melatonin group were. Melatonin-treated patients also had fewer side effects. Melatonin given with chemotherapy also improved the response of patients with advanced solid tumors such as metastatic breast cancer, gastrointestinal cancers, and head and neck cancers. Pairing melatonin with interleukin-2 brought higher rates of tumor response in non-Hodgkin's lymphoma, Hodgkin's disease, multiple myeloma, and leukemias, the Italian scientists reported in 2000. More recently, they have shown that melatonin improves outcomes when combined with conventional treatments for blood, breast, and colorectal cancers: for instance, 86 percent of patients with metastatic colorectal cancer who received melatonin in addition to the chemotherapy agent Camptosar (irinotecan) had significant tumor shrinkage or no further tumor growth compared with 44 percent of patients who received Camptosar alone. Moreover, melatonin has enabled the Italian scientists to use lower doses of highly toxic drugs such as interleukin-2 and Camptosar with no loss of effectiveness. Despite these remarkable results, in the United States melatonin is rarely used or even studied as a cancer treatment.[14]

Based on findings such as those described above, I recommend to my patients that they take a broad-spectrum formula of agents that have been found to strengthen the cancer-killing effectiveness of conventional therapy. It should include a combination of some or all of the following ingredients:

- 3 grams 80% omega-3, fish oil

- 1,000–2,000 mg black currant oil, source of important compounds such as gamma-linoleic acid

- 1,000–3,000 mg astragalus (spray-dried or freeze-dried extract)

- 1,000–1,500 mg quercetin (water-soluble form)

- 250–500 mg silymarin (standardized milk thistle extract)

- 100–250 mg L-theanine

- 3–20 mg melatonin (prolonged/time-release, taken at bedtime)

Be sure to work with your integrative practitioner to select agents and dosages that will be most appropriate for your situation.

CHAPTER 25

THE RADIATION
SUPPORT PROGRAM

Several years ago, I had two patients with oral tumors. Bill and Don each had surgery to remove the tumor, followed by extensive radiation therapy to the tumor site as well as to lymph nodes in the neck. Due to the dense network of nerves and vasculature in the mouth and neck, radiation there can cause devastating damage to the salivary glands, leaving patients with loss of taste and difficulty swallowing. Bill and Don hoped for the best.

But there was a crucial difference between the two. Don became a patient at our center only after he completed his radiation; Bill consulted us before and during his treatments at a nearby hospital. Don had no nutritional or other complementary treatments during his radiation. Bill adopted a nutrition program that emphasized whole-plant supplements to help offset the oxidative damage that radiation causes normal tissues. He also took the antioxidant drug Ethyol (amifostine), which reduces radiation damage to normal tissue and is known as a tissue-sparing agent.

When Bill asked his radiation oncologist about Ethyol, the doctor rejected it out of hand, saying he would be advising it if it worked. I gave Bill a stack of scientific literature, most of which demonstrated the potential value of Ethyol in cases like his, but the doctor tossed the papers onto his exam table and barked, "I already told you that I'd be using this if it had any clinical value." As I explained to Bill, my concern was not its efficacy, but a possibility for interference with treatment. Bill understood, but felt that for him the benefits outweighed the risks. So along with aggressive nutrition, Bill elected to receive Ethyol, using a programmable pump. Bill survived his radiation regimen with no severe burns and no major damage to his salivary glands or his ability to swallow. As I write, Bill has been cancer-free for more than ten years.

Don had a different experience. When he arrived at the Block Center after finishing his radiation, he had lost all salivary function and was unable to swallow. The radiation had burned his salivary glands beyond repair. Try as we did with nutrition, supplements, physical therapy, Asian fitness techniques, and mind-body approaches, we could not restore his ability to swallow, and other complications eventually took Don's life. I am convinced that Don would have suffered far less, and maybe would have lived longer, if his doctors had taken more aggressive steps to mitigate the toxic effects of his cancer treatment.

Innovative Tactics for Enhancing Radiation Therapy

▶ **Amifostine**
As Bill's story shows, this compound is among the more potent pharmaceutical cytoprotectors. Originally developed as part of a classified project sponsored by the U.S. Army to protect soldiers who might be exposed to radiation, it scavenges free radicals produced by either chemotherapy or radiotherapy. Clinical trials show that it significantly reduces a wide range of radiation side effects, especially damage to mucosal tissues (leading to mucositis, stomatitis, and dry mouth), which is common in treatment of head and neck and rectal cancers.

For several years there has been a controversy over whether the antioxidant effects of amifostine can protect tumor tissue as well as normal tissue from radiation. A 2006 analysis of fourteen individual trials involving 1,451 patients, as well as a 2007 study of six trials, concluded that amifostine protected against many radiation side effects, although there is a 2 percent chance that patients might fail treatment due to tumor protection. You and your doctor should discuss this risk if you want to use amifostine.[1] A new formulation nearly eliminates Ethyol's side effects.

▶ **Hyperbaric Oxygen Therapy**

Hyperbaric oxygen therapy (HBOT) is an accepted treatment for various forms of radiation damage and scarring. Tissue damage is sometimes the result of oxygen failing to reach certain tissues following radiation. In HBOT, you enter a chamber and breathe 100 percent oxygen under pressure. This allows oxygen to reach the damaged tissue. This can be especially important after radiotherapy to the brain, which can cause cognitive, memory, speech, and physical impairments. If you have suffered tissue damage after radiation treatment, ask your physician if treatment in a hyperbaric chamber might help you.[2] Be sure to consult with an expert in the field if you have previously had chemotherapy, since if you have had certain chemo drugs, including Adriamycin, HBOT cannot be given.

▶ **High-Tech Radiotherapy**

Vastly more precise than their predecessors, high-tech forms of radiation can eliminate tumors in spots such as the brain, lungs, and liver where traditional radiation produces serious collateral damage to normal tissues or is impossible to use altogether. For instance, whole-brain radiation can leave patients with cognitive and physical deficits; radiation to the lungs zaps so much normal tissue (as breathing and its attendant up-and-down motion of the chest causes healthy tissue to move into the X-rays' path) that it leads to sometimes irreversible lung damage. Now we can do better.

Stereotactic Radiosurgery. Stereotactic radiosurgery is a precise form of radiation that has been used mostly for brain and spinal cord tumors. There are different types, including the "gamma knife" for brain tumors. After careful pretreatment mapping of the brain and tumor (usually with magnetic resonance imaging, or MRI) to locate the tumor, the gamma knife targets tumors with beams of ionizing (gamma) radiation that meet precisely at the target, with little or no damage to surrounding tissues. What is so fabulous about the gamma knife is that it allows the surgeons to treat extremely small targets with a precision of one-tenth of a millimeter, minimizing the risk of damage to healthy tissue. In addition, your surgeon can block one or more of the converging radiation beams in order to prevent irradiating sensitive areas, such as the optic nerve. The proton beam and CyberKnife technologies are equally precise, in some cases vanquishing tumors that previously could never have been radiated or excised surgically.[3]

Radiofrequency Ablation. Radiofrequency ablation literally cooks tumors. A probe inserted into the cancerous organ delivers high levels of heat directed to the core of the tumor and destroys it. Originally used against liver cancer, and now with lung, bone, and other tumors as well, the technique can destroy tumors as large as nine centimeters and eliminate several tumors at different sites. We began utilizing this technique when it first came into use in the 1990s. At the time the average treatment took over an hour. Today our patients are able to receive treatment in four minutes, and leave the same day free of visible disease. This debulking technology may not cure cancer, but it buys the patient precious time not only to enjoy life but also to try new drugs, begin a recurrence prevention program or wait for the next breakthrough. Shrinking a tumor lets you move forward to strategies to help contain and eliminate microscopic disease. Be aware that not all physicians believe that radiofrequency ablation is a meaningful strategy, and not all situations are appropriate for this technique.[4]

Gated Radiation. Irradiating lung cancer can damage healthy tissue because breathing moves the tumor out of, and healthy tissue into, the path of the X-rays. Gated radiation adjusts for this problem and delivers radiation only when the tumor is in the X-ray field. It has been found useful in lung and other thoracic tumors, including in Hodgkin's disease. It is available at major hospitals including Stanford University, Fox Chase Cancer Center in Philadelphia, University of Pittsburgh Medical Center, Norris Cotton Cancer Center, and New York Presbyterian. The LOC website has an updated list of centers offering this therapy.[5]

Intensity-Modulated Radiation Therapy. In intensity-modulated radiation therapy (IMRT), computer-generated images tailor radiation doses to the size and shape of a tumor. The radiation beam is broken up into thousands of thin beams that enter the body at different angles, intersecting at the tumor with much less damage to surrounding normal tissues. Given its precision, IMRT allows delivery of higher radiation dosages with less damage and fewer side effects. In early trials, it has improved outcomes in prostate cancer and head and neck cancers. It is available at most major cancer centers.[6]

Neutron Therapy. Standard radiation uses X-rays, which are high-energy subatomic particles called photons. Some tumors, however, are radioresistant, meaning they respond poorly to photon therapy. In these cases neutron therapy is a viable alternative. It bombards the tumor with the subatomic particles called neutrons, which interact with the DNA in the nucleus of the cell. Clinical trials have shown neutrons to be more effective than photons for advanced prostate cancer and inoperable salivary gland tumors: after ten years, 70 percent of advanced prostate cancer patients treated with combined photon and neutron therapy were free of cancer, compared with 58 percent of those treated with photons only, while 56 percent of patients with inoperable salivary gland tumors were free of disease compared with 17 percent of those treated with photons. Advanced head and neck and prostate cancers are good candidates for neutron therapy, as are some inoperable cancers and recurrent cancers. You can find information on the cancers currently treated at www.neutrontherapy.niu.edu. As of this writing, neutron therapy is available at Northern Illinois University's program at the

Fermi National Accelerator Laboratory in Batavia, Illinois; the University of Washington in Seattle; and Harper Hospital in Detroit.[7]

Proton Therapy. Proton therapy uses the subatomic particles called protons and has been shown to be effective for small tumors located close to critical tissue such as brain tissue. In tumors in the base of the skull, 82 percent of patients treated with proton therapy were disease-free after five years, compared with 40 percent of patients treated with X-rays. If you have one of these rare cancers, ask your oncologist if you might benefit from proton therapy. It is available at the Indiana University Cyclotron Facility in Bloomington; Massachusetts General Hospital in Boston; and Loma Linda University Medical Center in Loma Linda, California.[8] New locations for both neutron and proton therapy will be added to www.lifeovercancer.com as they become available.

► **Hyperthermia**
The application of heat, medically called hyperthermia, can produce results similar to radiation. It is based on the finding that cancer cells are far more sensitive to destruction by heat than normal cells are, and that heat can increase cancer cells' vulnerability to chemotherapy (especially platinum drugs), and stimulates the body's anti-cancer defenses, especially cytokines. Hyperthermia can be delivered with devices that enable technicians to apply heat to accessible tumors (such as melanomas and head and neck cancers), in so-called loco-regional hyperthermia. It can also be applied to the entire body in what is called whole-body hyperthermia. In this approach, patients with organ tumors or metastatic disease enter a chamber that increases their body temperature to fever range (103–105°F) or higher (107–108°F). Hyperthermia, which usually takes six to seven weeks, does not cause the side effects that radiation can, including burns, tissue damage, and immune suppression. Whole-body hyperthermia is both approved and widely available in Europe; there are also a number of hyperthermia facilities, many offering only local hyperthermia, in the United

States. Ask your physician if you might be a good candidate for hyperthermia. You can find physicians who offer hyperthermia through the website of the International Clinical Hyperthermia Society, www.hyperthermia-ichs.org.[9]

Radiation Couplers

Radiation therapy delivers a powerful dose of X-rays to kill cancer cells. It is used most in the care of patients with early breast and prostate cancer. Most patients tolerate these treatments fairly well and may not need couplers to reduce side effects (especially if they are following a good diet and exercise program). But because the intensity of this radiation is many times stronger than that of diagnostic X-rays, it can harm normal cells, too, especially in patients with advanced cancers who are receiving palliative radiotherapy to shrink recurrent tumors. In this case, immune cells (lymphocytes) in particular may become impaired, making the body more vulnerable to other diseases. Other common side effects of radiation include fatigue, eating problems, emotional distress, nausea, vomiting, bloating, discomfort in the neck or throat, and skin changes such as itching, blistering, toughening, and darkening.

The good news is that you can ameliorate many, if not all, of these side effects through a combination of healthy diet, optimal supplementation, relaxation techniques, and other healthful lifestyle changes. Natural compounds may also increase the selective, cell-killing ability of radiotherapy, so that tumor cells die while normal cells survive. Those that thin the blood or stimulate circulation, for instance, may boost the efficacy of radiation by increasing blood flow through tumors: in order for radiation to kill cancer cells, there must be oxygen available nearby, and blood carries oxygen. I will discuss management of some common symptoms here. Also, you can refer back to the symptom management tips in Chapter 6, as well as the exercise recommendations in Chapter 9, for suggestions on how to manage symptoms.

Many radiation couplers act as antioxidants. A theoretical concern, not yet shown in research, is that this could be problematic in radiation therapy, which, even more than chemotherapy, uses free radicals to kill cancer cells, since antioxidants mop up free radicals. Indeed, a 2005 study found that while head and neck cancer patients given the antioxidants vitamin E and beta-carotene had fewer side effects from the radiation, they also had lower survival rates than patients receiving only dummy pills. This finding received major media attention; what received less attention was a 2008 follow-up analysis that showed that the excess mortality in this study occurred almost entirely among patients who smoked during radiation therapy, and not even among those who smoked before or after but stopped during therapy. This is not surprising, since earlier research had indicated a link between beta-carotene, smoking, and cancer.[10] This certainly implies that smokers should quit during their radiation therapy, but it also casts doubt on the concerns of oncologists that antioxidants will make radiation therapy less effective. I have not yet seen a review of this question that has adequately addressed the subject, although I feel the data currently lean in favor of antioxidants. A conservative position would be to omit antioxidant use during radiation when a real possibility of cure exists, but to consider it with palliative regimens, or when patients are not tolerating their treatments well.

Not all supplements and medications to relieve radiation side effects are antioxidants, however. And some supplements with antioxidant activity (such as EGCG, a green tea constituent) also have substantial anti-cancer activity independent of their antioxidant effects, which I feel makes them more acceptable, especially for patients who are having difficulty tolerating therapy. The following show promise for reducing the side effects of radiation.

• **Glutamine.** In a 2006 clinical trial, glutamine reduced the rate of mucositis in patients with head and neck cancers who were receiving chemoradiotherapy by 80 percent. It reduced their pain ratings by a factor of six. The glutamine was given intravenously, a form not sold in the U.S., but other studies show that glutamine taken orally is effective against other conditions, so it is worth considering for reducing the side effects of radiation.[11]

A radiation support formula should contain some of the following ingredients:

- 1,000–3,000 mg Three Sengs Decoction, spray-dried or freeze-dried extract (a Chinese medicine formula that includes Asian ginseng and other herbs).[12] (See the discussion of supplement quality at the LOC website for comments on imported herb formulas.)

- 500–1,500 mg EGCG (a concentrated green tea extract, should be at least 70 percent EGCG) to protect salivary glands, skin cells, and immune cells during radiation treatment. It also makes cancer cells more sensitive to the effects of radiation therapy in lab studies.[13]

- 300–600 mg soy isoflavones (40 percent genistein) may increase the sensitivity of tumor cells (but not normal cells) to radiation, especially lung, prostate, liver, and esophageal cancer cells.[14]

- 2,000–4,000 mg vitamin C (ascorbic acid) appears to improve the sensitivity of cancer cells to radiation.[15]

- 3–6 g fish oil (80 percent omega-3) increases the selective killing of cancer cells during radiation treatment. Omega-3s reduce the hypoxia, or localized oxygen deficiency, that makes cancer cells resistant to radiation.[16]

- 200–400 mg Siberian ginseng (also called eleuthero or eleutherococcus) standardized extract between meals protected general resistance and immune cells in breast cancer patients who received radiation.[17]

- 80–120 mg gingko biloba may protect immune cells, and possibly brain tissues, during radiation treatment.[18]

Be sure to work with your integrative practitioner to select agents and dosages that are most appropriate to your situation.

The effects of radiation depend on where it is targeted. Radiation to the abdomen and pelvis can cause radiation enteritis, which is characterized by inflammation of the intestines with severe diarrhea. If you develop this, avoid milk products and reduce your consumption of whole grains, nuts, seeds, most fruits (though it's okay if you cook and strain them to reduce fiber), greasy foods, raw vegetables, crunchy snacks, spicy foods, caffeine (coffee, tea, cola, chocolate, guarana herb preparations), alcohol, and tobacco. Among the products that may help with radiation enteritis are aged garlic extract (1,000–1,500 mg), selenium (200 mcg), pycnogenol (grape seed extract) (100–300 mg), vitamin A (5,000 IU), L-glutamine (10–30 g; may also help with oral mucositis from radiation), curcumin (1,500 mg), fish oil (3 g), and probiotics (5–10 billion live organisms of a high-quality probiotic product; some of the other products listed also have probiotic or prebiotic effects).[19]

Radiation to the chest or breast can inflame the esophagus, causing difficulty swallowing. The problem will go away after the treatment ends, though your treatment may be interrupted to allow the esophagus to heal. Eating soft foods will help, as will antacids, anesthetics, and following the Treatment Support diet found in Chapter 6, substituting shakes for some meals.

Radiation to the breast can result in a painful skin reaction: an ointment containing the herb calendula reduced this reaction, but aloe-containing ointments were not beneficial.[20]

Radiation to the head, neck, and mouth can cause fungal infections in the mouth in addition to the usual irritation of the mucous membranes. In this case, you may find relief with glutamine (5–10 g twice a day), green tea catechins (EGCG; 1,000 mg) and probiotics (5–10 billion live organisms).[21] If fungal infections persist, ask your doctor about nystatin or fluconazole.

CHAPTER 26

WHAT TO DO WHEN TREATMENT ENDS: GROWTH CONTROL AND CONTAINMENT IN THE FIRST YEAR THAT YOU'RE CANCER-FREE

Now that chemotherapy, surgery, or radiation is over, you're basically on your own."

Although this statement has many variations—"We'll see you in six months" or "You can get back to normal now"—the message is the same. If you are like many of the patients we see at the Block Center, hearing these words made you feel as if your fate was sealed by the completion (successful or unsuccessful) of conventional treatment. With no follow-up plan, you feel that all you can do is hope, pray, cross your fingers, or wait for the other shoe to drop. Is it any wonder that the end of treatment brings anxiety and a sense of loss?

There is a better way. Regardless of when we first see a patient at the center, we make a containment program a centerpiece of cancer treatment, for one simple reason: it can improve your odds of staying healthy and alive. This chapter outlines the basics of containing disease, whether visible (scans continue to show the presence of tumors) or invisible (your scans are clean, but there may be undetected micro-metastases in your body).

After the attack phase, you will be in one of three situations. If you still have visible disease but are unable to tolerate further therapy, the *rehabilitation* regimen described in Chapter 27 is appropriate for you; it will restore your strength so you can tolerate further treatment. If you are in otherwise good health but still have visible disease and have run out of further mainstream options, I recommend the *no stone unturned* approach in Chapter 28. If you are fortunate enough to have no visible disease remaining after the attack phase, you can follow the program in this chapter, *microscopic growth control*, for the first year after completing your conventional treatment. This chapter is aimed at bridging you into the long-term remission program in Chapter 29. Regardless of your situation, you should adhere to the Life Over Cancer diet, nutritional support supplements, exercise regimen, mind-spirit therapies, and terrain-modulating steps described in earlier chapters. When you make your internal biochemistry hostile to cancer, any residual cancer cells will be more likely to proliferate slowly if at all and less likely to send out metastatic off-shoots to distant sites. Remember, now that you are no longer receiving the cancer-killing treatments of radiation or chemotherapy, your containment strategy has to pack as much anti-cancer punch as possible. From the perspective of integrative oncology, this is a time to be particularly aggressive, especially since your residual cells may be more likely to be resistant to chemotherapy drugs if they do start to regrow.

Taking Treatment to the Molecular Level

Of all the recent advances in mainstream oncology, targeted molecular therapies have generated the most excitement, and for good reason: while far from foolproof, they promise to spare healthy tissue from the effects of anti-cancer drugs. Unlike standard chemotherapies, which attack dividing cells whether or not they are malignant, targeted therapies take aim only at cells that are multiplying uncontrollably—cancer cells.

They therefore are consistent with the main tenet of natural medicine: that we can intervene against cancer with gentler, safer treatments that leave your body and spirit intact. Although even targeted therapies have side effects—some quite significant—most are far less severe than chemotherapies.[1] If there is a targeted therapy for your cancer, your oncologist will make sure that proper tumor tissue samples are collected. These will be analyzed to see if your cancer cells contain the molecular target.

Targeted therapies are not perfect, however. They attack cancer's growth signals and growth pathways—but those are numerous. As a result, when a targeted drug prevents cancer cells from using one growth pathway, they can switch to a backup pathway, much as a hybrid car that runs out of gasoline switches to electric power. This is a big reason why targeted therapies have, by and large, failed to extend survival time by much: within a few months the malignant cells, having switched to a new growth pathway, are back to their lethal proliferative habits. In addition, different malignant cells in the same tumor are not identical. Some may use one growth pathway while others use another.[2]

That's why we need multiple strategies or multitargeting. If we block just one molecular pathway by which cancer cells proliferate or metastasize—even if it is the primary pathway—the cells will switch on another.[3] In mainstream oncology, this has meant searching for effective treatments that take aim at all of the cancer cells' growth pathways, either in succession or simultaneously. Most of today's targeted therapies still take aim at a single growth pathway, and their cost and toxicity are too great to take several at once. But research is moving quickly. The table opposite lists targeted therapies that have been approved as of this writing. I recommend that, along with your A-Team, you stay apprised of which targeted therapies have been approved, which are in clinical trials for which you may be eligible, and which ones you should bring to your doctor's attention. See www.clinicaltrials.gov for trial information, as well as for an updated list of targeted therapies and the cancers they have been approved for by the FDA.

TARGETED MOLECULAR DRUG THERAPIES FOR CANCER

Molecular Marker(s)	Targeted Drug	Comments
CD20 antigen	Bexxar (tositumomab)	Approved for use in follicular lymphoma patients who have been treated with chemotherapy and molecular target drugs.
CD20 antigen	Rituxan (rituximab)	Approved for use in B cell non-Hodgkin's lymphoma and B cell leukemia.
CD20 antigen	Zevalin (ibritumomab tiuxetan)	Approved for use in B cell non-Hodgkin's lymphoma.
EGFR (HERI)	Erbitux (cetuximab)	Approved for metastatic colon and rectal cancer and head and neck cancer.
EGFR (HERI)	Tarceva (erlotinib)	Approved for non-small-cell lung cancer and pancreatic cancer.
EGFR (HERI)	Vectibix (panitumumab)	Approved for colorectal cancer that has been previously treated.
HER2/neu	Herceptin (trastuzumab)	Approved for use in breast cancers with a specific genetic mutation, HER2/neu.
HER2/neu	Tykerb (lapatinib)	Approved for lung and breast cancers.

Molecular Marker(s)	Targeted Drug	Comments
Immune function, angiogenesis	Thalidomide, Revlimid (lenalidomide)	Approved for multiple myeloma, they appear to have several molecular targets.
Methyl transferase	Vidaza (5-azacytidine)	Approved for use in myelodysplastic syndrome.
mTOR	Torisel (temsirolimus)	Approved for use in renal cell carcinoma.
PDGF-r, c-Kit, bcr-abl	Gleevec (imatinib mesylate)	Approved for use in chronic myelogenous leukemia (CML) and gastrointestinal stromal tumor (GIST).
PDGF-r, VEGF-r, c-Kit, others	Sutent (sunitinib)	Approved for use in renal cell carcinomas and gastrointestinal stromal tumors.
PDGF-r, VEGF-r, c-Kit, Raf	Nexavar (sorafenib)	Approved for renal cell and liver cancers.
Proteasome inhibitor, bcl-2 overexpression	Velcade (bortezomib)	Approved for use in multiple myeloma.
VEGF	Avastin (bevacizumab)	Approved for use in non-small-cell lung cancer and metastatic colon or breast cancer.

Targeting Multiple Progression Pathways

Until effective drug cocktails come along, I believe that integrative cancer treatment offers the best way to hit multiple molecular targets simultaneously but with no toxicity. Some natural compounds, with scores or even hundreds of biologically active constituents, can hit multiple targets in cancer cells. Although, largely due to limitations in absorption, without pharmaceutical interventions they are not potent enough to cure cancer (especially advanced cancers) on their own. Whether you target growth pathways through one compound or many, logic suggests that the key is to hit as many tumor-specific targets and pathways as possible: blocking just one of cancer's growth pathways rarely keeps a tumor in check for long. Even lifestyle changes can alter the activity of genes that create these targets: a recent study of a low-fat vegetarian diet found changes in the activity of nearly five hundred genes, many of which had strong relationships to cancer processes.[4] This finding is of special interest in light of the discovery that individual tumors may have dozens of abnormal genes.

The multitargeting approach we use at the Block Center has as its foundation the terrain support program, so we keep your internal biochemistry as hostile as possible to cancer cells. We build on that with compounds that simultaneously target several important cancer growth pathways, hitting the disease with multiple therapies ranging from mainstream cancer drugs or radiation to natural compounds and herbal medicines. Nine processes are especially relevant to the microscopic growth-control program:

1. Those that allow a tumor to grow through rapid, uncontrolled cell **proliferation.**
2. Those that block malignant cells from undergoing **apoptosis** (programmed suicide). Normally, cells with precancerous mutations die by apoptosis; in some malignant cells, this suicide pathway is broken. Also, radiation and to some extent chemotherapy act by causing apoptosis,

but if the cancer cells have learned to resist apoptosis, these therapies will be ineffective.

3. Those that allow malignant cells to acquire **resistance** to treatment. Following chemotherapy or radiation many cells are killed while others resist and survive. With vulnerable cells eliminated, resistant cells have a clear field to proliferate, making billions of clones of themselves— all of which are, of course, more aggressive and also resistant. This is why recurrent cancers are often more difficult to treat.

4. Those that allow cancer cells to evade the **immune system,** which normally kills aberrant cells before they can proliferate into tumors, as explained in Chapter 16.

5. Those that allow malignant cells to grow blood vessels, which provide the nutrients they need. This process is called **angiogenesis,** and the promise of anti-angiogenesis is that tumor cells can hang around all they like, but without a blood supply they cannot proliferate.

6. Those that allow malignant cells to undergo **metastasis** or spread, which is the primary cause of treatment failure and mortality in cancer. By one estimate, metastases exist in about half of all cancer patients at diagnosis, and metastatic cancer—not the primary tumor—is responsible for 90 percent of cancer deaths.

7. Those that lead to defects in cell-to-cell **communication.** Normal cells stop proliferating when they sense similar cells nearby. Cancer cells either never receive this information or ignore it.

8. Those that keep cells from **differentiating,** or becoming specialized cells such as muscle, liver, or skin cells. Differentiation can stop proliferation.

9. Those that make cancer cells **immortal.** Normally, cells can undergo no more than fifty or so cell divisions before dying, but an enzyme called telomerase allows the cell to surpass this limit.

A number of conventional cancer drugs target these growth pathways. But so do natural compounds. Berries, for instance, have anti-angiogenic properties, which is one reason why they take center stage among the fruits in the Life Over Cancer diet.[5] In lab experiments strawberries, wild blueberries, bilberries, cranberries, and elderberries all inhibit the production of VEGF, a common growth pathway, and also prevent angiogenesis. The soy compound genistein also inhibits VEGF and angiogenesis, which may be one reason soy is associated with lower cancer rates.[6] There is also preliminary evidence (which I will keep up-dating on the LOC website) that some natural compounds can stimulate cells of the immune system to seek out and identify malignant cells: a lab study found that the active compound in ginseng has this effect, as does the active compound in aloe vera, acemannan.[7] Curcumin, the active ingredient in the spice turmeric, targets several of the nine progression pathways: it blocks the growth pathway stimulated by EGFR, helps induce apoptosis, and blocks the pathway leading to the growth of blood vessels needed to support metastasis. The effective dose is about 3 to 4 grams of turmeric daily, or 1,200–1,500 mg of cur-cumin or super-concentrates of turmeric.

I don't want you to think that all you need to do to cure your cancer is spice everything with turmeric. The doses that achieve the results described above, in lab studies of tumor cells growing in dishes as well as in lab animals injected with malignant tumors, may be far higher than you could get by simply using turmeric in food. On the other hand, several clin-ical studies are now using concentrated turmeric extracts (which can be safely taken in amounts up to 12 g daily), as well as combinations of turmeric with other multitargeted botanicals.[8] One of these studies, in patients with precancerous lesions of the prostate, is currently showing very interesting early results in retarding the development of cancers. My point is simply this: there exist natural compounds that target the same growth pathways as leading-edge pharmaceuticals. And that is why I make them a cornerstone of the Life Over Cancer tumor containment program.

Just as drug cocktails are a hot area of research in mainstream oncology, so combinations of anti-cancer compounds are some of the most exciting advances in integrative care. By combining compounds, we can take advantage of synergism, in which the effect of two agents is greater than the sum of each used separately—in this case, two plus two equals six or even eighteen. If multiple agents combine in a synergistic way, each can be used at a lower dose. Let me use green tea as an example of how synergism works. Green tea extract makes only a small difference in the growth of a particular strain of mouse tumors, decreasing average tumor weight from 152 mg to 147 mg. Grape seed extract and red pepper extract also have just small effects. But green tea extract plus grape seed extract combined shrinks the tumor to 68 mg. Green tea extract plus red pepper extract shrinks the tumor to 27 mg.[9]

These are just a couple of examples of nutraceuticals targeting cancer progression pathways. The table opposite shows some of our work matching nutraceuticals to the major progression pathways. It's easy to see why the versatile curcumin and green tea are so popular. Remember, though, that much of this research is preclinical—that is, it was done on lab animals and on cells growing in lab dishes, not on people, although some findings are based on human trials. And research on molecular targeting of natural agents is just beginning, so there is going to be a continual evolution of this list in coming years. But because the herbs and supplements have a wide margin of safety, we feel their use is justified in patients searching for additional non-toxic ways to contain tumor growth. We routinely develop protocols that increase the amounts of these compounds in our patients' diets.

Aggressive growth control strategies during the containment phase could help you hold on to your gains or even make further gains against any remaining tumors. At the Block Center, we believe that these strategies may help our patients in their battle to outlive their expected prognoses.

TARGETING PROGRESSION PATHWAYS WITH NUTRACEUTICALS

	Proliferation	Apoptosis	Resistance	Immune	Angiogenesis	Metastasis	Communication	Differentiation	Immortality
Curcumin[10]	X	X	X	X	X	X	X	X	
Green tea polyphenols[11]	X	X	X	X	X	X	X	X	X
Vitamin D[12]	X	X	X		X	X		X	X
Resveratrol[13]	X	X	X	X	X	X	X	X	
Grape seed extract[14]	X	X			X	X			
Reishi[15]	X	X	X	X		X			X
Maitake[16]	X	X		X		X			
Ellagic acid[17]	X	X	X		X	X		X	
Anthocyanins[18]	X	X	X		X	X		X	
Luteolin[19]	X	X			X	X		X	

CHAPTER 27

THE REHABILITATION PROGRAM: GETTING STRONG ENOUGH FOR TREATMENT

You may remember the story of my longtime friend Bill Dufty, who became deeply interested in a healthful diet and lifestyle after marrying the actress and natural-foods advocate Gloria Swanson and wrote the best-selling book *Sugar Blues*. Bill developed metastatic prostate cancer in his mid-seventies and was treated at the Block Center. At one point, after being away from our clinic for some time, he became extremely weak and gaunt and was unable to resume his prescribed chemo. "I hate to look in the mirror these days," he told our physical therapist. "I look like a prisoner of war. Where did I go?" Despite his enfeebled condition and inability to walk more than a few steps, Bill was able to mount a comeback by working intensively with our physical care staff, regaining sufficient strength to persist in his anti-cancer treatments and even walking two full miles daily during his chemotherapy visits. The regimen we developed for him became the Life Over Cancer rehabilitation program, whose goal is to strengthen patients enough to begin or resume treatment.

There are many reasons people with cancer become too debilitated to undergo the attack and growth-control strategies they need. Some, like Bill, become weakened due to advancing disease and other medical problems. Others are weakened by the acute toxicity of chemo or radiation. For many patients, malnutrition is both the result of their initial disease and the cause of a worsening of that disease. Inflammatory cytokines released by a tumor can trigger cachexia, and the side effects of drugs as well as stress and depression can cause a severe loss of appetite. Chemotherapy or tumor progression can bring on such severe nausea, vomiting, and diarrhea that you may derive no benefit from the food you manage to get down. Severe mucositis caused by radiation or chemotherapy can prevent you from eating. Chemotherapy can deplete essential nutrients, leaving you with a de facto deficiency disease.

Mary: Building Strength for Chemo

Mary, fifty-six, came to our clinic with cancer of the gallbladder, which is very hard to treat. The disease and its treatment had already damaged Mary's digestive system, leaving her extremely weak and cachectic. Conventional nutritional counseling had done her little good. While her weight was acceptable if a bit low, she had lost considerable muscle tone, was suffering from jaundice and fatigue, and had developed ascites, or excessive fluid in the abdomen, a sign of low protein reserves. Treating cancer under these conditions is nearly impossible. Yet without treatment, in her weakened condition the cancer was likely to take her life quickly.

Mary therefore began the Life Over Cancer rehab program, whose goal is to bring about sufficient clinical improvement to get you in shape to return to treatment, in Mary's case, chemotherapy. Within a week of starting our rehab program, Mary began to look and feel better. Her ascites and jaundice eased up, and by the second week her appetite and energy levels improved. Mary was able to resume chemotherapy.

If you are worn out and feel you can endure no more, my message is this: rehab can rebuild your strength enough to allow you to resume further treatment and give you a good chance at eliminating your residual disease. Over the years we have gotten many patients back into lifesaving or at least life-prolonging treatment. Our rehab program has six components, and since some of them may involve the use of prescription drugs, it is best to undertake such a program with the knowledge and support of your medical team.

Reducing the Inflammatory Response

Overcoming cachexia is a major problem for many cancer patients. The causes of cachexia are not entirely clear, but inflammatory cytokines secreted by tumors play a major role.[1] That's why when tumors are removed by surgery or shrunk to near nothingness by chemotherapy or radiation, cachexia often improves. Pancreatic, lung, colorectal, and renal cancers are more likely to cause cachexia, while breast and prostate cancer are less likely to cause it.

The first thing to do in combating cachexia is to quell the fires of inflammation that drive it. In general, the self-care steps outlined in Chapter 15 will help. But because cachexia is such a serious condition, I recommend undergoing lab tests to determine which inflammatory molecules are most elevated, as described in the medical partnership section of that chapter. Once you know what you are dealing with, you and your integrative practitioner can adapt your regimen accordingly. Options include any of the following, or a combination, depending on severity:

- A combination supplement that supports a healthy inflammatory response (see Chapter 15, page 337).

- Pure EPA or fish oil, 2 to 6 g daily, to help inhibit production of pro-inflammatory eicosanoids and cytokines.[2] Check the label of fish oil capsules to determine their EPA content. I recommend those that are at least 50 percent EPA. If you have difficulty digesting fish oil, try enteric-coated capsules.

- A mixture of some of the following: curcumin, holy basil, scutellaria, rosemary, ginger, and stinging nettle, which target the COX-2 enzyme, prostaglandin E2, NF-kappaB, and other inflammatory biochemicals.[3] For most patients, 1,000–3,000 mg of curcumin, 1,000–1,500 mg of standardized scutellaria extract, 10–20 mg of rosemary extract, 100–300 mg of ginger extract, and 1,500 mg of nettle extract can be taken daily.

- Vitamin C and vitamin E reduce NF-kappaB, which drives the inflammatory response.[4] For most patients, 1,000–1,800 mg of vitamin C and 200–400 mg of vitamin E can be taken daily.

- Ibuprofen also reduces inflammation. I recommend 400 mg three times a day. You may also take naproxen (500 mg twice a day). Take with food and watch for early signs of gastric bleeding (abdominal pain, fatigue, anemia, black stools).

Eating Enough and Eating Right

It may be that you are weak, tired, and wasting away because you are not taking in enough calories. Determining how many calories and how much protein and other nutrients you need every day in order to return to health is complicated, so I recommend asking your medical team for a nutritionist who can help you with this. Once you know your targets, you can implement a comprehensive plan for supplying protein, calories, and other nutrients. In the most serious cases, your physician will usually recommend an enteral formula, which can be drunk or delivered through a feeding tube. Though there are many commercial nutrition products, most contain high quantities of sugar, dairy products, and unhealthy fats, all of which can wreak havoc on your terrain, including worsening your inflammation levels. As I explained in Chapter 6, our center nutritionists have developed formulations that do not contain these cancer-promoting ingredients. The shake recipe in Chapter 6, page 131, is rich in calories and protein as well as micronutrients and phytochemicals. In addition, I recommend following the High-Intensity Nutritional Support diet described in Chapter 6, which contains high-calorie foods with an emphasis on high-quality concentrated protein such as fish, egg whites, soy, and whey.

Stimulating Your Appetite

Although many cancer patients experience a drastically reduced appetite that leads them to practically stop eating, this is usually temporary. If you have not been eating, or not eating enough, for more than a few days and are losing weight and muscle mass, reread the advice in Chapter 6 on stimulating your appetite. In particular, pay attention to the social dynamics of eating by making it a pleasant experience through colorful and attractive food presentations. Eating with other people also tends to improve appetite. Try eating several small meals a day; even people with no appetite find they can snack even when they can't stand the thought of a full meal. Vary food textures and odors; this may make what you see on your plate more appealing. If chemotherapy or illness has impaired your sense of taste or smell, even the most scrumptious food will leave you cold; work with a dietitian to cope with this problem, and look back at Chapter 6 for ways to adapt your diet in case of sensory loss or distortion. Eat at least a third of your daily calories at breakfast, when appetite tends to be greatest. Since the lack of appetite can leave you with no interest in preparing meals, try to get someone to do it for you, otherwise you risk falling into a vicious cycle: no appetite, no cooking; no cooking, no eating. Spice up your meals by adding tantalizing herbs such as tarragon. Some other possibilities:

- If you find that food seems to sit in your stomach like a cannonball, try chewing more thoroughly, take digestive enzymes such as bromelain or papain, or eat a small piece of pickled umeboshi plum.[5]

- Five or ten minutes of mild exercise, such as walking, half an hour before meals may stimulate appetite.

- If depression is causing you to have no appetite, tell your doctor, and discuss whether counseling, cognitive therapy, or herbal medication is appropriate.

- If the thought of eating makes you anxious, try to relax before meals using the relaxation response, progressive muscle relaxation, or other stress management techniques described in Chapter 11.

- Some traditional herbal teas that stimulate appetite are ginger, catnip, fennel, peppermint, and ginseng.

- Gentian extract, a constituent of "bitters," works for some patients.[6]

- A traditional Chinese medicine herbal formula for stimulating appetite is available at many health food stores. Look for the one called Bu Zhong Yi Qi Tang. Use 1,000–3,000 mg of a spray-dried extract. It should contain *radix astragali membranacei* (huang qi), *radix codonopsitis pilosulae* (dang shen), *sclerotium poriae cocos* (fu ling), *rhizoma atractylodis macrocephalae* (bai zhu), *radix angelicae sinensis* (dang gui), *rhizoma cimicifugae* (sheng ma), *radix bupleuri* (chai hu), *fructus amomi* (sha ren), *radix glycyrrhizae* (gan cao), *fructus germinatus oryzae sativae* (gu ya), and *fructus germinatus hordei vulgaris* (mai ya). Take one tablet a day, preferably on an empty stomach. (See the discussion of supplement quality on the LOC website for comments on imported supplements.)

- If your appetite is low because you are chronically nauseous, look back at the recommendations in Chapters 6, 9, and 24 on overcoming nausea. If those do not help, an antiemetic medication might. Similarly, if mucositis makes it too painful to eat or swallow, see the recommendations in Chapters 6 and 24 on treating mucositis.

- Megace (megestrol acetate) is a prescription drug given to cancer patients with cachexia to stimulate their appetite and help them gain weight.[7] The usual dosage is 400 to 800 mg/day. The prescription drugs Marinol (dronabinol) and Oxandrin (oxandrolone) may also be used.

Rebuilding Muscle

Muscle contains the immune-building amino acid glutamine, which can make your internal biochemistry more hostile to cancer. The program outlined in Chapter 9 is a good place to start. If you do not have access to a physical therapist you can help yourself tremendously by finding a sensitive trainer. Work on strength training (weight lifting) and other resistance exercise that can help you regain lean muscle mass. Recovery aerobic exercise in the form of interval training, discussed in Chapter 8, can help improve overall vitality. Fish oil also has muscle-building effects. And as a last resort, ask your physician about anabolic pharmaceuticals such as Oxandrin (oxandrolone).[8]

Boosting Immune Surveillance

The protein deficiency that typically results from loss of appetite and its attendant malnutrition can impair the immune system, making you more susceptible to recurrent and life-threatening infections. If you have a spiking fever, you will be in no condition to undergo the chemotherapy, surgery, or radiation that can extend your life. Look back at Chapter 16, on boosting your immune system. Astragalus extract (500–1,000 mg two or three times a day) and a mixture of echinacea, wild indigo, and baptisia (1 to 3 tablets two to three times a day), both of which are available in health food stores, have shown effectiveness at improving the functioning of immune cells.[9] We need more research on these extracts to clarify their usefulness.

Recovering from Emotional Stress and Fatigue

This is no time to neglect your mind and spirit, even as you focus on your body. Continue to implement the mind-spirit program in Chapters 10, 11, and 12 to increase emotional stamina.

You should follow this rehabilitation program until you can resume the normal activities of daily life and tolerate chemotherapy or other treatments appropriate for growth control or attack. And don't get discouraged—even tiny improvements can make a difference. Over the years, I have worked with patients who appeared far too weak to even consider a rehab program, but they bounced back in tiny steps, sometimes with only a minute of activity at a time repeated ten to twenty times a day. This has helped numerous bedridden patients to return to daily activities.

CHAPTER 28

LEAVING NO STONE UNTURNED: WHAT TO DO WHEN THERE'S "NOTHING LEFT TO DO"

I have already mentioned how I feel about doctors communicating hopelessness, telling cancer patients that "there is nothing more that can be done" or that they are "out of options." This usually occurs when patients still have visible disease (showing up on scans) after conventional treatment that has been unsuccessful. The message is, *We attacked your cancer with everything in our armamentarium, and it's still there, so we have to give up the battle.*

As I trust the preceding chapters have made clear, if you have maintained your strength and overall well-being, there is nearly always something else meaningful that can be done. You can follow the recommendations for Sphere 2 to make your terrain hostile to further cancer growth. You can follow the recommendations in Sphere 1 to make yourself as healthy as possible through diet, fitness, and mind-spirit techniques, and those in Chapter 27 to make yourself strong enough to undergo further or new treatments, which come along more and more frequently these days. In this chapter, I will explain why there are still meaningful strategies to try even if your doctor feels that further treatment would be of little value.

The approach that our center takes is based on our belief that anyone who wants to fight for his or her life, no matter what the odds, should be given every opportunity to do that. With my patients, I have always been an uncompromising realist, yet I have never given up on anyone. By using the widest array of tools and techniques, by convincing patients to confront the disease with vigor and a fighting spirit, and by working with patients to regain their physical, nutritional, and emotional resilience, I have seen patients win back their health and their lives. My "leave no stone unturned" philosophy explains why our center is so aggressive in monitoring and treating disease even after conventional treatment, and in searching for experimental or alternative options if mainstream therapies stop working.

Do you remember the story of Delores in Chapter 1? She had metastatic breast cancer, with 80 percent of her liver riddled with tumors. Her prognosis was beyond grim. But by following the Life Over Cancer program, she was able to hang on more than twice as long as predicted by statistics—at which point we were able to get her Herceptin. Delores was among the first patients in Illinois to get this drug outside of a trial. It melted away her disease. Had Delores not rejected the "nothing more we can do for you" message, she would not have survived long enough to receive this powerful drug, which gave her an additional four years of life. With this philosophy we have seen many patients like Delores who stabilized their tumor and controlled residual cancer cells for years beyond the usual expectations.

I therefore developed specific strategies for when chemotherapy or other attack-phase or growth-control therapies stop working. If you are in this situation, allow yourself the time and space to deal with the immediate shock and sadness. But then, with all the strength you can muster, get your A-Team and medical partner together and begin the arduous battle again. There are ways to get back on the road to recovery.

At around this point, some of you may be wondering whether it is right to "raise false hopes." For one thing, I do not believe these hopes are false. I, like many cancer specialists,

have seen way too many miraculous outcomes. For another, although I respect the views of physicians who worry that patients might pursue "futile" treatments rather than spend their
last days putting their affairs in order and saying good-bye,
there is no reason why people can't do both, being prepared
for the worst yet pursuing the best. I do encourage patients to
have their financial and other personal affairs in order even
early in their cancer journey, if they so choose, simply to shed a
burden from their minds so they can focus on their health.

Marilyn: Refusing to Give Up

Marilyn, a fifty-three-year-old housewife with three children,
heard the dread words "no further options" from her doctor
one day in March 2003. Three years before, during a routine
heart scan, doctors had found a nodule in her right lung that
turned out to be cancer. (Marilyn had smoked for thirty years,
until 1998.) Her surgeon found and removed a three-centimeter
adenocarcinoma, as well as a four-millimeter tumor that showed
the cancer had spread locally. It had not, however, spread to
Marilyn's lymph nodes. Her doctors sent Marilyn home, with
only three-month checkups as their follow-up plan.

Three years later, a scan found a 1.5-centimeter nodule in
Marilyn's lung. This time she had non-operable non-small-cell
lung cancer, and it had spread to both lungs, her diaphragm,
and her bones, from which it was encroaching on her spinal
cord, causing serious pain. Marilyn reported hearing from her
oncologist, "The cancer is back, it is inoperable, and there's
nothing we can do. If you want, you could try chemotherapy,
but it won't do much for you." In March 2003, with multiple
new metastases in both lungs, a liver lesion, and cancer in her
ribs, Marilyn's doctors recommended hospice care.

But Marilyn refused to give up. Instead of enrolling in hospice, she came to the Block Center in June 2003, signing herself
out of the hospital against her doctor's advice. It was clear she
had several major challenges: one was that she had lost more

than thirty pounds over the preceding ten weeks, mostly because the pain had diminished her appetite to the point where she had been eating next to nothing. We therefore started her immediately on a rehabilitation program, as outlined in the preceding chapter, to help her regain lean muscle and get in shape to tolerate further treatment. This entailed pain medication so she could regain her appetite, the appetite-stimulating drug Marinol (dronabinol), and the anti-inflammatory Aleve (naproxen) to assist with reversing her cachexia. We instructed Marilyn to begin eating more protein and calories, plus high-dose fish oil and a rebuilding product like the shake I describe in Chapter 6. She took a multivitamin designed for cancer patients and a concentrated green drink to build her stores of micronutrients, phytochemicals, and calories. As her pain diminished and the rebuilding program took effect, Marilyn's appetite returned.

In order to tailor her treatment regimen, we performed Sphere 2 laboratory testing. It showed low serum levels of lutein and vitamin C, high morning and evening cortisol levels, low evening melatonin levels, high serum fibrinogen, and astronomical levels of the inflammatory marker C-reactive protein (15,000 compared with a normal level of less than 1.2). These results indicated severe inflammation and an inverted pattern of stress chemistry, exacerbating her cachexia and pain. Low levels of several antioxidants and cancer-fighting phytochemicals suggested oxidative stress. We started Marilyn on an aggressive anti-inflammatory and stress chemical rebalancing program: pantothenic acid, vitamin C, and cold-processed whey protein for improving stress chemistry and protein levels; off-label Celebrex to tame the fires of inflammation; fish oil and a broad-spectrum antioxidant formula to squelch free radicals and restore antioxidants. Over the next four months her levels of C-reactive protein fell like a rock, and by March 2004 all of her Sphere 2 lab tests were normal. She even increased her weight from 118 to 133 pounds. As soon as Marilyn began regaining strength, we referred her for radiation therapy, which she tolerated well. She took Siberian ginseng extract as a radiation coupler (as discussed in Chapter 25), since it can maintain energy levels and support immune function.

Marilyn was also strong enough to resume an innovative attack therapy. We considered several experimental and alternative options, run by exceptional scientists in and outside the U.S. After much discussion, and having improved her condition, we elected to give her carboplatin and gemcitabine weekly, as well as Zometa (zoledronic acid) monthly to treat bone metastases. As a chemotherapy treatment coupler, we chose high-dose melatonin (20 mg a day), which has been studied in combination with chemotherapy for advanced lung cancer patients.[1] As difficult as this chemotherapy regimen can be, the only side effect she experienced was minor fatigue. The real payoff came in December 2003, when CT and bone scans showed that a tumor that had been six centimeters across was almost gone, and another tumor ten centimeters across had shrunk by 90 percent. Her liver lesion was now too small to measure. Over the next few months, Marilyn's scans continued to show marked improvement, with her multiple lung metastases nearly cleared.

At this point we segued from the aggressive attack therapies and began a growth control plan. We used the new targeted therapy Iressa (gefitinib) (which, unfortunately, has since been withdrawn from the market). We also put Marilyn on a molecular support formulation, composed of several of the nutraceuticals listed in the chart on page 507, with the aim of inhibiting proliferation pathways. As I write, Marilyn continues to manage her cancer as a chronic illness three and a half years after being told that hospice was her only option.

The Question of Scientific Proof

The message I hope you take from Marilyn's story is not that everyone will necessarily have the success that Marilyn has had, but rather that every person who wants to fight for his or her life, no matter the odds, should be given the opportunity. You may hear criticisms that the therapies in a "no stone unturned" approach are not based on randomized controlled trials. I certainly believe that integrative medicine, no less than conventional medicine, should be evidence-based. But by definition, if your oncologist tells you that there is nothing more he or she can do for you, it means there is nothing in the conventional arsenal that can help you. That leaves, by default, agents or therapies that for one reason or another—generally economic—have not been tested in clinical trials. In many cases, the reason is that they are natural compounds; since these cannot be easily patented, no company can make much profit from them, and therefore no company has any incentive to spend the hundreds of millions of dollars necessary to obtain regulatory approval. Other compounds have been used for centuries, often in Chinese or other traditional medicine systems, but have only gotten as far as in vitro or animal testing, since they only recently came to the attention of interested scientists. I certainly agree that it is problematic to offer drugs whose safety has not been proved. But when it comes to well-known natural agents that have been used for centuries, the risk of harm is very low, or maybe almost zero, and the possibility of benefit is greater than zero. In cases where zero is what is left of conventional options, anything better than zero looks good. Ironically, among the thousands of cancer patients our center has treated are a growing number of physicians; although many admit to rejecting therapies for their own patients for "lack of evidence," as patients themselves they embraced these integrative strategies. Suddenly, waiting years for clinical trials—despite their great value and importance—didn't seem so smart.

Let's now turn to the five categories of no-stone-unturned therapies that you can consider during this phase of your care. All meet my three criteria of (1) having been proved safe, through either clinical studies or a long track record of use, (2) having at least some evidence of effectiveness, and (3) having a favorable cost/convenience ratio.

Off-Label Use of Pharmaceuticals

The use of drugs that have been approved by the FDA, but for another purpose, is called off-label use. If I prescribe the cholesterol-lowering statins for cancer treatment, for example, that is an off-label use.

I chose that example because statins may indeed play an important role in cancer therapy. They block an enzyme called HMG-CoA reductase, and this lowers production of several proteins essential for cell proliferation and thus the progression of cancer. For instance, statins block the activity of the *ras* oncogene, which is important in esophageal cancer as well as colon cancer, breast cancer, and other cancers. Statins also have other effects such as encouraging apoptosis (cell suicide) and increasing susceptibility of cancers to treatment in lab studies.[2] Whether statins actually slow tumor growth or metastasis remains to be proved, but some experiments to date are encouraging: studies find that statins inhibit the growth of multiple myeloma, malignant melanoma, breast cancer, pancreatic cancer, and other cancers in the lab. Advanced liver cancer patients given statins survived twice as long as control patients, a randomized trial in Japan found, and a 2007 trial suggested that a statin may overcome drug resistance in multiple myeloma.[3] So if a patient has multiple myeloma and is out of options, I would certainly consider as one option prescribing a statin for her alongside her drug protocol, in hopes of overcoming resistance and initiating a response. (Because statins deplete coenzyme Q_{10} from your muscle cells, particularly your heart, I advise patients on statins to take at least 30 mg of coQ_{10} per day, and 200 mg or considerably more if they are taking any heart-damaging medications such as Adriamycin or Herceptin.)

Off-label drugs could be particularly valuable during the growth-control phase by making your terrain as hostile as possible to malignant cells. For example, a 2004 study in the journal *Cancer* reported that a combination of the diabetes drug Actos (pioglitazone) and the COX-2 inhibitor Vioxx (rofecoxib), which help to control blood sugar and inflammation, respectively, along with a weekly low-dose oral chemotherapy drug, shrank tumors or stabilized their growth in patients with advanced cancers.[4] Although Merck pulled Vioxx off the market in 2004, other COX-2 inhibitors such as Celebrex work by the same mechanism. The FDA has recently warned that Actos may worsen heart failure.

COX-2 inhibitors are a good example of treatments that can be used off-label. It takes years to complete randomized clinical trials on whether an existing drug makes a difference when combined with chemotherapy. In the meantime, there is ample evidence that cancer patients stand to gain from inhibiting the COX-2 enzyme, since the inflammatory chemicals it spawns play a major role in blocking the effectiveness of chemotherapy and radiation. This is why I urge you to ask your physician about off-label options. You can also check www.lifeover cancer.com for a list of off-label strategies, such as:

- Naltrexone (a prescription drug used to counter narcotics overdose and to help patients recover from addiction to heroin and other opiates) in a very small dose of 4.5 mg at bedtime, to activate Th1 cancer-fighting immune cells and apoptosis of cancer cells while binding opiate receptors that can stimulate cell replication.[5]

- Tetrathiomolybdate (TM, used to treat Wilson's disease) to inhibit angiogenesis.[6] TM keeps copper levels too low for angiogenesis. Very low copper levels may cause anemia, so careful monitoring is needed.

- Calcitriol, the most active form of vitamin D and of particular interest in prostate cancer.[7] Another form of vitamin D, alfacalcidol, resulted in prolonged remission in glioblastoma patients.

Vaccines and Immune Therapies

Vaccines and immune therapies are mostly useful for containing growth rather than shrinking visible tumors. The basic idea is to take tumor cells—your own or those from a patient with the same kind of cancer—and develop antibodies to the cells' surface proteins (called antigens). These antibodies can then be injected back into you, and attack malignant cells. Other cancer vaccines in development contain tumor antigens themselves, or crushed tumor cells known as tumor lysates. To get a sense of the promise of cancer vaccines, consider just one recent study, in which patients with the brain cancer glioblastoma, which has a particularly poor prognosis, were given the Newcastle vaccine, prepared by infecting their tumor cells with the Newcastle (chicken) virus, which does not cause disease in humans. After one year, 91 percent of the patients were still alive (compared to 45 percent of those with the same cancer who did not receive the vaccine), 40 percent survived two years (compared to 11 percent in the control group), and 4 percent became long-term survivors (compared to zero in the control group).[8]

Cancer vaccines have been most successful with cancers that are more immune-sensitive, such as melanomas and kidney cancers. The most advanced cancer vaccines available today are for malignant melanoma; Melacine given with low-dose interferon recently had good results in a clinical trial.[9] You can find clinical trials of cancer vaccines at www.clinicaltrials.gov, a website sponsored by the National Cancer Institute.

We have referred patients to doctors in Germany and Israel who are doing especially innovative work. We maintain an interest in the most forward-looking international clinics, which are using immune, gene, pheresis, donor lymphocytes, and other innovative therapies. You can find more about these clinics on the LOC website.

Immune therapies can be very useful for some patients whose tumor shrinks, but does not disappear, in response to the front-line attack strategies, or in whom residual malignant cells hang on. In these cases, it sometimes happens that all you need to drive the cancer into remission is a strengthened immune response. For example, the immune modulator BCG is a mainstay in the treatment of bladder cancer but is little more than a preparation of crushed bacteria that basically revs up the immune system; we are also investigating bacterial vaccines at the Block Center.[10] There is also a great deal of research into immune adjuvants.[11] These are cellular growth factors (such as interleukin-2) that pump up immune responses. In patients with residual tumor, this could translate into tumor shrinkage. In patients in remission, these strategies could translate into an anti-tumor immune response that is strong and persistent enough to prevent recurrence.

Targeted Molecular Therapies

Targeted molecular therapies, as discussed in Chapter 26, take aim at the particular growth pathways that malignant cells use to proliferate, but spare normal cells. As this field expands, we are learning that targeted therapies are not specific to particular cancers—such as breast, lung, or prostate—but to particular genetic or molecular abnormalities that can exist within cancer

EXAMPLES OF NATURAL MOLECULAR TARGET MODIFIERS

Marker	Nutraceuticals
COX-2	Curcumin, fish oil, ginger, *Scutellaria baicalensis*[13]
IGF-I	Lycopene, genistein, quercetin[14]
MDR	Rosemary extract, fish oil, indole-3-carbinol[15]
VEGF	Luteolin, apigenin, milk thistle[16]
p53	Green tea (EGCG), genistein[17]
EGFR	Curcumin, resveratrol, grape seed extract[18]
ras	Garlic, limonene, tocotrienols[19]
HER2/neu	Green tea, olive oil[20]
PTEN	Indole-3-carbinol, soy isoflavones[21]

cells of many types. For instance, Herceptin has been approved for metastatic breast cancer, and it may ultimately be shown to improve treatment for, say, stomach cancer, which also tends to over-express the HER2/neu molecule.[12]

Check the website www.clinicaltrials.gov to see which targeted therapies are in clinical trials, especially drugs approved for one type of cancer (which have already shown some degree of safety and efficacy) but are being investigated for efficacy against other types—yours. Don't assume your doctor has had time to review all of the latest clinical trials available to you. Bring what you find to your physician and ask if a trial seems right for you. This is another reason to have a sample of your tumor preserved (as discussed in Chapter 22): if a new targeted therapy emerges, you will be able to have your sample tested to see if the molecule that drives the growth of your tumor is targeted by the new drug. Even before a new drug is approved to target your cancer's growth pathway, you may find treatments available in other countries.

There are natural compounds that can target these pathways as well. At the Block Center we test patients for a variety of targets that can be addressed by natural agents; a small sample is shown in the table on the previous page. Including natural agents in your anti-cancer arsenal lets you multitarget a tumor in a safe way. If you have had your tumor analyzed to identify its chief growth pathways, this gives you and your expert advisers still more options.

Reasonable and Responsible Alternative Therapies

By "alternative therapies," I mean treatments not approved for any purpose in the United States and not the focus of serious scientific investigation in the United States. Several herbal agents are increasingly used in cancer clinics in other countries, and some, such as the Chinese herb *Scutellaria barbata*, have been studied in clinical trials. More often than not, however, an alternative therapy gains popularity among patients because of a claim of a theoretical mechanism that might have a clinical benefit. What should you do if you come across an alternative therapy that you think might be worth trying? You certainly would not be alone if you did try it: up to 60 percent of cancer patients may turn to these therapies at some point, usually without telling their doctors. If there is evidence that the agent is safe, and if it has a plausible mechanism of action and has demonstrated some efficacy in clinical or pre-clinical research, it is not unusual for me to support patients who choose to try it, especially when conventional treatments have stopped helping. I strongly encourage patients who choose an alternative therapy to continue with mainstream diagnostics such as scans and tests of tumor marker levels, and careful monitoring with a knowledgeable cancer specialist.

If you go this route, remember that some supplements can adversely interact with conventional medications, which makes it important to discuss your use of alternatives with your doctor. Yes, many patients worry that their doctor will not be supportive or, worse, will scold or belittle them; certainly, many physicians have some work to do when it comes to communicating about this issue. If you decide that you want to use an alternative therapy alongside conventional treatment but are afraid to tell your doctor, try to find a more open practitioner, or at least discuss it with a pharmacist, a nurse, or another health practitioner who may be more approachable, and be sure to ask about possible drug interactions. To be fair, however, it is important to keep in mind that the vast majority of physicians will provide valuable information and are communicating their genuine concerns. Their advice shouldn't be rejected simply because of personal dogmas. Rather, your choices should grow out of informed decisions that have been carefully thought through.

Review the scientific research on alternatives with your medical partner. Some are backed by rigorous science; some have decades or even centuries of use behind them. Be cautious with those that have only a limited record of use in people. While the Internet may give you many leads, it may also set you up to be scammed, or worse, endanger your life, so don't go for just any alternative treatment you discover there. There are excellent sources of updated information on alternatives, including assessments of the science behind them. One of these is a website run by the National Cancer Institute called the PDQ Cancer Information Summaries on Complementary and Alternative Medicine (www.cancer.gov/cancertopics/pdq/cam). Another good source is the Moss Reports, by Ralph Moss (www.cancerdeci sions.com). Other authoritative sources are listed on the LOC website.

Let me give you a sense of the kind of alternatives I would consider reasonable and responsible. Without knowing your specific needs, I am unable to make any particular recommendations about these, but I point them out as examples of the type of assessment you can do as part of leaving no stone unturned.

- Mistletoe has been used by physicians in Europe, particularly Germany, since 1920. The preparation called Iscador consists of fermented extracts of European mistletoe (*Viscum album*) and has been shown to have anti-cancer and anti-metastatic properties when tested on cells of lung, breast, bladder, and several other types of cancer growing in lab dishes. In animal experiments, mistletoe compounds called lectins have been shown to kill cancer cells, stimulate anti-cancer immune defenses (especially natural killer cells), and block tumor growth. According to a 2003 review, eight controlled clinical trials have now demonstrated significant improvements in survival for cancer patients receiving mistletoe preparations. This remains a controversial conclusion, however, in part because the best-designed studies did not show any benefits in survival.[22]
- Ukrain is a semi-synthetic derivative from the herb greater celandine combined with a conventional cancer drug, thiotepa. Administered intravenously, it is licensed as a drug in parts of the former Soviet Union. A number of clinical studies have reported that Ukrain can slow the progression of pancreatic tumors and extend the remission of patients with this cancer. In a 2002 clinical trial, for instance, patients with advanced

pancreatic cancer who received Ukrain and the chemotherapy drug Gemzar (gemcitabine) had double the median survival time of patients who received Gemzar alone. However, a 2005 review of these studies found them to be of dubious quality, and treatment costs some $3,800 per week.[23] Also, I have had patients who came to my clinic already taking Ukrain who have suffered serious side effects. This illustrates the tricky balancing act you will face in evaluating alternative therapies.

• Intravenous vitamin C in high doses has shown some success against a variety of cancers for which conventional chemotherapy had been unsuccessful. Although IV vitamin C remains controversial, scientists at the National Cancer Institute have found that at very high doses it killed cancer cells with a pro-oxidative mechanism, by triggering production of hydrogen peroxide, but did not harm normal cells. A recent report on two patients who had good results after taking intravenous vitamin C alongside their chemotherapy triggered a randomized trial in ovarian cancer, now in progress in Kansas. Another recently completed early-stage trial of intravenous vitamin C did not show any tumor regression. The LOC website includes updates on clinical trials using intravenous vitamin C and other important alternatives.[24]

• MSC, obtained from fermented wheat-germ extract, has promising preclinical activity. Small clinical trials also indicate significant increases in survival, but larger trials are needed to confirm these data. This example illustrates something you will find repeatedly with alternative therapies: it sounds promising, but requires better studies to make claims for it credible.[25] On the other hand, aside from the expense, the risks appear to be low.

• Oleander, however, may expose you to high risks of toxicity if it is obtained from the wrong source. This plant has several anticancer activities. Research shows its abilities to induce apoptosis, boost immune response, inhibit angiogenesis, and drop the inflammatory biochemical NF-kappaB. Promising extracts exist, including one presently in clinical trials.[26] A physician may be able to arrange to get a product from an approved pharmaceutical laboratory, in which the toxic but cancer-killing compounds are at safe levels. See the LOC website for further information.

Traditional Medicine Systems

Traditional medicine systems are those that were developed millennia ago in China, India, the Middle East and elsewhere. Their long history means that the compounds they use are generally safe and potentially effective. There are also responsible practitioners of a tradition of herbal medicine based on the herbs of Europe and other countries, often called Western herbalists.[27] If you want to go this route, it is best to seek the help of a traditional Chinese medical practitioner, preferably an M.D. with extensive training in this tradition, or seek an herbalist who has training and professional certification. He or she can tell you about herbs that can support the body's natural resistance to tumor growth and that help reduce side effects. You can find a practitioner through one of the colleges of Oriental medicine in the United States, independent clinics such as the Pine Street Clinic in San Anselmo, or the American Society of Medical Acupuncture (www.medicalacupuncture.org). Western herbalists in the United States can be located through the American Herbalists Guild (www.americanherbalistsguild.com). As always, be sure to find an expert to advise you whether a traditional compound interacts adversely with any mainstream treatments you are also receiving. Also be sure that your traditional practitioner supports your continuing commitment to your conventional and integrative cancer care.

As you can see from the strategies discussed above, there is a reason I am including them in a chapter on leaving no stone unturned. The evidence for their efficacy against cancer is limited but tantalizing, and there are many more of them. As long as you understand that in general there is a low level of scientific support for these therapies, if your cancer is advancing and showing little or no response to either mainstream treatments or those I discuss earlier in this book, you should certainly feel comfortable in counseling with an integrative medicine expert and together evaluating alternative treatment options. My hope and expectation is that both the quality of research on alternative therapies and patients' abilities to access reasonable alternatives will improve in the future.

CHAPTER 29

THE REMISSION MAINTENANCE PROGRAM

If you are like most patients whose attack phase eliminated all visible tumor, your physician offered congratulations, said he or she would see you in three to six months for diagnostic scans or blood tests to make sure the tumor had not grown back or spawned metastases—and that's it. No drugs to maintain remission (unless you were prescribed a hormonal blocking therapy, usually for breast or prostate cancer, or rarely, a targeted therapy). No diet plan. No fitness plan.

This, I do not recommend.

Even complete remission is not necessarily synonymous with *cure*. (Today, some 60 percent of cancer patients are cured, but these are mostly patients with cancers that were caught very early and cases in which surgery really is a cure. These include very early melanomas that don't invade the deeper layers of skin, and solid tumors that are very small and/or contained or encapsulated in the lungs, breast, colon, prostate, bladder, or other organs.) A patient in remission may still harbor malignant cells (ones that were resistant to chemotherapy or radiation, and therefore survived the attack phase) that not even the best diagnostic technologies can detect. This is why some patients who have achieved a complete remission sometimes suffer a recurrence months or years later. I wish I could tell you that the conventional five-year milestone of being disease-free really is synonymous with a cure. But it's not. As you may recall from the introduction, my grandmother's breast cancer recurred with metastases in distant organs more than two decades after her initial treatment. This chapter can tell you how to lower recurrence risks through what I call *remission maintenance*.

First, take heart. If your attack strategies were so effective that no visible tumor remains, this is definitely cause for celebration. Understandably, you may want to retreat psychologically to a "cancer-free" zone and never think about your disease again. What you need to do now is keep residual, invisible cells from proliferating. Even millions of malignant cells, as long as they never get together and form a dangerous tumor, will not threaten your life or your health. If you received adjuvant chemotherapy to rid the body of microscopic cancer cells, you already have a leg up. But not even adjuvant therapy is a guarantee, and for some advanced cancers it is not nearly enough. That is why we recommend an ongoing comprehensive program of diet, supplements, exercise, mind-spirit care, and anti-tumor therapies. At the Block Center, we help patients find peace and confidence in proactive strategies so that each time they have a scan or another diagnostic test to see if the cancer has returned they do not feel like they are just waiting for the other shoe to drop. As opposed to "watchful waiting," I encourage what I call "active participating," a remission maintenance plan that bolsters your energy, brightens your health, and protects against a return of your cancer. I want you engaged in preventing a recurrence in order to get the full benefit from your months of treatments. After all, you've gone through the ordeals of surgery, chemo, radiation, or all three. You deserve to never see cancer again.

Let me give you a sense of what a difference "active participating" rather than "watchful waiting" can make. One cancer that is often managed by just the latter is early-stage prostate cancer, since it seldom develops into full-fledged disease. But in one very recent study, scientists had thirty-one men with early-stage prostate cancer try "active participating" instead. Rather than holding on to old habits, the men switched to a diet built around low-fat, mostly plant-based, whole foods; learned stress management; engaged in moderate exercise; attended support groups; and took soy supplements, fish oil, vitamins C and E, and selenium. The scientists compared samples of prostate tissue taken before and after the men began this regimen. As they reported in 2008, oncogenes as well as genes involved in insulin-like growth factor 1 (which promotes malignancies), tumor formation, and fat metabolism all became less active. After two years, men who had adopted these lifestyle changes were significantly less likely to need conventional prostate cancer treatment than men who had not. Even something as simple as relaxation techniques can alter genes involved in cancer's return: genes controlling the generation of mutation-causing free radicals and metabolic pathways leading to inflammation became less active in patients who were trained in relaxation techniques compared with those who were not, another 2008 study found. The result was a biochemical terrain that grew less and less hospitable to cancer—exactly what you want for maintaining a remission.[1] New studies that analyze many genes in cancer cells have found that in the most common cancers multiple genes are abnormal—up to 60 abnormal genes in some cancer types. This makes the potential relevance of these lifestyle studies—and your own efforts in carrying out the LOC program—even more exciting.

Aggressive Monitoring

At the Block Center, we believe in staying ahead of cancer. That means frequent monitoring of patients' status with lab tests and imaging to detect early signs of disrupted biochemistry or a recurrence of disease, especially in the year or two after remission, since the earlier we catch a problem, the more likely we are to be able to nip it in the bud. Being "diagnostically aggressive" may allow us to be less invasive therapeutically. In the first years after remission, therefore, I recommend:

- Clinical visits with your oncologist, at least every three to four months in the first year and every six months for the next few years

- Scans and blood tests of tumor markers every three months

- Complete blood count and chemistry test every three months

- Nutrition status, including weight changes, body composition, and albumin levels, every three months

- Internal terrain monitoring, as listed in Chapters 14 to 19, every three to six months for the terrain factors that are most problematic

Suppressing Dormant Tumor Cells

Remember, you can live a perfectly healthy life even with millions of malignant cells in your body—as long as they do not begin proliferating and metastasizing. If you have already adopted the Life Over Cancer Sphere 1 and 2 programs, you don't need to do much more than you're already doing. Refer back to Chapters 6, 9, and 12, each of which contains programs for remission, emphasizing ways to make these lifestyle changes easy to implement and enjoyable. I also recommend that you continue taking supplements that target the growth pathways that fueled your form of cancer, as explained on page 527. If your disease was caught very early or was one of the types for which surgery really is a cure (as mentioned on page 532), you may not have any residual microscopic cancer cells, in which case you may only need basic support (see Chapter 5): the supplements, diet, and fitness programs may be enough to reduce the risk of a new cancer, by making your internal terrain and tumor microenvironment hostile to malignancies.

Soy and Breast Cancer

Breast cancer patients who are in remission face a question specific to their condition: if your cancer was estrogen-receptor-positive (ER+ in pathology reports), can you safely eat soy? Soy, of course, contains substantial amounts of the isoflavones genistein and daidzein, which act like estrogens and attach to estrogen receptors, leading to fears that they might trigger breast cancer anew. But soy isoflavones activate these receptors very weakly, so their estrogenic effect is small. In a dozen studies in which women were given soy isoflavones, the compounds did not affect the rate at which breast cells divide, meaning they are unlikely to stimulate breast cancer.[2]

My current assessment of this research is that both premenopausal and postmenopausal women with ER+ tumors can safely eat soy foods such as tempeh and tofu about two or three times per week. However, until more research is available I do not recommend that these women take isoflavone supplements, which are sold to help control hot flashes and supply phytoestrogens at levels much higher than dietary levels. Women who are taking tamoxifen, Aromasin (exemestane), Arimidex (anastrozole), or Femara (letrozole) should also avoid isoflavone supplements. Women with ER- breast cancer should be fine taking soy foods and soy isoflavones. Additionally, premenopausal breast cancer patients with higher estrogen levels, whether ER+ or – should have no added risk by consuming soy. In fact, as noted above, soy isoflavones would act as weak estrogens and thus would decrease overall estrogen exposure by blocking the binding of normal estrogen with receptors. However, in ER+ postmenopausal women, including those younger women pushed prematurely into menopause from surgery or chemotherapy, soy isoflavone supplementation may stimulate estrogen receptors and thus adversely encourage cellular replication. I suspect as the research continues we will find that both soy foods and soy isoflavones are not a problem for women with ER+ breast cancer. In the meantime, I advise caution.

Reducing the Risk of Secondary Cancers

Cancer patients can be at higher risk of developing a second cancer—not a recurrence, but an entirely new disease—years after treatment has eradicated their disease. These cancers are called second primaries, and may appear because your terrain has become hospitable to malignancies. An example is head and neck cancer, in which up to 23 percent of patients may develop new cancers, often in the lung. Both the initial cancer and the second cancer are usually a result of heavy tobacco or alcohol use, which has affected multiple organs. Treatment itself may increase your risk of developing another tumor, as is the case with treatment for childhood leukemia.[3] To avoid second primaries, you should follow the basic Life Over Cancer diet. I also recommend chemopreventive agents, nutrients, and pharmaceuticals that suppress the growth of particular types of cancer cells and may thus reduce risk of both tumor recurrence and second primaries, or that are major constituents of foods associated with reduced recurrence risk in population studies. Oxidative stress may be an underlying cause of these, and you should thus review Chapter 14.

The nutraceuticals in the table below are either specific nutrients such as vitamin A or a grouping of related phytochemicals, many of which were discussed in the diet chapters. Phytochemicals are compounds occurring in the pigments of the vegetables and fruits you consume. Consuming a wide array of richly colored vegetables and fruits will give you a good foundation for implementing the table below, but you may also need to take some of these phytochemicals in supplement form. *Glucosinolates* comprise phytochemicals found in cruciferous vegetables and can be found in concentrated supplement form under such names as indole-3-carbinol, DIM, sulforaphane, and PEITC. *Flavonoids* are found in colorful fruits and vegetables and include compounds such as quercetin, rutin, and anthocyanidins. *Isoflavones* are found in high concentrations in soy and many other legumes; they can be found in concentrated supplements under such names as genistein, daidzein, and biochanin A. The eight *tocopherols* and *tocotrienols* constitute natural vitamin E;

CHEMOPREVENTIVE NUTRACEUTICALS AND PHYTOCHEMICALS

Type of Cancer	Glucosinolates	Flavonoids	Isoflavones	Vitamin A	Vitamin D	Tocopherols/tocotrienols	Selenium	Curcuminoids	Green Tea	Organosulfurs	Flax Lignans	Calcium	Carotenoids
Breast[4]	X	X			X	X		X	X		X		
Prostate[5]	X	X	X		X	X	X			X			X
Lung[6]	X	X		X	X								
Melanoma[7]		X		X	X			X	X				
Pancreatic[8]			X		X			X	X				
Colon[9]	X	X			X	X	X	X	X	X		X	
Brain[10]							X	X					
Ovarian[11]		X	X						X				
Endometrial[12]	X		X	X	X								
Leukemia[13]				X	X	X			X				
Lymphoma[14]		X			X		X		X				

rice bran oil contains the full complement of vitamin E whereas most supplements contain only one form, alpha-tocopherol. *Organosulfurs* from vegetables such as garlic and onions can be found in concentrates under the names allicin, ajoene, diallyl disulfide, S-allylcysteine, and S-allylmercaptocysteine. *Carotenoids* are in many red, yellow, and green vegetables and include alpha- and beta-carotene, lycopene, and lutein. Find the type of cancer you are in remission from, and for reducing risks of recurrence read across to find the nutraceutical most likely to impede development of another cancer.

The following table shows some of the food sources for these phytochemicals. Use these along with the guidelines in Chapters 4, 5, and 6 to help structure your dietary choices in remission.

FOOD SOURCES OF CHEMOPREVENTIVE SUBSTANCES

Phytochemical/ Nutraceutical	Food
Glucosinolates	Broccoli, cauliflower, brussels sprouts, cabbage
Flavonoids	Onions, apples, green/black tea, grapes
Isoflavones	Soy, red clover
Vitamin A	*See* Carotenoids, important precursors of vitamin A
Vitamin D	Salmon, mackerel, sardines, tuna
Tocopherols/ tocotrienols	Vegetable oils, wheat germ, almonds, rice bran oil, oats, barley, rye
Selenium	Brazil nuts, tuna, cod, eggs
Curcuminoids	Turmeric
Green tea	Green tea
Organosulfurs	Garlic, onions, leeks, green onions, shallots
Flax lignans	Flaxseed
Calcium	Greens, salmon, tofu, broccoli, beans
Carotenoids	Carrots, squash, sweet potatoes, apricots

Detoxification

We live in a toxic world. U.S. industries release about 2.3 billion pounds of toxic chemicals a year, but even that represents only 5 percent of the chemical pollution we are exposed to. Workplaces continue to expose employees to toxic compounds, and our foods are loaded with pesticides, herbicides, and numerous chemical additives. Even plastic food containers can leach carcinogens into what we eat. Although the science is not yet complete, there are suggestions that toxic chemicals may promote the development or persistence of cancer. Breast cancer patients have higher organochlorine levels in their body fat than controls, as do pancreatic cancer patients, especially those who have the K-*ras* mutation. On-the-job exposure to pesticides and other toxins appears to be linked to cancer development. Toxins in the body may stimulate inflammatory reactions, raise oxidative stress, and impact the immune system, all terrain factors that may prime you for a recurrence. Clearly, then, a remission-maintenance program (as well as a cancer prevention program) should include minimizing exposure to carcinogens and toxic chemicals. The Life Over Cancer diet helps you do this, since it reduces consumption of fats that are major sources of pesticides and oxidants, as well as meat that contains hormones and other growth factors, and recommends organic produce, which is free of pesticides. Following are more specific suggestions, and you can find others on the LOC website.

Choosing Food

- Choose organic foods, especially for staples. See www.food news.org for the Environmental Working Group's "dirty dozen" list of the most contaminated foods, and avoid their nonorganic versions.

- Wash fruits and vegetables thoroughly, using a pesticide-removing spray, which can be found in health food stores. (Apple cider vinegar may also work.)

- Substantially reduce or avoid mercury-laden fish such as swordfish, tuna, shark, and marlin. Avoid fish from fresh-water lakes, which tend to be high in industrial chemicals. Wild and farmed Chilean and Pacific salmon have fewer carcinogenic pollutants than farmed Atlantic salmon.

- Limit or avoid alcohol.

- Avoid irradiated foods.

- Chew food well to prevent a buildup of half-digested food toxins in the stomach and intestines, including ammonia from protein and alcohol from carbohydrates. You can also increase your digestive efficiency by taking bitter herbs such as goldenseal or gentian, which increase the secretion of digestive enzymes, or by taking enzyme supplements such as bromelain, which digests protein, and amylase and lipase, which digest carbohydrates and fats.

- Choose detoxifying foods such as cruciferous vegetables (brussels sprouts, broccoli, cauliflower, cabbage, kale, and their relatives), onions and related vegetables (garlic, shallots, green onions), sea vegetables (alaria, dulse, kombu, kelp, hijiki, nori), fish, legumes; occasional servings of omega-3 eggs, sprouts (broccoli and alfalfa), powerfood concentrates, whey protein, turmeric, milk thistle, odorless garlic, resveratrol, kelp tablets, and the enzyme supplements bromelain and papain.

Drinking Water

- Drink six to eight glasses of water a day. The kidneys filter toxins from your blood, and the best way to support them is by maintaining adequate fluid intake. Half of your water intake can come from non-caffeinated herbal tea or juice.

- Drink safer water (see tips in Chapter 5 and on the LOC ⓘ website). An excellent option is to use a home filtering system for your drinking water.

- Consider filtering shower and bath water, since common contaminants such as chlorine, trihalomethanes, and industrial chemicals can be inhaled and absorbed through the skin. A ten-minute hot shower or a thirty-minute bath exposes you to more volatile organic compounds than drinking a gallon of tap water. Such filters cost about $50 to $100. Turn on the exhaust fan or open a window when you shower or bathe to release vaporized contaminants.

In Your Home

- Air in modern airtight buildings can have two to five times the level of pollutants of outdoor air, and sometimes more than a hundred times, according to the Environmental Protection Agency. Ventilate your home by opening windows, and open a window or turn on the exhaust fan when cooking with a gas stove, which can emit pollutants, such as 1,8-dinitropyrene, 2-nitrofluorene, and benzopyrene, that induce breast and other cancers in lab animals.

- Avoid "air fresheners," and fill your home with plants, which absorb pollutants.

- Use least-toxic, unscented cleaners or make your own. See www.eartheasy.com/live_nontoxic_solutions.htm and other websites.

- Try not to buy particleboard, pressed wood, or synthetic carpet, all of which release toxic compounds.

- Minimize use of dry cleaning with perchloroethylene, a probable carcinogen. Select environmentally safe dry cleaners instead. Wash new clothes before wearing.

- Do not use indoor pesticides or insecticide strips, and treat flea-ridden pets with herbal remedies.

- Test your home for radon, a carcinogenic gas.

- When painting or using solvents, have adequate ventilation.

- Eliminate mold growing in your house.

In Your Yard

- Avoid or minimize use of chemical insecticides, herbicides, and fungicides.

- If you hire a pest control or lawn care company, make sure it uses integrated pest management, a non-pesticide approach.

Does sustaining remission mean adhering to these programs forever? Well, one consideration is that a healthy diet, a clean, chemical-free home and work environment, and a fitness regimen can help improve your odds of keeping your cancer from returning and are good for staving off other diseases as well, including cardiovascular disease and diabetes. It is my hope that you will indeed adopt them for good. But whether you continue taking supplements and nutraceuticals depends on your risk of recurrence and what way of life you are comfortable with. Once you have an idea of your risk of recurrence, which your doctor can help you gauge, you must decide how aggressive you wish to be in preventing a recurrence. Whether you are at particularly high risk of recurrence or not, though, maintaining an optimal terrain with Sphere 2 along with the basics of the Sphere 1 diet and lifestyle interventions definitely belongs in your life. Eating a diet that will make your body less hospitable for cancer, finding a practical and pleasurable way to include regular physical activity in your schedule, removing toxic chemicals from your home and workplace, and working toward enlarging your emotional strength and spirit will all help you with your ongoing choice of life over cancer.

THE GIFT OF TIME
AND HOPE

Many of my patients, while acknowledging the adversities they face, still describe their cancer as a surprising opportunity, one that helped them to appreciate what is truly important in life including a greater appreciation for their relationships, a deeper regard for self-discovery, an enlarged scope of meaning and purpose, and a deeper connection to faith or awe in living. A diagnosis of cancer can remind us that we don't have unlimited time and help us to reengage in living and rediscover what and who are most important in our lives. Cancer can strip away our armor, uncovering what is both meaningful and genuine in our lives. While work is necessary and important, I cannot recall any patients telling me they wished they had spent more time at their job. Yes, of course, some wished they had completed this project or that: a book, a play, a home, or a trip to Italy. But mostly, my patients expressed a wish to have repaired injured or lost relationships earlier, and to have spent more tender and sensitive time laughing and sharing with those they love. Whether under the strain of diagnosis or in the arduous days of treatment, I have witnessed many patients find the courage and strength to confront past regrets or reach out to those they have hurt, forgive those who have hurt them, and find profound healing. My patients tell me their diagnosis changed them, making them more spiritual, more sensitive, and more compassionate toward themselves, toward others, and toward their—and our—world. I've heard countless patients say, "I've lived more in the past six months than I've lived in the last six decades."

Take the case of Freddy (Chapter 14). A hard-driving businessman, Freddy was diagnosed in 2001 with kidney cancer and liver metastases. His family was told to take him home and forgo further treatment, since he had less than six months to live. Instead, Freddy assertively sought out a nutritional intervention, and visited the Block Center to get instruction in the LOC program, as we coordinated chemotherapy treatment plans with his oncologist in Argentina. After going into remission, Freddy obtained an experimental vaccine treatment, and remains free of disease today. He told me, "There has been a 100 percent change in my life. I was completely materialistic, and getting cancer really helped me see things from a different point of view. When you see what and who we really are, you understand there is so much more than just things. It is our relationships with ourselves, with God, with our families, and even our relationship with our own minds that is what is real."

Yet conventional approaches to cancer care can be so fixated on the disease that the patient's emotional well-being and the healing power of hope are overlooked. What I have learned is that regardless of the so-called odds, there are patients who overcome them. I have shared with you stories of survivors in addition to statistics to show that people do survive, often against daunting odds. My purpose has been to offer you genuine hope, because it is hope that provides fuel for your healing. Let me remind you of what some of the patients in this book heard from their doctors and what actually happened.

• Maryann (Chapter 4) was sent home after her initial surgery and told that they "got it all," but with no plan for how to keep it that way. Her cancer recurred and metastasized. Today, after over two decades with metastatic breast cancer, she is alive, well, and free of disease. For me, Maryann's case exemplifies why a growth control plan should be standard care. Cancer is a microscopic and molecular disease, not simply a macroscopic disease, so engaging in a program to avoid a recurrence is essential. And it should be routine, not a hard-to-find resource that patients must seek out on their own.

• Joe Horcher (Chapter 18) was told by one of his early doctors that "diet had nothing to do with anything." His reaction was: "I'll do whatever it takes!" He told his wife to throw out the pork roast she was cooking and immediately started the LOC program. Diagnosed with metastatic prostate cancer and bone lesions, he is today, at eighty-four years old, alive and active some twenty years later.

• Doug (Chapter 20) is a young adult patient of mine who frustratingly insisted, "I just want my old life back." Doug had been given a terminal prognosis for an incurable brain cancer, with six months to live. As an avid mountain biker, he so much wanted to return to his old life and stop his treatment. And although that old life was never to fully return, he now acknowledges that life is even better. While his cancer changed him forever, his health has returned and he remains cancer-free, well, and mountain-biking regularly a full fourteen years after being given a death sentence.

• Gladys (Chapter 6) was told: "We're sorry, there's nothing more that can be done for you." Despite severe weight loss and this poor prognosis for inoperable metastatic pancreatic cancer, she started the LOC program and is active, well, and disease-free two decades later.

• Marilyn (Chapter 28) had progressive inoperable metastatic lung cancer when her doctor said, "There's nothing we can do." Rather than entering a hospice as he suggested, Marilyn adopted a comprehensive LOC program and improved enough to stop chemotherapy. It is now seven years since her diagnosis, four and a half years since major metastases, and no hospice is in sight.

I certainly do not mean to imply that every patient who follows our program has an amazing breakthrough. Many cancers, especially metastatic ones, are still considered incurable and I have held too many patients' hands in the last days and hours of their lives. But no one has the right to tell you that you'll be one of the unlucky patients whose disease is not cured: you could just as easily be among the fortunate ones, patients that I consider the realization of hope.

As is true for all cancer centers, of course, we have patients with less favorable outcomes. Our staff spends much time and effort helping these patients to feel as well as possible and to explore multiple paths toward emotional wholeness, to living strong, well, and tenderly even if in decline. We find that an integrative program offers a healing experience that can occur and be profound regardless of outcome or survival.

Without surefire cures for so many cancers, no one has earned an exclusive on cancer care. I believe we therefore have a responsibility to maintain an open mind about possible solutions. As our understanding improves, people with cancer are offered new grounds for realistic optimism, better ways to attack cancer, as well as to redress the biochemical, metabolic, and genetic imbalances that support the disease. This should give you a sense of authentic hope and a reason to bank health. The more you do, the more options will be open to you.

Many of our patients want to give back something for the gift of time they were given by therapies that extended their lives far beyond what the statistics led them to expect. With this in mind, I want to tell you a story that exemplifies for me the transformative potential of cancer. One of my patients, Randy Lopez, says his cancer turned him into a "crusader." Told at age thirty-four that he had five months to live once his scans showed that his colon cancer had spread to his liver and that he should be looking into hospice, Randy instead sought out the Block Center. Chronotherapeutically delivered chemotherapy and a full nutrition and supplementation program helped him tolerate a regimen containing a drug (irinotecan) notorious for side effects. Randy's scans cleared up, and he is free of cancer ten years later. After his success with our program, his wife Beatrice left her law practice for her great love, cooking. With a deep appreciation for the important role diet played in Randy's recovery, Beatrice started a catering company creating foods that were both nutritionally sound and delicious. Randy took his expertise from the world of marketing to help run the Colon Cancer Alliance. As Beatrice told us, "No one who meets Randy or listens to him laugh and talk would guess that he had spent over seven years in a raging battle for his life. We are fighting a daily war to keep him from becoming one of the thousands of Americans who yearly succumb to colon cancer. We know that the statistics say we're fighting an uphill battle, but it is with a deep resolve that we fight—not only to win Randy's own war against America's second-leading cancer killer, but also to help as many others as possible. Randy wants to help them beat the disease or, better yet, avoid falling victim to its clutches in the first place."

A cancer diagnosis is the emotional equivalent of an earthquake. Your relationships, dreams, career, family life, self-image, and concepts of health and longevity are rocked. Few people can come through this experience without feeling fractured, like broken pieces of china, needing considerable glue to carefully put the pieces of their lives back together. This is the time for new thinking, new ways of being, new options, and a newly meaningful fabric of relationships with your friends and family. How you pick up the pieces will determine whether you find meaning and peace through the experience. You'll experience fear and anguish, but that does not mean that your life must be dominated by relentless feelings of distress. Every day, people overcome cancer and other diseases that medical science once called incurable. We've learned that patients can move through the cancer experience with hope, purpose, meaning, faith, strengthened relationships, and a renewed sense of awe and spirit.

Ideally, an integrative oncology program should help you not only to achieve a sustained remission but also to heal the various aspects of your life and help you live in a fully engaged and vital way. That is why coming out the other end of this experience with a life transformation, like so many of the patients you have read about, may in a small way help reconnect you to what is really important.

If you were my patient, I would sit down beside you, and to-gether we would explore how you can sustain your hope and revitalize your reason for being. Our center would help you devise an action plan that combined tumor-killing approaches with self-care strategies to regenerate your anti-cancer defenses. I would bring you into a community of helpers and healers who would optimize your health and guide and support you throughout your ordeal. And I would encourage you to develop a team of your own, to help you make the experience one of healing and connectedness.

Cancer is only a part of your story, a part that I believe can feel smaller and smaller, until it is no longer a major player in your life. It is my hope and prayer that this book and the program and experience it grew out of will motivate and equip you to make important steps toward healing, and bring you to a full and complete recovery.

A NOTE ON REFERENCES
AND RESOURCES

Complete reference notes for each chapter, keyed to the superscript numbers in the text, are posted at www.lifeover cancer.com, together with a description of how to use the PubMed online database to retrieve articles and abstracts. Please be aware that most of the reference numbers in the book chapters are supported by two or more articles, books, or websites.

The website also includes continuously updated resources to support the Life Over Cancer program. For a full description, see pages 47–48, and look for the icon (i) in the text.

ACKNOWLEDGMENTS

While I express below my indebtedness to many of the people who have been crucial to the evolution of our work and this book, in this limited space it is not possible to fully acknowledge each person who has contributed. I thus want initially to honor and recognize all of those whose influence and efforts have not been mentioned.

I owe a great debt to many patients, colleagues, friends, and family who sadly are no longer alive to witness the publication of this book:

To my cherished grandmother, if not for the unfortunate suffering you endured, I very well may have chosen a different path. Your battle with breast cancer was my catalyst for searching out better ways to combat malignant disease.

To my blessed father-in-law, Allan Harris: You were among Penny's and my staunchest supporters. From the beginning you believed—and encouraged our belief—when there was only an early vision of what might be possible.

To Dr. Robert Mendelsohn, your steadfast support and guidance opened an arena to think freely and creatively, and to dream—and gave direction and an "anything's possible" mindset to my medical career.

To Bill Dufty, for your friendship and your fresh flow of ideas, and for helping me originate and give rise to an "integrative" language when there simply was none.

To Dr. Paul Raccah, for opening a door to prayer, righteousness, and inspired living where deep meaning and purpose are rooted.

To my dear brother, Russell, for opening a door to play. Your very essence and gentle soul helped bring *life* to otherwise difficult times. Your untimely death is a neverending reminder of life's importance.

To Dennis Roth: Your friendship was far too touching and far too short. Your tireless efforts to save Jeff and all those who sought your help are a reminder of the power of what one single life can accomplish. You are a model I will always treasure and a reminder of *why* to dream.

To Rell Sunn, the best long boarder ever: For living everyday with the unwavering belief that our lives can be a journey of fun, mystery, and discovery, even when the surf—and life—are flat.

May each of your memories be a blessing.

To Penny Block, Ph.D.: As my partner in every sense of the word, you have worked side-by-side with me—with passion and vision—in developing a system of care that can help bring about true health as well as freedom from disease, and you have been essential to the evolution of this book.

To Sharon Begley: With your high-level experience and extraordinary skills as a science editor and writer, along with your sensitivity and heart, you have helped to ensure that this book is a solid and truly meaningful guide to *Life Over Cancer.*

To Toni Burbank (and the entire team at Bantam): Your belief and perseverance in seeing the project through, your editing expertise, guidance, and astute insistence that this book speak directly to patients, their families, and friends have made it far more accessible and genuinely helpful to those in need.

To Muriel Nellis and your staff at Literary and Creative Artists Agency, Inc.: Your unwavering support, full encouragement, knowledge, and direction have been an essential force in helping me to bring *Life Over Cancer* to fruition.

To Leni Kass, for your tenacity, enduring commitment, generous contributions, and undaunted belief in the work, in us, and in the change it could bring about. You and your friendship have contributed immeasurably.

To Dr. Charlotte Gyllenhaal, Mark Myers, and Mark Mead, for your years of commitment and unstinting effort in helping research and wrestle many concepts of this manuscript, and for bringing new insights to the clinical program on which it is based. I remain grateful to each of you for your friendship and your immeasurable dedication.

To Julie Fulton and Amanda Koch, your expertise and careful thinking increased the rigor and professionalism of this book while making it more usable and easier to grasp.

To Dina Warner and Dave Parmenter, your ongoing support, friendship, encouragement, and substantial input helped form the thinking and sharpen the content behind this manuscript.

To Dr. Andrew Weil, for your friendship, encouragement, and thoughtful support, and for your tireless efforts in transforming medicine into a more humane art of caring and true integration.

To Dr. Robert Newman, for your years of friendship, wise counsel, and insight, your thoughtful vetting of *Life Over Cancer,* and your expert collaboration in nutraceutical research projects with the goal of achieving more effective treatments and better patient outcomes.

To Dr. Jacob Shoham, for your sensitive clinical advice and your helpful input as we planned the *Life Over Cancer* manuscript, and for your efforts with us in researching whole-systems and nutritional therapies, all the while maintaining a keen focus on the soul of patient care.

To Dr. Mark Renneker, for your friendship and unfaltering support: Yes, I, too, wondered if the book would ever emerge out of challenging waters. Our running clinical dialogue, whether at ASCO, crossing the Drake Passage, or off to the next remote surf spot, has led to expanded thinking, wider options, and possibilities, resulting in more comprehensive treatment planning.

To my colleagues Dean Les Sandlow, Dr. David Mayer, Dr. Yee-Kin Ho, Dr. Phyllis Bowen, Dr. Norman Farnsworth, Dr. Mark Potter, and Dr. Nipa Shah at the University of Illinois at Chicago, for your continued support, effort, and attention, which have provided me the research and educational environments to carry this work beyond our clinic.

To my clinical associates Dr. Mike DeLaTorre, Dr. Deva Nathan, Dr. Nora Bucher, and Jennifer Ellis: Each of you embodies the philosophy of the Block Center with your full commitment to integrative treatment, life-affirming communications, and noteworthy dedication to true patient care.

To our team of compassionate and knowledgable nurses, physical therapists, massage therapists, dietitians, mind-spirit clinicians, and other integrative specialists. Each of you has been hand-picked because you emanate the spirit of genuine care. While I am grateful, it is our patients who have reaped the full benefits.

To Jeanette Cordero, for your skills, talents, and years of dedication: Your true contributions to our professional work are simply incalculable.

To our administrative team of Neil Udovich, Linda Bourdosis, Shana Ocasio, and David Eddy: You are at the core of the Block Center. You have each been essential in helping us put our shared dream and mission of providing the best clinical care possible into an achievable vision for every patient who walks through our doors.

To the full staff at Block Center: You have each been instrumental in helping carry the dream of better solutions to those battling to recover health and wellness.

To Dr. Michael Lerner and the entire Commonweal Community: For your support in bringing together a group of dedicated, integrative healers and practitioners. Our shared vision and friendship continues to be both a blessing and a source of inspiration.

To Dr. Ralph Moss, for your continuing friendship and encouragement, your many years of investigating cancer issues, providing patients with a resource for information, an ongoing discussion of options, and your diligent efforts in a global search for meaningful therapies.

To Dr. William Hrushesky, Dr. Wayne Jonas, Dr. Robert Nagourney, and Dr. Jeffrey White, for your support and friendship and for your drive and determination in introducing innovative thinking, important research, and new approaches to cancer medicine.

Through the course of my medical education, postgraduate training, subsequent clinical research, and clinical practice, there have been many colleagues and friends whose valuable lessons and support I want to acknowledge. These include: Donald Abrams MD, Jeff Baumann MD, Anton Bilchik MD, David Blask MD, Mark Blumenthal, Barry Boyd MD, Brian Bouche MD, Michael Broffman LAc, Terrence Bugno, MD, Phil Carlson, Iqbal Chaudrey PhD, Lorenzo Cohen PhD, Alastair Cunningham PhD, Henry Dreher, Mayer Eisenstein MD, Eilhys England, Joseph Espat MD, Fred Ettner MD, Leo Galland MD, Ian Gawler OAM, Jeremy Geffen MD, Jim Gordon MD, Steven Greer MD, Bill Gushwan, Michael Hamblin MD, Paul Harch MD, Avery Hart MD, Arika Hirsch MD, Ron Hoffman MD, Judith Jacobsen MD, Jon Kabat-Zinn PhD, Mitchel Kaminsky MD, Richard Kane MD, Aaron Katz MD, Kara Kelly MD, Will Kennedy MD, John Knaus DO, Fredi Kronenberg PhD, Larry Kushi PhD, Victoria Kut MD, Elena Ladas MS, RD, Bo In Lee LAc, Roberta Lee MD, Larry LeShan PhD, Jochen Lorch MD, Tom Newmark, Christiane Northrup MD, Alfred Neugut MD, Dean Ornish MD, Candace Pert PhD, David Perlmutter MD, Jack Pfeiffer MD, Azra Raza MD, J. Peter Rosenfeld PhD, David Rosenthal MD, Martin Rossman MD, Julia Rowland PhD, Daniel Rubin ND, Gordon Saxe MD, Rachel Naomi Remen MD, Stephen Sagar MD, Mark Schacht MD, Paul Schulick, Victor Sierpina MD, Mark Shusterman MD, Stephanie Simonton-Atchley PhD, Bill Spears, Kevin Starr MD, William Steinmann MD, Leo Stolbach MD, Gwen Stritter MD, Sensei Akira Tohei, Peter Tothy MD, Debu Tripathy MD, Lydia Temoshok PhD, Nicholas Vogelzang MD, and Al Yung MD. To these as well as my many other professors, teachers, colleagues, and guides in oncology, medicine, and integrative disciplines, I acknowledge my great debt and appreciation.

To the team at Sage Publications, for according me the honor of editing the very first journal in the field of integrative oncology, *Integrative Cancer Therapies,* and to the staff members and the advisory and editorial boards, all of whom helped to establish a highly respected publication in this important, emerging field of medical care.

Most important, I want to recognize and express my deep appreciation to the many patients who have taught me so much about the true nature of courage and determination. Their energy and spirit are the real roots and soul of *Life Over Cancer.*

INDEX

ABOUT THE AUTHOR

Keith I. Block, M.D., is an internationally recognized expert in integrative oncology. Referred to by many, including Dr. Andrew Weil, as the "father of integrative oncology," Dr. Block combines cutting-edge conventional treatment with individualized and scientifically based complementary and nutraceutical therapies. In 1980 he cofounded the Block Center for Integrative Cancer Treatment in Evanston, Illinois, the first such facility in North America, and serves as its medical and scientific director.

Although Dr. Block has been at the forefront of integrative oncology throughout his career, this field was formally recognized by the launching of *Integrative Cancer Therapies (ICT)*. In 2000 Dr. Block was invited by Sage Science Press to be the founding editor in chief of this peer-reviewed journal, the first medical journal devoted to exploring the research and science behind integrative oncology. Recently, *ICT* was accepted by Thomson Scientific for inclusion in the Science Citation Index Expanded™.

Due to Dr. Block's work in integrative oncology, in 2005 he was appointed to the National Cancer Institute's Physician Data Query (PDQ) Cancer CAM Editorial Board, where he continues to serve today.

Dr. Block is currently director of integrative medical education at the University of Illinois College of Medicine at Chicago. Additionally, he is the scientific director of the Institute for

Integrative Cancer Research and Education, where he collaborates with colleagues at the University of Illinois in Chicago, the University of Texas M. D. Anderson Cancer Center in Houston, and Bar-Ilan University in Israel. Dr. Block is also on Dr. Andrew Weil's faculty at the Arizona Center for Integrative Medicine, the University of Arizona College of Medicine.

After receiving his medical degree from the University of Miami School of Medicine, Dr. Block completed a medical residency at Illinois Masonic Medical Center, an affiliate of the University of Illinois College of Medicine at Chicago. Dr. Block went on to study and train in medical acupuncture, Chinese medicine, medical hypnotherapy, mind-body medical systems, and conventional and alternative nutrition, including parenteral and therapeutic nutrition. The latter was core to Dr. Block's development of a nutritional oncology regimen. For example, one of Dr. Block's early contributions to the field of integrative oncology was the first dietary exchange system for cancer and optimal health.

In the late 1980s Dr. Block was selected to participate as a committee member and medical consultant for the first advisory panel on Unconventional Treatments for the U.S. Congressional Office of Technology Assessment (OTA). This panel was convened to review efficacy, safety, and other critical concerns pertaining to alternative cancer treatments and was seminal in the formation of the Office of Alternative Medicine, which later became the National Center for Complementary and Alternative Medicine. At the request of the OTA, Dr. Block submitted an extensive review of his work on a "middle-ground approach to cancer treatment." This was the first public introduction to an integrative cancer treatment model.

In conjunction with his research team, during the early 1990s Dr. Block devised a systematic set of assessments to identify biochemical disruptions and, later, molecular defects. These evaluations were more comprehensive than traditional testing, and enabled Dr. Block to use pharmaceuticals and nutraceuticals as multitargeted interventions in order to individualize each patient's treatment plan. He also introduced the concept of nutraceutical coupling with conventional protocols. The intent of this work is to enhance treatment response and reduce treatment-related side effects.

By the mid-nineties Dr. Block recognized the potential treatment benefits and diminished toxicity made possible by timing the administration of chemotherapy to synchronize with medication characteristics, cancer cell division patterns, and each patient's biological clock. After evaluating a large number of multisite clinical studies, he introduced chronomodulated chemotherapy to his patients, making the Block Center one of the first U.S. clinics to provide this innovative approach.

Dr. Block has published more than seventy-five scientific papers and numerous articles relevant to nutritional and integrative oncology. Recent papers were published in *Cancer Treatment Reviews* 2007, *International Journal of Cancer* 2008, *Molecular Interventions* 2008, *Journal of National Cancer Institute* 2008, and *The Breast Journal* 2009.

His model of individualized integrative oncology continues to set the standard for the practice of this comprehensive approach to cancer treatment in the United States.

THE BLOCK CENTER
FOR INTEGRATIVE
CANCER TREATMENT

In 1980, Keith Block, M.D., and Penny Block, Ph.D., founded the Block Center for Integrative Cancer Treatment, the first center of its kind in the United States. From the inception, their mission has been to provide the kind of care they would each hope to receive should they ever be faced with a diagnosis of cancer. The center's innovative approach combines the best of conventional cancer treatments with research-based therapies tailored to each patient's unique medical needs. These interventions include therapeutic diet, selective supplementation, stress-care strategies, and prescriptive exercise programs. Together, these treatment regimens are aimed at restoring biological integrity and laying the foundation essential to an enduring recovery.

The spa-like setting of this Evanston, Illinois, clinic includes a cancer chemotherapy unit with private chemo suites; a demonstration kitchen where patients and staff enjoy healthy foods prepared by the Block Center's dietitians, accompanied by nutrition education; a life-strategies meeting area; a full physical therapy space; quiet rooms for massage, training in yoga, and related fitness systems; and individual as well as family consultation rooms. To support each patient's care, the team is comprised of board-certified oncologists and internists, physician assistants, oncology nurses, mind-spirit clinicians, psychologists and social workers, registered dietitians, physical therapists, licensed massage therapists, instructors in Asian fitness systems, medical researchers, and other integrative care specialists.

In the mid 1990s the Block Center introduced an innovative and unique method for the administration of chemotherapy. This approach, chronomodulated chemotherapy (chronotherapy), uses special programmable pumps that infuse chemotherapy when cancer cells are actively dividing and healthy cells are at rest. Extensive research of chronotherapy has demonstrated enhanced treatment response, improved outcomes, and diminished side effects.

To address the specific medical needs that can arise during each phase of a patient's care, the Block Center implements seven strategic interventions:

Integrative Treatment Support—coupling specific herbs or
   nutraceuticals with conventional drugs to help improve
   treatment response

Side Effect Deterrence and Relief—using a combination of
   appropriate medications and nutraceuticals, mind-spirit
   techniques, and noninvasive technologies for addressing side
   effects such as fatigue and nausea, and using infrared laser
   therapy to counter neuropathy

Pain Management—conventional pain medication along
   with a tailored program of physical therapy, body work
   and massage, acupuncture, innovative and advanced
   technologies including micro-electrical nerve stimulation,
   mind-spirit techniques, an anti-inflammatory diet, and
   anti-inflammatory nutraceuticals

Rehabilitation and Rebuilding—implementing a systematic
   program of physical therapy, an anti-inflammatory food
   regimen, appropriate supplementation, and mind-body
   support to recover physical, biological, and psychological
   stamina

Leaving No Stone Unturned—assessing and implementing appropriate experimental options, research-supported off-label drugs, nutraceutical interventions, and reasonable and responsible use of alternatives

Recurrence Prevention and Remission Maintenance— employing a select group of post-treatment strategies tailored to the particular disease and status of each patient to minimize the potential for a return of disease

Medical Detoxification—using a research-supported set of noninvasive detox methods to help rid the body of residual metabolites from accumulated chemicals

The Block Center's approach to cancer care begins with a thorough medical work-up and detailed patient assessments that, in addition to routine labs, include biochemical and molecular profiling and nutritional, physical, and quality-of-life evaluations. These data provide the information used to create each person's individualized plan of care. This personal tailoring is a distinguishing feature of the Block program.

The Block Center for Integrative Cancer Treatment
1800 Sherman Avenue
Evanston, IL 60201
Phone: 847-492-3040
www.blockmd.com